D0528997

HIV and Psychiatry

Training and Resource Manual

Second Edition

Edited by

Kenneth Citron, M.D.

Marie-Josée Brouillette, M.D.

Alexandra Beckett, M.D.

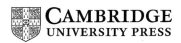

CAMBRIDGE
UNIVERSITY PRESS

CAMBRIDGE UNIVERSITY PRESS
Cambridge, New York, Melbourne, Madrid, Cape Town, Singapore, São Paulo

CAMBRIDGE UNIVERSITY PRESS
The Edinburgh Building, Cambridge CB2 2RU, UK

www.cambridge.org
Information on this title: www.cambridge.org/9780521009189

© Cambridge University Press 2005

This book is in copyright. Subject to statutory exception
and to the provisions of relevant collective licensing agreements,
no reproduction of any part may take place without
the written permission of Cambridge University Press.

First published 2005

Printed in the United Kingdom at the University Press, Cambridge

Typeface in 10.5/14pt Minion   *System* Advent 3B2 8.07f [PND]

A catalog record for this book is available from the British Library

Library of Congress Cataloging in Publication data

ISBN-13 978-0-521-00918-9 paperback
ISBN-10 0-521-00918-9 paperback

Cambridge University Press has no responsibility for the persistence or accuracy of URLs for external or
third-party internet websites referred to in this book, and does not guarantee that any content on such
websites is, or will remain, accurate or appropriate.
Every effort has been made in preparing this book to provide accurate and up-to-date information that is in
accord with accepted standards and practice at the time of publication. Nevertheless, the authors, editors and
publisher can make no warranties that the information contained herein is totally free from error, not least
because clinical standards are constantly changing through research and regulation. The authors, editors and
publisher therefore disclaim all liability for direct or consequential damages resulting from the use of
material contained in this book. Readers are strongly advised to pay careful attention to information
provided by the manufacturer of any drugs or equipment that they plan to use.

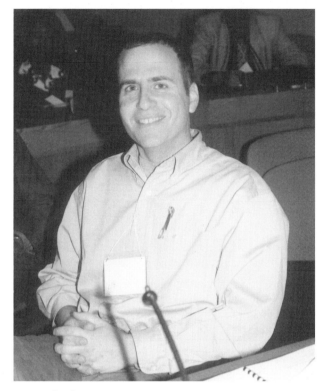

Kenneth Citron

In June 2004, we were all saddened by the death of Ken, at the early age of 45. He had been struggling for over a year with a very difficult illness. We lost an extraordinary man.

Ken was a skilled teacher, consultant, and colleague, who always put connecting and relationship first. He had a gift for friendship, discretion, and collaboration, and was always approachable. His sense of humor and relaxed manner were part of his style. The way he had of assuming the best about people was inspiring. All this was balanced with his being a devoted husband, father, sibling, and son. Soon after he was diagnosed with a brain tumor, numerous friends and collaborators offered their help; his reply reflected his approach to life:

People say "If there's anything I can do to help . . ."
So I thought about that and what I would like is the following . . .
I would like you all to spend the next weeks enjoying your loved ones, your partners, children, and others you care about. Just really show them, and tell them how much you love them and appreciate them. I think that would help me the most.

He will be sorely missed by all of us.

Allan Peterkin
Marie-Josée Brouillette

Contents

Contributors

Kimberly R. Jacob Arriola, M.P.H., Ph.D.
Assistant Professor
Rollins School of Public Health of Emory
University
Atlanta, GA, USA

Kenneth Ashley, M.D.
Assistant Professor of Psychiatry and
Behavioral Sciences,
Albert Einstein College of Medicine
Attending Psychiatrist at Beth Israel Medical
Center in New York City, NY, USA.

Andrew C. Blalock, Ph.D.
Department of Psychology,
Georgia State University
Atlanta, GA, USA

Ronald L. Braithwaite, Ph.D.
Professor, Department of Community
Health and Preventive Medicine,
Morehouse School of Medicine,
Atlanta, GA, USA

William Breitbart, M.D.
Professor of Psychiatry
Weill Medical College of Cornell
University
Chief, Psychiatry Service

Department of Psychiatry and Behavioral
Sciences
Attending Psychiatrist
Pain and Palliative Care Service
Department of Neurology
Memorial Sloan-Kettering
Cancer Center
New York, NY, USA

Robert P. Bright, M.D.
Assistant Professor of Psychiatry,
University of North Carolina
Attending Psychiatrist
Carolinas HealthCare System
Charlotte, NC, USA

Marie-Josée Brouillette, M.D.
Assistant Professor of Psychiatry,
McGill University
Consulting Psychiatrist,
Immunodeficiency Program
McGill University Health Center,
Montréal, Canada

Larry K. Brown, M.D.
Professor
Bradley/Hasbro Research Center
Department of Psychiatry
R.I. Hospital and Brown University
Providence, RI, USA

Jose Catalan, FRCPsych
Honorary Senior Lecturer, Imperial College
School of Medicine, University of London
Consultant Psychiatrist,
Central North West London Mental Health
NHS Trust,
London, UK

Glenn Catalano, M.D.
Professor, Department of Psychiatry and
Behavioral Medicine, University of South
Florida College of Medicine
Medical Director of Psychiatry,
Tampa General Hospital,
Tampa, FL, USA

Annunziata Ciafrone, M.D.
Assistant Consultation Psychiatry Unit
Cotugno Hospital,
Naples, Italy

Kenneth Citron, M.D.[†]
Assistant Professor of Psychiatry
University of Toronto
Staff Psychiatrist, Clinic for HIV-Related
Concerns
Department of Psychiatry, Mt. Sinai
Hospital, Toronto, Canada

Francine Cournos, M.D.
Professor of Clinical Psychiatry
Columbia University College of Physicians
and Surgeons
Deputy Director, New York State
Psychiatric Institute, New York, NY, USA

Peter DeRoche, M.D.
Assistant Professor of Psychiatry
University of Toronto
Director, Clinic for HIV-Related
Concerns,
Department of Psychiatry, Mt. Sinai
Hospital, Toronto, Canada

Francisco Fernandez, M.D.
Professor and Chairperson
Department of Psychiatry and Behavioral
Medicine
University of South Florida College of
Medicine
Tampa, FL, USA

Frank Hector Galvan, Ph.D., L.C.S.W.
Assistant Professor
Department of Psychiatry and Human
Behavior
Charles R. Drew University of Medicine
and Science
Los Angeles, CA, USA

Sheryl M. Hakala, M.D.
Child Fellow, Department of Psychiatry
and Behavioral Medicine
University of South Florida College of
Medicine,
Florida, FL, USA

Mark Halman, M.D.
Assistant Professor of Psychiatry,
University of Toronto
Director, HIV Psychiatry Program
St. Michael's Hospital, Toronto, Canada

Barbara Hedge Ph.D.
Director of Clinical Psychology Training,
Department of Psychology,
University of Waikato,
New Zealand

Richard Herman, M.A.
Co-Director, HIV Prevention Training
Columbia University HIV Mental Health
Training Project Research Scientist, New
York State Psychiatric Institute, New York,
NY, USA

Heather Hunter, B.A.
Department of Psychology
University of Kansas
Lawrence, KS, USA

Peter E. Kassel, Psy.D.
Assistant Professor of Psychiatry
Harvard Medical School
Staff Psychologist, Massachusetts
Institute of Technology Medical
Department, Private Practice in Brookline,
MA, USA

Thomas N. Kerrihard, M.D.
Director, Psychiatry and Mental Health
Services
AIDS Healthcare Foundation, Los Angeles,
CA, USA

Stephen Knowlton, Ph.D.
Licensed Psychologist
Private Practice in Somerville and Boston,
MA, USA

Stephanie Le Melle, M.D.
Assistant Clinical Professor of Psychiatry
Columbia University College of Physicians
and Surgeons, New York, NY, USA

Howard Libman, M.D.
Associate Professor of Medicine
Harvard Medical School
Director, HIV Services, Healthcare
Associates
Beth Israel Deaconess Medical Center
Boston, MA, USA

Kevin J. Lourie, Ph.D., L.M.H.C.,
Director of Youth and Family Services,
East Greenwich, RI, USA

Julie D. Maggi, M.D., M.Sc.
Assistant Professor of Psychiatry
University of Toronto
Staff Psychiatrist
Mental Health Service
St. Michael's Hospital
Toronto, Canada

J. Stephen McDaniel, M.D.
Professor, Department of Psychiatry and
Behavioral Sciences
Emory University School of Medicine
Atlanta, GA, USA

Karen McKinnon, M.A.
Director, Columbia University HIV Mental
Health Training Project
Research Scientist, New York State
Psychiatric Institute,
New York, NY, USA

Giuseppe Nardini, M.D.
Assistant Director,
Consultation Psychiatry Unit,
Cotugno Hospital, Naples, Italy

Cassandra F. Newkirk, M.D., CCHP
Mental Health Director at Riker's Island
Penitentiary,
Prison Health Services, Inc.
East Elmhurst, NY, USA

Lori A. Panther, M.D., M.P.H.
Assistant Professor of Medicine
Harvard Medical School
Beth Israel Deaconess Medical Center
Division of Infectious Diseases
Boston, MA, USA

Maryland Pao, M.D.
Deputy Clinical Director,
Intramural Research Program
National Institute of Mental Health
Department of Health and Human
Services
Bethesda, MD, USA

Sean B. Rourke, Ph.D.
Associate Professor of Psychiatry,
University of Toronto
Director of Research, Mental Health Services
St. Michael's Hospital, Toronto, Canada

Cécile Rousseau, M.D.
Associate Professor of Psychiatry
McGill University
Director, Transcultural Child Psychiatry
Team
Montréal Children's Hospital, Montréal,
Canada

**David J. Roy, O.C., O.Q., LL.D.(H.C.),
S.T.L., Ph.L., Dr. Theol.**
Research Professor, Faculty of Medicine,
Université de Montréal
Director, Center for Bioethics
Institut de Recherche Clinique de Montréal,
Montréal, Canada

Sanjay M. Sharma, M.D., M.B.A.
Assistant Professor
Department of Psychiatry and Behavioral
Sciences
Emory University School of Medicine
Atlanta, GA, USA

Nancy L. Sheehan, B.Pharm, M.Sc.
HIV Pharmacotherapy Specialist

McGill University Health Centre
Montréal, Canada

Lorraine Sherr
Professor of Clinical and Health
Psychology
Head of Health Psychology Unit
Department of Primary Care and
Population Sciences, Royal Free and
University College School of Medicine,
London, UK

Fabrizio Starace, M.D.
Director, Consultation Psychiatry and
Behavioural Epidemiology Service
Cotugno Hospital, Naples, Italy

Andrea Stolar, M.D.
Assistant Professor,
Department of Psychiatry and Behavioral
Medicine, University of South Florida
College of Medicine
Staff Psychiatrist, Women's Program,
Bay Pines Veterans Administration
Medical Center,
Bay Pines, FL, USA

Terry Tafoya, Ph.D.
Executive Director, Tamanawit, Unltd.,
Seattle, WA, USA

Cynthia J. Telingator, M.D.
Instructor in Psychiatry
Harvard Medical School
Training Director Division of Child and
Adolescent Psychiatry
Cambridge Hospital/Cambridge Health
Alliance, Cambridge, MA, USA

Preface

It was in 1996. The manuscript for the first edition of this Training Manual, produced under the auspices of Health Canada and the Canadian Psychiatric Association, was being completed. Many clinicians caring for HIV-infected individuals were becoming demoralized. The nucleoside reverse transcriptase inhibitors (NRTIs), the only class of antiretrovirals available at the time, were failing to make a significant impact on mortality. The full implication of the development of resistance to these medications was being felt.

Then, a second class of antiretroviral agents, the protease inhibitors (PIs) became available. Clinical trials were initiated and, at the International AIDS Conference held in Vancouver (Canada) in 1997, it became clear that a turning point had been reached. Antiretrovirals from different classes, used in combination, were exerting a very significant impact on mortality among HIV-infected individuals (Figure 0.1). Clinically, the result was striking. The waiting rooms of HIV clinics were the theaters of astonishing scenes. Patients on the brink of death were putting on weight and regaining stamina. Enthusiasm among patients and clinicians alike was palpable.

Psychiatrists too, were enthused. There was a sense that the psychological and neuropsychiatric burden associated with this infection would significantly decrease. Almost 10 years down the road now, it has become clear that the need for psychiatric care has far from decreased. As patients live longer, psychological and psychiatric difficulties negatively impact on quality of life.

The efficacy of Highly Active Antiretrovial Therapy (HAART) has a price: strict adherence to a complex medication regimen. The management of psychiatric problems is crucial in fostering the adherence required to achieve full viral suppression. Pharmacotherapy has become complicated by the fact that several medications used in HIV care have the potential to interact significantly with psychotropic medications. The development of cognitive difficulties remains a concern. Patients still have to contend with multiple stressors while trying to achieve a balance between immediate gratification and long-term planning in the face of a prognosis

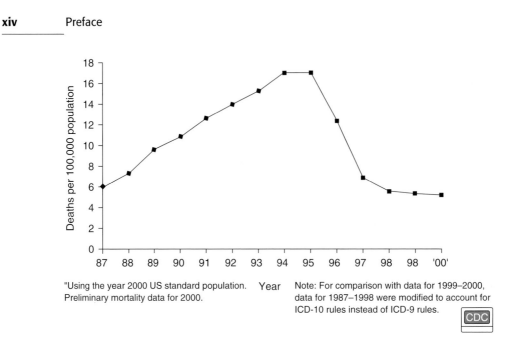

Figure 0.1.   Trends in age-adjusted rate of death due to HIV infection, USA, 1987–2000. Available at www.cdc.gov/graphics/mortalit.htm.

that remains uncertain. The epidemic is moving into new populations, requiring from care providers different approaches and new sets of skills.

In order to help the psychiatrist face these new challenges, a second edition of the Training Manual has become a necessity. The purpose of the book, hence the format, has not changed. Several medical schools and continuous medical education programs are turning to case-based learning as this method facilitates the acquisition of knowledge in a manner that is meaningful for clinical application. This case-based manual is meant to be a training tool that will equip the psychiatrist or other practitioners with the knowledge base necessary to provide competent psychiatric and psychosocial care to individuals infected with HIV. The information is structured around vignettes and flows in much the way questions would arise in practice.

The knowledge in this area is progressing at a rapid pace. With the background information provided in this text, clinicians will be able to make sense of the literature should they choose to later perfect their knowledge of the area.

For this second, international edition, we have put together an exceptional group of contributors with years of expertise in the field. We have asked them to distill the huge amount of information available in order to extract what they consider to be the essential knowledge for the practicing psychiatrist or mental health practitioner. Once again, we have benefited from the expertise of Jean Bacon, professional writer, to ensure optimal flow of the information and consistency in style throughout the chapters. We are confident that you will find the information both accessible and highly informative.

1

Medical overview

Lori A. Panther, M.D., M.P.H.[1] and Howard Libman, M.D.[2]

[1] Assistant Professor of Medicine, Harvard Medical School, Beth Israel Deaconess Medical Center,
Division of Infectious Diseases, Boston, MA
[2] Associate Professor of Medicine, Harvard Medical School, Director, HIV Services, Healthcare Associates,
Beth Israel Deaconess Medical Center, Boston, MA

Introduction

The first report of acquired immunodeficiency syndrome (AIDS) appeared in the June 5, 1981, edition of *Morbidity and Mortality Weekly Report*. It described five men who had sex with men (MSM) diagnosed with *Pneumocystis carinii* pneumonia (PCP). In 1984, researchers reported the discovery of a retrovirus, now known as Human Immunodeficiency Virus, type 1 (HIV-1), associated with AIDS. In 1986, researchers described a second strain, HIV-2, which shares 42% genetic homology with HIV-1 but is less virulent. Based on genetic sequence analysis, scientists have concluded that HIV-1 originated in the African chimpanzee and HIV-2 in the African sooty mangabey.

What is the epidemiology of HIV infection?

World

According to recent estimates, 40 million people worldwide are infected with HIV, and 3 million have died of AIDS in the past year.

Sub-Saharan Africa has been most severely affected, with the highest prevalence in Botswana, South Africa, and Zimbabwe. In Botswana, 36% of the adult population is infected with HIV. By the end of 1999, an estimated 10.7 million African children had lost one or both of their parents to AIDS.

Asia has also been affected by the epidemic. Thailand experienced a dramatic increase in heterosexually acquired HIV cases in the mid-1980s. About 80% of injection drug users (IDUs) in China are HIV seropositive, and the epidemic in the heterosexual population in India is growing rapidly.

In Eastern Europe, injection drug use is the main means of acquiring HIV. Ukraine has reported the majority of cases. Given the sociopolitical instability of this region, the epidemic is expected to increase.

HIV and Psychiatry. A Training and Resource Manual, Second Edition, ed. Kenneth Citron, Marie-Josée Brouillette, and Alexandra Beckett. Published by Cambridge University Press. © Cambridge University Press 2005.

In Latin America and the Caribbean region, HIV infection rates continue to increase over time, with a risk behavior profile similar to that of the USA (see below).

Globally, the HIV epidemic has disproportionately affected socially and economically disadvantaged persons. Frequent migration and low literacy rates have also impeded access to health care. While the availability of medical therapy has decreased the number of deaths attributable to HIV infection in the USA, Western Europe, and Brazil, antiretroviral drugs are not affordable in many developing countries, and the healthcare infrastructure required to properly monitor patients and maximize medication adherence does not exist.

Despite the lack of universal access to medications, some developing countries have reported decreases in HIV incidence after initiating intensive prevention programs. In Thailand, Uganda, Zambia, and Senegal, public education about safer sex, clean needle use, sexually transmitted disease (STD) prevention and treatment, and prenatal care has shown promise in curbing the spread of HIV infection.

USA

The first cases in the USA were primarily MSM. Over time, however, the epidemic has spread to injection drug users (IDUs), who contract HIV via contaminated drug equipment, and women, whose main risk behavior is heterosexual contact. A small but significant proportion of early HIV cases were in blood transfusion recipients and infants born to HIV-infected mothers but, with the screening of the blood supply and the widespread use of antiretroviral therapy in HIV-seropositive pregnant women, the incidence of infection attributed to these risk factors has decreased over time. In recent years, there has been an increased frequency of new cases of HIV infection in MSM of color, and the rate of heterosexual acquisition in women has been steadily rising.

AIDS incidence in the USA rose rapidly through the 1980s, peaked in the early 1990s, and then declined. As of December, 2001, 816,148 people with AIDS had been reported to the Centers for Disease Control and Prevention (CDC), and 57% of them had died. An estimated 40,000 new cases of HIV infection occur in the USA each year. Because of greater longevity, more people are alive with an AIDS diagnosis than ever before.

How is HIV transmitted?

Sexual

The overall risk of HIV transmission associated with unprotected sexual activity is estimated to range from 0.3 to as high as 30 in 1000 (Table 1.1). However, the per-episode risk associated with a specific sexual act has been difficult to quantify. Unprotected receptive anal intercourse is thought to be the highest risk sexual

Table 1.1. Estimates of per-contact risk of HIV infection

Activity	Risk
Needle-Sharing	6/1000 to 30/1000
Occupational Needle Stick	1/300
Receptive Anal Sex	8/1000 to 30/1000
Receptive Vaginal Sex	2/1000 to 8/1000
Insertive Anal or Vaginal Sex	3/10,000 to 10/10,000
Receptive Oral Sex	Unknown

Adapted from Table 1–2 in Libman H, Makadon HJ, eds. HIV, *Therapy Series, American College of Physicians, Philadelphia, PA, 2003.*

activity followed by unprotected receptive vaginal intercourse. Few data exist about the degree of risk associated with insertive anal or vaginal intercourse. In general, male-to-male and male-to-female transmission is more efficient than female-to-male and female-to-female transmission. Seroconversion as a result of oral sex has been reported, and recent information suggests that there is a tangible risk associated with this activity. The correct and consistent use of latex condoms can significantly reduce the risk of HIV transmission during anal, vaginal, and oral sex.

Injection drug use

The overall risk of HIV transmission associated with injection drug use is comparable to that of unprotected sexual activity, ranging from 6–30 in 1000. Needles and syringes are the primary drug equipment involved in transferring HIV-infected blood between drug injectors. Drug treatment and needle exchange programs are the most effective means of reducing HIV transmission in IDUs. However, if these are not accessible, IDUs should be instructed not to share drug equipment or to disinfect it prior to use with bleach.

Maternal–fetal

Approximately 70% of maternal–fetal transmissions occur in the peripartum period. Perinatal transmission rates in untreated mother–infant pairs vary geographically, with a 15–30% transmission rate in the USA, 13–15% in Europe, and 40–50% in Africa. Fetal passage through the birth canal is associated with most peripartum transmission through exposure to maternal blood. In 1994, a large study of zidovudine (ZDV, AZT) monotherapy in mother–infant pairs was stopped after interim analysis because ZDV decreased perinatal transmission rates from 25.5% to 8.3%. Although cesarean section has been shown to further decrease the perinatal transmission rate, its role in mothers whose viral load is suppressed on antiretroviral therapy has not been elucidated. HIV-infected mothers are discouraged from nursing because of a 3.5–10.3% transmission risk, with the higher rate associated with a longer duration of breast-feeding.

Other considerations

Options for the HIV-seronegative woman who wishes to conceive with an infected partner are currently under investigation. Sperm washing, which involves removal of HIV from sperm prior to artificial insemination, is the most popular choice for risk reduction. The CDC has advised against sperm washing because of concerns about safety, but the procedure is currently being used in European countries with success.

There is no risk of HIV transmission from non-intimate household or routine work exposures. During phlebotomy or other invasive procedures, all patients should be managed using universal precautions regardless of their HIV serostatus.

The risk of HIV transmission in healthcare workers after exposure to HIV-infected blood is 0.3% per percutaneous exposure and 0.09% per mucous membrane exposure. The risk associated with body fluids other than blood has not been quantified but is thought to be substantially lower. The risk of transmission is increased with the inoculation of a large quantity of blood, visible blood on the device to which the worker was exposed, exposure to a needle that was inserted directly in a vessel, exposure to a hollow-bore needle, deep injury, and exposure to blood or secretions from an HIV-infected person with a high viral load. Postexposure prophylaxis (PEP) consists of a short course of antiretroviral therapy after a high-risk exposure. In general, PEP consists of 4 weeks of antiretroviral therapy instituted as soon as possible after exposure. For most exposures, a two-drug regimen, usually ZDV and lamivudine (3TC), is used. If the exposure is to a person thought likely to harbor resistant virus, a third agent, often indinavir or nelfinavir, is added. Non-occupational PEP, which might be used following rape or condom failure, consists of the same regimens.

What is the pathogenesis of HIV infection?

HIV is a cytopathic virus, composed of a central cylindrical core of RNA surrounded by a spherical lipid envelope. Through the binding of the HIV envelope glycoprotein gp120 to the receptor present on the surface of CD4+ T lymphocytes, the virus fuses with the cell membrane. Once within the cytoplasm of the host cell, the envelope of the virus is shed, and its contents are released. It is then that reverse transcription occurs: DNA is made from the viral RNA template, and the viral DNA inserts itself into the host cell genetic material. Infected cells remain in a dormant state for a variable period of time. When activation occurs, the proviral DNA transcribes genomic and messenger RNA. After viral proteins are synthesized, new virions are assembled and bud from the infected cell. For budding virions to become functional,

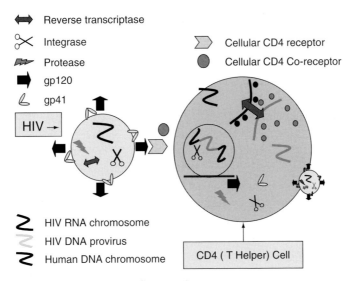

Figure 1.1.   Schematic of HIV/CD4 cell interaction.

processing by a viral protease is required. Once this processing has been accomplished, the virions circulate until they identify new target cells (Figure 1.1).

How is a diagnosis of HIV infection made, and how is HIV infection classified?

A diagnosis of HIV infection is made by testing a patient for antibodies specific to HIV. Timing of the testing is important. HIV antibodies are not detectable using the standard serologic tests (i.e., enzyme-linked immunosorbent assay [ELISA] and Western blot [WB]) until approximately 3 weeks after infection. As part of antibody testing, the patient should receive standardized pretest and post-test counseling (see Appendix 1). HIV viral load testing, which is a direct measurement of HIV in the plasma, should never be used for the initial diagnosis of a suspected chronic infection because false-positive low titer results (usually < 2000 copies/ ml) have been reported in acute non-HIV-related illnesses.

The CD4 cell count correlates highly with the progression of HIV disease and is the main surrogate marker for immunologic function. The CDC classification system for AIDS is based on the patient's CD4 cell count and clinical history: AIDS is defined as a CD4 count less than 200 cells/mm^3 or a history of opportunistic infections and malignancies that occur in the context of HIV infection (Table 1.2).

Without effective antiretroviral therapy, the average decline per year in CD4 count is 75 to 100 cells/mm^3. However, there is a great deal of variability among patients and in a given patient over time. A normal CD4 count is generally greater than 500 cells/mm^3 in healthy people, but it may be as low as 350 cells/mm^3. Although opportunistic infections usually do not occur with CD4 counts of

Table 1.2. Indicator conditions for case definition of AIDS

Candidiasis of bronchi, trachea, lungs or esophagus

Cervical cancer, invasive

Coccidioidomycosis, disseminated or extrapulmonary

Cryptococcosis, extrapulmonary

Cryptosporidiosis, chronic intestinal

Cytomegalovirus disease (other than liver, spleen, or lymph nodes)

Encephalopathy, HIV-related

Herpes simplex: chronic ulcer(s) or bronchitis, pneumonitis, or esophagitis

Histoplasmosis, disseminated or extrapulmonary

Isosporiasis, chronic intestinal

Kaposi's sarcoma

Lymphoma: Burkitt's, immunoblastic or primary (in brain)

Mycobacterium avium complex or *M. kansasii*, disseminated or extrapulmonary

Mycobacterium tuberculosis, any site

Pneumocystis carinii pneumonia

Pneumonia, recurrent

Progressive multifocal leukoencephalopathy

Salmonella septicemia, recurrent

Toxoplasmosis of brain

Wasting syndrome, HIV-related

Adapted from Box 1.1 in Libman, H. and Makadon, H. J., eds. *HIV, Therapy Series.* American College of Physicians, Philadelphia, PA, 2003.

greater than 500 cells/mm^3, conventional bacterial infections, herpes simplex virus (HSV), varicella-zoster virus (VZV), thrush, tuberculosis (TB), Kaposi's sarcoma (KS), generalized lymphadenopathy, and chronic skin conditions may be seen as the count declines (Figure 1.2). A CD4 count of less than 200 cells/mm^3 indicates significant immunodeficiency with increased risk for serious opportunistic infections, such as PCP, toxoplasmosis, and cryptococcal meningitis. Patients with a count of less than 50 cells/mm^3 are also at risk for cytomegalovirus (CMV) and *Mycobacterium avium* complex (MAC) infection and for lymphoma. The highest risk for death in HIV-infected patients is in those with a CD4 count less than 50 cells/mm^3.

What are the clinical manifestations of HIV infection?

The clinical manifestations of HIV infection are listed in Table 1.3.

Primary HIV infection

At 2–6 weeks after exposure, the most common symptoms are fever, fatigue, rash, headache, lymphadenopathy, and pharyngitis. Neurologic manifestations of primary

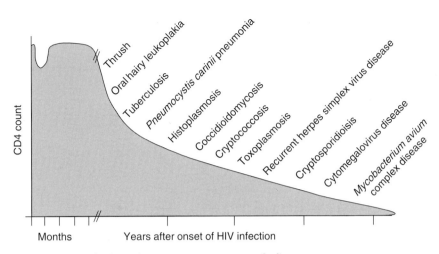

Figure 1.2.   Opportunistic infections that occur as CD4 counts decline.

infection include aseptic meningitis, myelopathy, radiculopathy, peripheral neuro-pathy, meningoencephalitis, and Guillain–Barré syndrome. Between 40% and 90% of HIV-infected people can recall an illness suggestive of primary HIV infection. The syndrome of primary or acute HIV infection should be suspected in anyone who presents with an atypical or prolonged viral illness or an unexplained mononucleosis syndrome. A negative HIV antibody test in the presence of a high (i.e., > 50 000 copies/ml) viral load is diagnostic of primary HIV infection.

Latency period

After primary HIV infection, there is a period of clinical latency before patients develop an AIDS-defining diagnosis. The latency period lasts 2 years in 5% of patients, 6 years in 20–25% of patients, and 10 years in 50% of patients. The single best predictive laboratory test for progression to AIDS is the HIV viral load measurement: a viral load of less than 10 000 copies/ml predicts the development of AIDS in fewer than 32% of patients at 6 years of follow-up, and a viral load of greater than 30 000 copies/ml predicts AIDS in 80%. Using both the CD4 count and HIV viral load values is even more helpful in determining an individual patient's prognosis.

Oral and skin manifestations

Oral lesions can occur throughout the course of HIV infection. Thrush and angular cheilitis are forms of oral candidiasis. Oral hairy leukoplakia is caused by the Epstein–Barr virus and is usually asymptomatic. Oral ulcerations are common in HIV disease and can be aphthous or caused by HSV or CMV. A severe and progressive form of gingivitis, acute necrotizing ulcerative gingivitis (ANUG),

Table 1.3. Clinical manifestations of HIV disease

Primary HIV infection
Latency period
Oral
  Candidiasis
  Hairy leukoplakia
  Herpes simplex virus
  Cytomegalovirus
  Aphthous ulcers
  Gingivitis
  Kaposi's sarcoma
Skin
  Seborrheic dermatitis
  Bacterial folliculitis
  Eosinophilic folliculitis
  Herpes simplex virus
  Varicella-zoster virus
  Molluscum contagiosum
  Human papillomavirus
  Bacillary angiomatosis
  Kaposi's sarcoma
  Persistent generalized lymphadenopathy
Pulmonary
  Community-acquired pneumonia
  Pneumocystis carinii pneumonia
  Tuberculosis
  Kaposi's sarcoma
  Lymphoma
Gastrointestinal
  Esophagitis
  Cholangiopathy
  Hepatitis (A,B,C)
  Pancreatitis
  Diarrhea
  Wasting syndrome
Multi-organ system disease
  Cytomegalovirus
  Mycobacterium avium complex
  Lymphoma
Neurocognitive and neurologic
  Progressive multifocal leukoencephalopathy
  Toxoplasmosis

Primary CNS lymphoma
Cryptococcosis
Vacuolar myelopathy
Demyelinating polyradiculopathy
Peripheral neuropathy
HIV encephalopathy

often requires debridement and antibiotics. Oral nodules may represent KS, lymphoma, warts, or salivary gland enlargement.

The skin is commonly involved in HIV disease. Reactivation of VZV infection ("shingles") is often one of the earliest cutaneous manifestations. Molluscum contagiosum is caused by a poxvirus and presents as centrally umbilicated papules. Nodules, abscesses, ulcers, or lymphadenitis can manifest from histoplasmosis, cryptococcosis, and KS, as well as *Penicillium marneffei*, nontuberculous myco-bacteria, and *Bartonella* infections. Human papillomavirus causes anogenital warts as well as cervical and anal dysplasia and carcinoma. Persistent generalized lymphadenopathy occurs in 50–70% of HIV-infected patients early in the course of disease and can recrudesce in patients who have initiated combination anti-retroviral therapy as their CD4 counts recover.

Pulmonary manifestations

Pulmonary complications are a leading cause of morbidity and mortality in people with HIV infection. Of these, community-acquired pneumonia (CAP) is the most common and is caused by the usual respiratory pathogens. PCP was the first reported opportunistic infection. Most patients with PCP have a CD4 cell count less than 200 cells/mm^3. Tuberculosis and multidrug-resistant TB (MDRTB) are reported more frequently in AIDS. Although MAC and CMV are sometimes isolated from lung specimens in patients with HIV-associated respiratory illness, they are rarely the causative pathogens. Pulmonary KS and Hodgkin's and non-Hodgkin's lymphomas manifest in the chest as intrapulmonary nodules or med-iastinal or hilar lymphadenopathy.

Gastrointestinal manifestations and multi-organ system disease

Esophagitis presenting as dysphagia and odynophagia can be caused by *Candida albicans*, CMV, or HSV, and is one of the more common gastrointestinal mani-festations occurring in advanced HIV disease. Less frequent causes of esophageal symptoms include KS and lymphoma. AIDS cholangiopathy can be caused by CMV, *Cryptosporidium* species, microsporidial organisms, *Isospora belli*, or MAC, and is associated with very high alkaline phosphatase levels. People with HIV infection are at risk for hepatitis A (HAV), B (HBV), and C (HCV). Patients co-infected with HIV and HCV are at risk for accelerated development of cirrhosis and increased mortality. Drug toxicity (e.g., ddI [didanosine], pentamidine) is the usual cause of pancreatitis. Diarrhea is common in people with HIV infection and most often related to infection or drug toxicity. HIV wasting syndrome, defined as loss of greater than 10% of baseline body weight associated with chronic diarrhea, weakness, or fever in the absence of a known cause, was one of the earliest recognized manifestations of AIDS. Opportunistic infections and malignancies including CMV, MAC, and lymphoma can cause multi-organ system disease in people with HIV infection.

Neurocognitive and neurologic manifestations

Neurocognitive and neurologic diseases are most prevalent in advanced HIV disease. Opportunistic infections and malignancies of the brain occur most often in patients with a CD4 cell count of less than 100 cells/mm^3. Progressive multifocal leukoencephalopathy (PML) manifests as slowly progressive neurocognitive deterioration associated with paresis, apraxia, aphasia, vertigo, ataxia, and/or diplopia. Brain MRI shows multiple non-enhancing white matter lesions adjacent to the cerebral cortex. Cerebral toxoplasmosis, caused by the parasite *Toxoplasma gondii*, generally presents subacutely with headaches, seizures, and/or focal neurologic findings. Computerized tomography with contrast or magnetic resonance imaging (MRI) scan shows multiple ring-enhancing lesions in the cortex, basal ganglia, or thalamus. Diagnosis is made by demonstration of serum antibodies to *T. gondii* and characteristic findings on neuroradiologic imaging. Primary central nervous system lymphoma (PCNSL) is a rapidly advancing brain malignancy manifesting as acute neurologic decompensation with imaging studies showing deep white matter lesions with weak contrast enhancement. Lesions associated with toxoplasmosis may be radiologically indistinguishable from those of PCNSL. Other opportunistic pathogens that can result in focal brain lesions in HIV disease include *Cryptococcus neoformans*, *Mycobacterium tuberculosis*, *Nocardia* species, and *Aspergillus* species. Diagnosis of these infections requires cerebrospinal fluid (CSF) examination and sometimes brain biopsy.

Meningoencephalitis is generally acute or subacute in presentation and most commonly caused by the fungus *C. neoformans*. Less frequent etiologies include the encapsulated bacteria *Neisseria meningitidis*, *Streptococcus pneumoniae*, and *Hemophilus influenzae*; and the viruses CMV, HSV, and VZV. Symptoms of meningoencephalitis include fever, headache, altered mental status, and meningismus. Diagnosis is generally made by CSF examination and appropriate microbiological studies.

Vacuolar myelopathy, which occurs in advanced HIV disease, is characterized by loss of motor function in the lower extremities. Dementia may or may not accompany the symptoms. The diagnosis is based on clinical grounds, but CSF examination is recommended to rule out treatable conditions.

Peripheral neuropathy is well described in HIV disease and can be caused by medication toxicity, opportunistic infections, or HIV itself. Medications associated with peripheral neuropathy include the antiretroviral drugs ddI, ddC (zalcitabine), and d4T (stavudine). Symptoms often slowly improve once the offending agent is discontinued. Autoimmune motor polyneuropathies manifest as Guillain–Barré syndrome or an acute or chronic demyelinating polyneuropathy. A rapidly progressive ascending mixed polyradiculopathy can occur from CMV infection of the nerve roots and spinal cord, manifesting as back pain, bowel and bladder dysfunction, and ascending loss of sensation and motor function. Myopathy has been described in association with HIV disease; ZDV was a frequent cause earlier in the epidemic, but its incidence has decreased since the standard drug dosage was reduced.

Cognitive impairment related to HIV infection has been the subject of much research investigation. Ten to twenty per cent of HIV-infected patients have some degree of cognitive impairment. HIV-associated cognitive/motor complex (HACM) is a subcortical dementia, a continuum of disorders resulting from the direct effects of HIV on the central nervous system, ranging from mild cognitive symptoms to a nearly vegetative state. Neuroradiologic imaging studies and CSF sampling is generally performed to rule out other causes of dementia. HIV viral load levels in the CSF have been shown to correlate with the severity of symptoms. Treatment with combination antiretroviral therapy has been variably effective in reducing HACM symptoms.

Other medical conditions that can result in altered mental status in people with HIV infection include metabolic disorders, such as drug toxicity, anemia, dehydration, hypoxemia from lung disease, hypoadrenalism, and significant kidney or liver dysfunction. Most of these are associated with advanced HIV disease. See Table 1.4 for medications that may produce neuropsychiatric side effects.

What is involved in the initial evaluation of a patient with HIV disease?

History

A detailed history is essential in the initial evaluation of HIV-infected patients. Practitioners should:
- Elicit past medical and family medical histories, as well as constitutional symptoms and localized complaints on review of systems.
- Ask specific questions regarding a history of STDs, viral hepatitis, TB exposure and skin testing, Pap smear results in women, and immunizations.

Table 1.4. Neuropsychiatric side effects of drugs used to treat HIV infection and related medical conditions

Drug class	Drug	Target condition	Side effects
NRTIs and NtRTI			
NRTIs	Zidovudine (ZDV, AZT)	HIV	Headache, malaise, confusion, insomnia, mania, seizures
	Didanosine (ddI)	HIV	Peripheral neuropathy, mania, seizures, insomnia, headache, dizziness
	Zalcitabine (ddC)	HIV	Peripheral neuropathy, fatigue, seizures, headache
	Stavudine (d4T)	HIV	Anxiety, insomnia, mania, seizures, headache
	Lamivudine (3TC)	HIV	Insomnia, malaise, headache, neuropathy, depression
	Emtricitabine (FTC)	HIV	Headache
	Abacavir (ABC)	HIV	Insomnia, headache, dizziness, fatigue
NtRTI	Tenofovir (TDF)	HIV	Headache, asthenia
NNRTIs			
	Nevirapine	HIV	Somnolence, fatigue, headache
	Delavirdine	HIV	Headache, fatigue
	Efavirenz	HIV	Confusion, nightmares, depression
PIs			
	Saquinavir	HIV	Asthenia, paresthesias, peripheral neuropathy
	Ritonavir	HIV	Asthenia, circumoral paresthesias, malaise, insomnia
	Indinavir	HIV	Asthenia, headache, dizziness, aseptic meningitis

Drug class	Drug	Target condition	Side effects
	Nelfinavir	HIV	Headache, poor concentration
	Amprenavir	HIV	Headache, circumoral paresthesias, depression
	Fosamprenavir	HIV	Headache, insomnia, fatigue
	Lopinavir/ritonavir	HIV	Headache, insomnia, asthenia
	Atazanavir	HIV	Headache
EIs	Enfuvirtide	HIV	Peripheral neuropathy, anxiety, insomnia, fatigue
Prophylactic agents	Trimethoprim-sulfamethoxazole	PCP and toxoplasmosis prophylaxis	Depression, appetite loss
	Dapsone	PCP prophylaxis	Peripheral neuropathy, tinnitus, psychosis, insomnia, headache
	Atovaquone	PCP prophylaxis	Headache, insomnia, paresthesias, anxiety
	Pentamidine	PCP prophylaxis	Confusion, emotional lability, hallucinations
	Azithromycin	MAC prophylaxis	Headache, dizziness
	Clarithromycin	MAC prophylaxis	Headache
Antivirals	Acyclovir	HSV, VZV	Visual hallucinations, confusion, thought insertion, insomnia
	Famciclovir	HSV, VZV	Headache, fatigue
	Valacyclovir	HSV, VZV	Headache, aseptic meningitis, dizziness
	Ganciclovir	CMV, HSV, VZV	Headache, paresthesias

Table 1.4. (cont.)

Drug class	Drug	Target condition	Side effects
	Valganciclovir	CMV	Headache, insomnia, peripheral neuropathy, paresthesia
	Foscarnet	CMV, HSV, VZV	Paresthesias, seizures, confusion, hallucinations
	Interferon	Hepatitis C, hepatitis B, Kaposi's sarcoma	Depression, confusion, myalgias, headache
Antifungals			
	Fluconazole	Candidiasis, cryptococcosis	Dizziness, seizures
	Amphotericin B	Cryptococcosis, histoplasmosis	Delirium, peripheral neuropathy, diplopia
Antimycobacterials			
	Isoniazid (INH)	Tuberculosis	Depression, hallucinations, paranoia, anxiety
	Rifampicin	Tuberculosis	Headache, dizziness, fatigue, paresthesias, CSF xanthochromia
	Pyrazinamide	Tuberculosis	Seizures, hyperthermia
	Ethambutol	Tuberculosis, MAC	Peripheral neuropathy, headache, dizziness, mania, hallucinations, psychosis
	Quinolones	Tuberculosis, MAC	Delirium, seizures, depression, psychosis

NRTIs = nucleoside reverse transcriptase inhibitors; NtRTIs = nucleotide reverse transcriptase inhibitors; NNRTIs = non-nucleoside reverse transcriptase inhibitors; PIs = protease inhibitors; EIs = entry inhibitors; PCP = *Pneumocystis carinii* pneumonia; MAC = *Mycobacterium avium* complex; HSV = herpes simplex virus; VZV = varicella-zoster virus; CMV = cytomegalovirus.

- Pay careful attention to travel in areas endemic for specific opportunistic infections when reviewing the patient's social history. Someone who has spent time in developing countries, is using or has used alcohol or drugs, or has been homeless is at a higher risk for TB exposure.
- Ask about pets – cats carry the risk of transmission of toxoplasmosis and bartonellosis, and reptiles carry the risk of gram-negative rods including salmonellosis.
- Take a sexual history, focusing on use of barrier methods and the importance of disclosure of one's HIV serostatus to sexual partner(s).
- Counsel patients who are active IDUs on proper cleaning of shared drug equipment.
- Assess the patient's mental status to screen for neurocognitive impairment and depression.

Physical examination

Because HIV infection and its complications may involve nearly every organ system, the practitioner should perform a comprehensive physical examination, with special focus on the skin, mouth, anogenital region, and central nervous system. Skin and mucous membranes should be examined for the manifestations described above, and all peripheral lymph node chains should be palpated. Women should have a cervical Pap smear. All patients should receive a thorough neurologic examination to assess for global or focal disorders. Patients with a CD4 count less than 100 cells/mm^3 should be referred for a baseline dilated ophthalmologic examination to check for CMV retinitis.

Laboratory studies

Baseline laboratory studies in the HIV-infected patient are listed in Table 1.5
- Repeat HIV antibody testing for patients who present without valid documentation of a positive HIV antibody test.
- Perform the CD4 cell count and HIV viral load at each of the first two visits to establish a baseline. The CD4 count is a surrogate marker for degree of immune function and is used to determine whether antiretroviral therapy and opportunistic infection prophylaxis are indicated. The normal range is 350–1100 cells/mm^3. By contrast, the HIV viral load provides an indication of the pace of immunologic deterioration over time and is used to determine whether antiretroviral therapy is indicated and to assess its effectiveness. A higher baseline viral load portends more accelerated disease. Methodologies include the branched DNA (bDNA) and PCR assays. The usual range of HIV viral load testing is less than 50 copies/ml to greater than 100 000 copies/ml.

Table 1.5. Baseline laboratory studies in the HIV-infected patient

CD4 cell count
HIV viral load
Complete blood and differential counts
BUN/creatinine, liver function tests
Glucose, lipid profile
Toxoplasmosis serology
Hepatitis A, B, and C serologies
Syphilis serology (RPR or VDRL)
Purified protein derivative (PPD)
Pap smear
HIV resistance test*

*Indicated in context of recent seroconversion
Adapted from Box 2.6 in Libman, H. and Makadon, H. J., eds. *HIV, Therapy Series*. American College of Physicians, Philadelphia, PA, 2003.

- Consider viral resistance testing in the patient with recently acquired HIV infection to facilitate the selection of antiretroviral drugs.
- Conduct baseline laboratory studies including a complete blood count, serum blood urea nitrogen (BUN), and creatinine, liver function tests to assess vital organ function, fasting glucose and lipid panel.
- If dapsone or sulfonamides are to be used in the course of therapy, obtain a qualitative assay for glucose-6-phosphate dehydrogenase (G6PD) level since a deficiency of this enzyme can lead to hemolysis in the presence of these agents.
- To look for exposure to various infectious diseases, order additional tests such as a toxoplasmosis serology, hepatitis A, B, and C serologies, syphilis serology (RPR or VDRL), and skin test (PPD) for TB exposure (a positive test in an HIV-infected person is ≥ 5 mm of induration). If the RPR and confirmatory test is positive and the patient has neurologic symptoms/signs or has had syphilis for longer than 1 year, a lumbar puncture is indicated to rule out central nervous system involvement.

How is HIV infection managed?

General management considerations for HIV disease are guided by the CD4 cell count and HIV viral load (Table 1.6). Specific issues include:
- the institution and maintenance of combination antiretroviral therapy and prophylactic therapies against opportunistic infections
- management of side effects and complications from these therapies
- education of patients regarding disease status and therapeutic advances.

Table 1.6. Management of HIV disease stratified by CD4 cell count

CD4 cell count	Management of HIV disease
> 350/ mm^3	Initiate antiretroviral therapy if patient is symptomatic or pregnant after addressing factors that could negatively affect adherence
	Consider initiation of antiretroviral therapy if patient is asymptomatic with a high (>55 000 copies/ml) viral load, has HIV seroconversion syndrome, or acquired HIV infection within prior 6 months
	If above criteria are not met, monitor patient off antiretroviral therapy
	Initiate TB prophylaxis in patient with positive PPD
	Address immunizations and other healthcare maintenance issues
350–200/mm^3	Initiate antiretroviral therapy if patient is symptomatic or pregnant after addressing factors that could negatively affect adherence
	Consider initiation of antiretroviral therapy if patient is asymptomatic, has HIV seroconversion syndrome, or acquired HIV infection within prior 6 months
	Maintain antiretroviral therapy in patient who is already receiving it with modification of regimen as necessary based upon effectiveness and tolerability
	Initiate TB prophylaxis in patient with positive PPD
	Address immunizations and other healthcare maintenance issues
200–50/mm^3	Initiate antiretroviral therapy in all patients after addressing factors that could negatively affect adherence
	Maintain antiretroviral therapy in patient who is already receiving it with modification of regimen as necessary based upon effectiveness and tolerability
	Initiate PCP prophylaxis*
	Initiate TB prophylaxis in patient with positive PPD
	Address immunizations and other health care maintenance issues
< 50/mm^3	Initiate antiretroviral therapy in all patients after addressing factors that could negatively affect adherence
	Maintain antiretroviral therapy in patient who is already receiving it with modification of regimen as necessary based upon effectiveness and tolerability
	Initiate or maintain PCP prophylaxis*
	Initiate prophylaxis for MAC infection
	Initiate TB prophylaxis in patient with positive PPD
	Address immunizations and other healthcare maintenance issues

PCP = *Pneumocystis carinii* pneumonia; MAC = *Mycobacterium avium* complex; TB = tuberculosis.
*Alternative prophylaxis for toxoplasmosis should be initiated in the patient with CD4 count < 100 cells/mm^3 and positive toxoplasmosis serology who is not receiving TMP–SMX for PCP prophylaxis.

Antiretroviral therapy

Principles of use

Recommendations for the management of HIV disease have evolved with the development of laboratory techniques that enhance monitoring of viral activity, the availability of an increasing number of antiretroviral drugs, and emerging information on long-term complications. Anatomic (brain and genital tract) and physiologic (latent CD4 lymphocytes) reservoirs of HIV are not eradicated with currently available drugs. Therefore, the goal of antiretroviral therapy is to achieve viral suppression to the greatest extent possible for as long as possible in order to preserve and ultimately restore immune function.

Based upon published guidelines, antiretroviral therapy is generally recommended if the patient is symptomatic (from an opportunistic disease or other significant HIV-related condition), has a CD4 count of less than 350–200 cells/mm^3, or is pregnant (Table 1.6). Clinical benefit has been demonstrated in controlled trials only for patients with a CD4 count of less than 200 cells/mm^3, but many clinicians offer therapy at the 350/mm^3 threshold. Antiretroviral therapy should be considered if the patient is asymptomatic with a CD4 count of greater than 350 cells/mm^3 and a high (>55 000 copies/ml) viral load, has HIV seroconversion syndrome, or acquired HIV infection within the prior six months. Before starting antiretroviral medications, factors that could have a negative impact on adherence should be reviewed. Regularly missed doses will render a drug regimen ineffective by leading to the development of viral resistance. Every effort should be made to address active substance abuse, alcohol abuse, or significant psychological problems, all of which may interfere with a patient's ability to take medications reliably.

There are currently 20 approved antiretroviral drugs used in various combinations to treat HIV infection (Table 1.7). The four classes are the nucleoside and nucleotide reverse transcriptase inhibitors (NRTIs and NtRTIs), non-nucleoside reverse transcriptase inhibitors (NNRTIs), protease inhibitors (PIs), and entry inhibitors (EIs). A standard initial regimen includes two NRTIs *and* either an NNRTI or a PI.

Ritonavir is used more often as adjunctive therapy at reduced dosage to boost the trough level of other PIs by inhibiting their metabolism, rather than as an antiretroviral drug in full dosage. In general, three-NRTI regimens are not advised because of decreased effectiveness when compared with the others listed (Table 1.8).

Adherence

Approximately two-thirds of patients started on combination antiretroviral therapy achieve an undetectable HIV viral load. Patient adherence to medical

Table 1.7. Preferred and alternative drug regimens for ARV treatment-naïve patients

NNRTI-based regimens	
Preferred	EFV + 3TC + (ZDV or TDF or d4T) (except in pregnant women or in women with pregnancy potential)
Alternatives	EFV + 3TC + ddI (except in pregnant women or in women with pregnancy potential)NVP + 3TC + (ZDV or d4T or ddI)
PI-based regimens	
Preferred	LPV/RTV + 3TC + (ZDV or d4T)
Alternatives	APV + RTV + 3TC + (ZDV or d4T)IDV + 3TC + (ZDV or d4T)IDV + RTV + 3TC + (ZDV or d4T)NFV + 3TC + (ZDV or d4T)SQN + RTV + 3TC + (ZDV or d4T)

Adapted from US Department of Health and Human Services Guidelines: www.aidsinfo.nih.gov

Table 1.8. Antiretroviral agents used to treat HIV infection

Drug	Dosing recommendations (≥ 60 kg)	Side effects
Nucleoside and nucleotide reverse transcriptase inhibitors (NRTIs and NtRTIs)		
Zidovudine (ZDV, AZT)	300 mg bid	Nausea, headache, bone marrow suppression
Didanosine (ddI)	400 mg qd	Peripheral neuropathy, pancreatitis
Zalcitabine (ddC)	0.75 mg tid	Peripheral neuropathy, oral ulcers
Stavudine (d4T)	40 mg bid	Peripheral neuropathy
Lamivudine (3TC)	150 mg bid	No significant side effects
Emtricitabine (FTC)	200 mg qd	Headache
Abacavir (ABC)	300 mg bid	Rash; also hypersensitivity reaction of fever, diarrhea, and/or dyspnea (can be fatal if the drug is discontinued and restarted)
Tenofovir (TDF) (nucleotide)	300 mg qd	Nausea, diarrhea
Non-nucleoside reverse transcriptase inhibitors (NNRTIs)		
Nevirapine	200 mg bid	Rash, hepatitis
Delavirdine	400 mg tid	Rash

Table 1.8. (cont)

Drug	Dosing recommendations (≥ 60 kg)	Side effects
Efavirenz	600 mg qd	Rash, vivid dreams, neurocognitive symptoms
Protease inhibitors (PIs)		
Saquinavir	1600 mg bid	Diarrhea, nausea
Ritonavir	600 mg bid (full dose); 100–200 mg bid (adjunctive dose)	Nausea, diarrhea, perioral numbness
Indinavir	800 mg tid	Nephrolithiasis, nausea, diarrhea, indirect hyperbilirubinemia
Nelfinavir	1250 mg bid	Diarrhea, nausea
Amprenavir	1200 mg bid	Rash, diarrhea, nausea
Fosamprenavir	1400 mg bid, or if combined with ritonavir, 1400 mg qd + 200 mg ritonavir qd, or 700 mg bid + 100 mg ritonavir bid	Nausea, vomiting, diarrhea
Lopinavir/ritonavir	400 mg/100 mg bid	Nausea
Atazanavir	400 mg qd	Diarrhea, nausea, vomiting, indirect hyperbilirubinemia
Entry Inhibitors		
Enfuvirtide	90 mg sc bid	Injection site reactions

therapy is key; they are required to take several medications at specific times, under certain strict dietary conditions. When patients miss more than 10% of their doses, the likelihood of achieving maximal viral suppression decreases and the risk of viral resistance increases. Factors that have a negative impact on adherence should be addressed before starting antiretroviral therapy and monitored during treatment (see Table 1.9).

Table 1.9. Negative prognostic factors for medication adherence

Lack of education about HIV disease
Denial, anxiety, or depression
Current alcohol or drug use
Poor social situation
Inadequate health insurance
Number of medications prescribed/pills per day
Frequency of dosing
Stringent dosing requirements
Presence of side effects or long-term toxicities
Poor clinician–patient relationship

Adapted from Box 2.8 in Libman, H. and Makadon, H. J., eds. *HIV, Therapy Series.* American College of Physicians, Philadelphia, PA, 2003.

Table 1.10 shows an example of a moderately complex treatment regimen.

Resistance

HIV is a highly changeable virus, and under the selective pressure of antiretroviral therapy, mutations in the HIV genome can occur, making it less susceptible to specific drugs. Some mutations confer cross-resistance to other drugs within the same class. In cases where HIV resistance is suspected, the practitioner should order an HIV genotype or phenotype test (Table 1.11).

The genotype test provides a genetic "blueprint" of the predominant viral strain, and the phenotype test offers a drug-sensitivity profile. Both tests identify medications to which the virus is resistant. Genotype testing is more readily available and less costly than phenotype testing but provides an indirect measure of susceptibility. Both tests examine only the predominant viral strain isolated, and may miss resistant "quasi-species."

Modification of regimen

In cases of drug ineffectiveness or toxicity, practitioners may have to modify antiretroviral regimens. Specific criteria for changing therapy because of drug failure include:

- less than 0.5–0.75 log reduction in viral load by 4 weeks after initiating therapy or less than 1 log reduction by 8 weeks
- failure to achieve full suppression of viral load 4–6 months after initiation of therapy

Table 1.10. An example of a moderately complex treatment regimen

Medication	7h00 Breakfast	11h00 (1 hour before lunch)	12h00 Lunch	19h00 Dinner	23h00 Bedtime
Didanosine (Videx EC™) 400 mg capsules Take 1 hour before or 2 hours after a meal Do not take with other medications		1 capsule			
Lamivudine (Epivir®) 300 mg tablets Take 1 tablet once a day	1 tablet				
Lopinavir / ritonavir (Kaletra™) 133 mg / 33 mg per capsule Take capsules every 12 hours with a meal	4 capsules			4 capsules	
Efavirenz (Sustiva®) 600 mg tablets Take 1 tablet once a day at bedtime. Avoid taking with a high-fat meal					1 tablet
Atovaquone (Mepron®) 750 mg / 5 mL Take 5 mL every 12 hours for PCP prophylaxis	5 mL			5 mL	
Azithromycin (Zithromax®) 600 mg tablets Take 2 tablets once a week on Sunday for MAC prophylaxis				2 tablets every Sunday	

Table 1.11. Recommendations for use of drug resistance assays

Use of assay	Comments
Recommended	
Virologic failure during combination antiretroviral therapy	Role of resistance?
Suboptimal suppression of viral load after starting antiretroviral therapy	Maximize the number of active drugs in the new regimen
Acute HIV infection (if treatment is to be started)	Determine if drug-resistant virus was transmitted; change regimen accordingly
Consider	
Chronic HIV infection before starting therapy	Assays may not detect minor resistant species; consider if significant probability of transmitted drug-resistant virus
Not usually recommended	
After discontinuation of drugs	Resistance mutations may become minor species in the absence of selective drug pressure
Plasma viral load < 1000 copies/ml	Resistance assays unreliable if viral load is low

Adapted from US Department of Health and Human Services Guidelines: www.aidsinfo.nih.gov

- detectable viral load after initial full suppression or a three-fold increase in viral load after a nadir in the level
- a declining CD4 cell count or clinical deterioration regardless of viral load response.

Side effects attributable to a single drug can be addressed by substituting an equivalent agent. However, in a patient with treatment failure, it is preferable to change all three agents. In some cases, especially in the patient who has experienced many side effects from medications and/or has had extensive prior exposure to antiretroviral drugs, continuing a partially effective regimen may be preferable to discontinuing antiretroviral therapy.

Long-term toxicities

In addition to specific toxicities from individual drugs, some patients experience lipodystrophy syndrome on combination antiretroviral therapy, especially regimens containing d4T and/or PIs. This syndrome consists of body morphology changes (deposition of fat in abdomen, breasts, and neck; loss of fat in face and extremities), metabolic complications (hyperlipidemia, glucose intolerance/

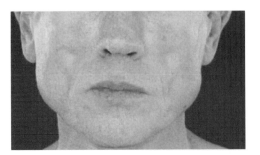

Figure 1.3.   Lipodystrophy syndrome: facial wasting. Reprinted with permission from Carr A, Cooper DA: "Images in clinical medicine; lipodystrophy associated with an HIV-protease inhibitor." *New England Journal of Medicine* 339: 1296,1998.

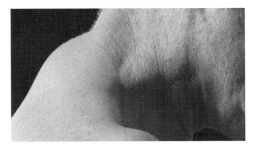

Figure 1.4.   Lipodystrophy syndrome: "Buffalo Hump." Reprinted with permission from Carr A, Cooper DA: "Images in clinical medicine; lipodystrophy associated with an HIV-protease inhibitor." *New England Journal of Medicine* 339: 1296,1998.

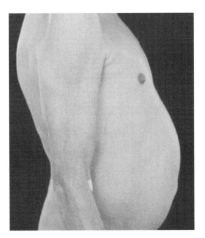

Figure 1.5.   Lipodystrophy syndrome: fat deposition in abdomen and fat loss in extremities. Reprinted with permission from Carr A, Cooper DA: "Images in clinical medicine; lipodystrophy associated with an HIV-protease inhibitor." *New England Journal of Medicine* 339: 1296,1998.

diabetes mellitus), or both (Figures 1.3, 1.4, and 1.5). Its epidemiology and pathogenesis are not yet fully understood, and its optimal management is unknown.

Lactic acidosis with a variety of clinical manifestations (peripheral neuropathy, pancreatitis, myopathy, steatosis with liver failure) has been described in patients on NRTI-based regimens. Routine screening for this condition in asymptomatic individuals is not recommended. However, in patients on NRTI-based regimens who have unexplained constitutional or gastrointestinal symptoms, practitioners should consider a venous lactate level. Premature osteopenia/osteoporosis and avascular necrosis of the hips have also been reported in HIV-infected patients on long-term antiretroviral therapy.

New therapeutic modalities

The optimal time to initiate antiretroviral therapy and compare different types of regimens is being investigated, as are:

- simplification of an initial HAART regimen to reduce pill burden and reduce number of long-term side effects
- the role of therapeutic drug monitoring (measuring their plasma levels)
- strategies for choosing second and subsequent drug combinations in patients with resistant viral strains.

Cross-resistance within the three classes of antiretroviral drugs leaves limited therapeutic options for heavily pretreated patients. Several new drugs in these classes are currently under investigation, but it remains to be seen whether they will prove to be less cross-resistant. New therapies, based on an improved understanding of the pathogenesis of HIV disease, are also being developed, including: cytokine-receptor inhibitors, integrase inhibitors, immunotherapy, cytotoxic T lymphocytes directed against HIV components, and vaccine preparations.

Opportunistic infection prophylaxis

Principles of use

Because successful combination antiretroviral therapy can reconstitute and preserve the immune system, the incidence of opportunistic infections has decreased. However, practitioners are advised to prescribe antimicrobial prophylaxis for HIV-infected patients with a CD4 cell count below established thresholds. (See Table 1.12 for recommended prophylactic antimicrobial drugs and immunizations.) A distinction should be made between primary prophylaxis (preventing the first episode of an opportunistic infection), and secondary prophylaxis (preventing recurrence of an opportunistic infection after initial therapy) (Table 1.12).

Table 1.12. Primary prophylaxis against opportunistic infections

Pathogen	Indication	Regimen
Pneumocystis carinii	CD4 count < 200 cells/mm^3	Trimethoprim-sulfamethoxazole or dapsone or atovaquone or aerosol pentamidine
Toxoplasma gondii	CD4 count < 100 cells/mm^3 and positive IgG antibody test	Trimethoprim-sulfamethoxazole or dapsone + pyrimethamine + leucovorin or atovaquone
Mycobacterium avium complex	CD4 count < 50 cells/mm^3	Azithromycin or clarithromycin or rifabutin
Mycobacterium tuberculosis, isoniazid (INH)-sensitive	Positive PPD or contact with active tuberculosis	INH + pyridoxine × 9 months
Mycobacterium tuberculosis, isoniazid (INH)-resistant	Positive PPD and probable contact with isoniazid-resistant tuberculosis	Rifampicin or rifabutin × 4 months
Multidrug-resistant tuberculosis (MDRTB)	Positive PPD and probable contact with MDRTB	Consult local public health authorities

Pathogen	Indication	Prophylaxis/Vaccine
Varicella-zoster virus (VZV)	Exposure to primary VZV infection or shingles in a patient with no history of primary VZV infection or documented negative VZV antibody test	Varicella-zoster immune globulin within 48 h of exposure
Streptococcus pneumoniae	All patients with CD4 $\geq$ 200 cells/mm^3	Pneumococcal vaccine $\times$ 1
Hepatitis B virus	All patients who are HBcAb negative	Hepatitis B vaccine at 1, 2 and 6 months
Hepatitis A virus	All MSM and patients with chronic hepatitis B or C	Hepatitis A vaccine at 1 and 6 months
Influenza virus	All patients	Inactivated trivalent vaccine $\times$ 1 on a yearly basis

Discontinuation of prophylaxis

Practitioners can discontinue prophylaxis under the following circumstances:

- primary and secondary PCP prophylactic therapies and primary toxoplasmosis prophylaxis in patients whose CD4 cell count rises above 200 cells/mm^3 for at least 3 months on combination antiretroviral therapy
- secondary toxoplasmosis prophylaxis if the patient is asymptomatic, has completed the course of initial therapy, and has a CD4 count greater than 200 cells/mm^3 for at least 6 months
- secondary prophylaxis for disseminated MAC infection, CMV infection, and cryptococcosis if the patient is asymptomatic and has no evidence of active disease, has completed a specified course of therapy, and has a CD4 count of greater than 100 cells/mm^3 for at least 6 months.

Conclusion

As the HIV epidemic enters its third decade, important advances have been made in understanding its epidemiology, virology, and immunology, and in developing more effective antiretroviral therapies and the means to monitor them. Prevention and treatment of opportunistic infections have also improved significantly over time. Although drug treatment is not readily available in many underdeveloped countries, steps are being taken to address this difficult issue.

Preventing HIV infection – developing a vaccine or encouraging and fostering behavior changes that reduce the risk – remains a great challenge.

SUGGESTED READING

Antman, K. and Chang, Y. Kaposi's sarcoma. *New England Journal of Medicine*, **342** (2000): 1027–38.

Bartlett, J. G., ed. *Hopkins HIV Report*. Bimonthly publication of Johns Hopkins University AIDS Service, Baltimore, MD.

Centers for Disease Control and Prevention. Revised classification system for HIV infection and expanded surveillance case definition for AIDS among adolescents adults. *Morbidity and Mortality Weekly Report*, **41** (1993) (RR-17).

Centers for Disease Control and Prevention. Guidelines for preventing opportunistic infections among HIV-infected persons. *Morbidity and Mortality Weekly Report*, **51** (2002) (RR-8): 1–52. Available at http://www.aidsinfo/nih.gov/guidelines

Cotton, D. J., ed. *AIDS Clinical Care*. Monthly publication of the Massachusetts Medical Society, Waltham, MA.

Greenspan, D. and Greenspan, J. S. Oral manifestations of HIV infection. *AIDS Clinical Care*, **9** (1997): 29–33.

Hirsch, M. S., Brun-Vezinet, F. and D'Aquila, R. T. Antiretroviral drug resistance testing in adult HIV-1 infection: recommendations of an International AIDS Society – USA Panel. *Journal of the American Medical Association*, **283** (2000): 2417–26.

Kahn, J. O. and Walker, B. D. Acute human immunodeficiency virus type 1 infection. *New England Journal of Medicine*, **339** (1998): 33–9.

Libman, H. and Makadon, H. J., eds. *HIV, Therapy Series*. Philadelphia, PA: American College of Physicians, 2003.

Mellors, J. W., Munoz, A., Giorgi, J. V. *et al.* Plasma viral load and CD4+ lymphocytes as prognostic markers of HIV-1 infection. *Annals of Internal Medicine*, **126** (1997): 946–54.

Moe, A. A. and Hardy, W. D. *Pneumocystis carinii* infection in the HIV-seropositive patient. *Infectious Disease Clinics of North America*, **8** (1994): 331–64.

Porras, B., Costner, M., Friedman-Kien, A. E. and Cockerell, C. J. Update on cutaneous manifestations of HIV infection. *Medical Clinics of North America*, **82** (1998): 1033–80.

Stenzel, M. S., Carpenter, C. C. The management of the clinical complications of antiretroviral therapy. *Infectious Disease Clinics of North America*, **14** (2000): 851–78.

United States Department of Health and Human Services. *2003 USPHS/IDSA Guidelines for the use of Antiretroviral Agents in HIV-Infected Adults and Adolescents*. Rockville, MD: HIV/AIDS Treatment Information Service, 2003. Available at http://www.aidsinfo/nih.gov/guidelines

Yeni, P. G., Hammer, S. M., Carpenter, C. C., *et al.* Antiretroviral treatment for adult HIV infection in 2002: updated recommendations of the International AIDS Society-USA Panel. *Journal of the American Medical Association*, **288** (2002): 222–35.

WEB SITES

Aegis http://www.aegis.com
AIDSInfo: US Department of Health and Human Services http://www.aidsinfo.nih.gov
The Body http://www.thebody.com
Centers for Disease Control and Prevention http://www.cdc.gov/nchstp/hiv_aids/pubs/facts.htm
HIV InSite http://hivinsite.ucsf.edu
JAMA HIV/AIDS Information Center http://www.ama-assn.org/aids
The Johns Hopkins AIDS Service http://www.hopkins-aids.edu
National AIDS Education and Training Centers http://www.ucsf.edu/warmline/aetc.html
National Library of Medicine http://sis.nlm.nih.gov/aidswww.htm

Cognitive disorders in people living with HIV disease

Julie D. Maggi, M.D., M.sc.[1], Sean B. Rourke, Ph.D.[2]
and Mark Halman, M.D.[3]

[1] Assistant Professor of Psychiatry, University of Toronto, Staff Psychiatrist, Mental Health Services, St. Michael's Hospital, Toronto, Canada
[2] Associate Professor of Psychiatry, University of Toronto, Director of Research, Mental Health Services, St. Michael's Hospital, Toronto, Canada
[3] Assistant Professor of Psychiatry, University of Toronto, Director, HIV Psychiatry Program, St. Michael's Hospital, Toronto, Canada

Introduction

Cognitive complaints are common in HIV disease. Over the course of the HIV epidemic, researchers have come to understand a great deal about cognitive difficulties associated with HIV disease. HIV enters the central nervous system shortly after infection and has a predilection for subcortical brain areas. As the disease progresses, proinflammatory neurotoxins that cause cell injury and cell dysfunction are released. As a result, many people with HIV disease begin to experience difficulties in cognitive functioning. Given the morbidity associated with cognitive disorders for people living with HIV disease, it is essential that practitioners accurately assess changes in mental status. Diagnosis must be grounded in a thorough history and careful psychiatric, mental status, neurologic examination, and where available, neuropsychological examination. Assessment must consider the patient's clinical stage as well as laboratory markers of immune dysfunction and viral burden.

What causes the cognitive dysfunction associated with HIV infection?

The pathophysiologic mechanism that leads to cognitive dysfunction is unclear, but is thought to be related to HIV replication in the brain, activation of HIV-infected brain microglial cells, liberation of inflammatory neurotoxins (e.g., cytokines, Tumour Necrosis Factor), and impairment in natural host repair mechanisms, ultimately resulting in a level of neuronal dysfunction, injury, or death. The areas most affected are the subcortical brain regions and the fronto-striatal circuitry

HIV and Psychiatry. A Training and Resource Manual, Second Edition, ed. Kenneth Citron, Marie-Josée Brouillette, and Alexandra Beckett. Published by Cambridge University Press. © Cambridge University Press 2005.

(Cummings, 1990; Parks *et al.*, 1993; Wesselingh *et al.*, 1994; Tyor *et al.*, 1995; Grant and Adams, 1996; Masliah *et al.*, 1997; Tan and Guiloff, 1998).

More broadly, cognitive complaints in HIV disease can be attributed to the interactions between HIV-strain factors and host factors. The host factors that can have an impact on a person's cognitive signs and symptoms include:

- the person's systemic condition
- biological vulnerability to cognitive disorders
- neuropsychiatric effects of medications used to treat HIV disease
- premorbid primary psychiatric disorders
- substance-related disorders
- the psychological impact of a life-threatening illness.

The interaction of all these factors can be challenging to understand.

What nomenclature is used to describe the neurobehavioral disorders that occur in HIV infection?

> Other terms used to describe HIV-associated dementia complex in the literature:
> HIV-associated dementia
> AIDS dementia complex
> HIV encephalopathy
> AIDS encephalopathy
> Subacute encephalitis
> AIDS-related dementia
> Terms used to describe HIV-associated minor cognitive motor disorder:
> HIV-associated mild neurocognitive disorder
> HIV-associated neurocognitive disorder

In 1991, the American Academy of Neurology AIDS Task Force published criteria to describe two neurobehavioral disorders that occur in HIV infection:

(1) HIV-associated dementia complex (HADC) and
(2) HIV-associated minor cognitive motor disorder (MCMD).

Collectively, these two disorders are referred to as HIV-associated cognitive/motor complex (HACM). The main differences between the disorders are the severity of the neuropsychological impairment and the degree of impairment in daily living.

- In HADC, neuropsychological deficits are moderate to severe and cause marked interference with day-to-day function.
- In MCMD, neuropsychological deficits are mild and cause only mild functional impairment.

What is the prevalence of HADC and MCMD?

The prevalence of HADC and MCMD has been difficult to determine due to the range of criteria used in definitions and the differing measurement instruments. According to studies conducted in the pre-HAART era, the rates of neurocognitive impairment on objective neuropsychological testing increased across successive disease states. That is, rates of neuropsychological impairment for persons in more advanced Center for Disease Control and Prevention disease categories were higher than those in less advanced categories. The reported rates of cognitive impairment prior to the introduction of HAART were 35% in asymptomatic patients, 44% in mildly symptomatic patients, and 55% in patients with AIDS (Heaton and Grant 1995; White *et al.*, 1995).

In the pre-HAART era, about 15–19% of people with clinically defined AIDS would develop HADC (McArthur *et al.*, 1993). With HAART, that number has dropped. A recent study showed that for 6% of those diagnosed with AIDS, HADC was their AIDS-defining illness (Dore *et al.*, 1999). MCMD is thought to be present in approximately 20–25% of people with HIV disease, and that has remained fairly constant both prior to and after HAART (Grant and Martin, 1994; Neuenburg *et al.*, 2002).

What are the characteristics of HACM?

HACM is characterized by impairment in cognitive functioning, particularly attention, processing speed, new learning, and executive functions. This pattern is similar to other subcortical dementias such as the ones resulting from Huntington's disease or Parkinson's disease. Higher cortical dysfunctions such as aphasia and agnosia are usually absent, until the end stage of the disease. Impairment in motor functioning can also occur, with complaints of difficulty with handwriting, clumsiness, unsteadiness of gait, hyperreflexia, motor slowing, and deficits in motor control.

> Common subjective complaints made by patients experiencing HACM include:
> "I am having difficulty focusing."
> "I have trouble concentrating when someone is giving me instructions."
> "I can't work as fast as I used to."

To be diagnosed with HACM, a patient must have a verifiable change in cognitive ability that affects her or his capacity to work or perform other activities of daily living. A deficit in either motor function or affect and behavioral function can also exist but may tend to occur more in HADC. The change must persist for at least 1 month and cannot be attributed to another cause such as an opportunistic infection. Some patients with HIV disease may have neuropsychological impairment on testing, with no apparent impact on their day-to-day functioning. These patients are not given a diagnosis of HACM. Current investigations are under way in HIV research centers to determine whether these atypical presentations represent subclinical or early HIV-associated complications.

Depression and anxiety are common in people with HIV, and a key component of the psychiatric assessment is to discern whether a patient's cognitive complaints are due to an underlying cognitive disorder secondary to HIV-related brain disease (HACM), secondary to a major depression, or attributable to a combination of both processes.

Case study: A woman with minor cognitive motor disorder

Clair is a 37-year-old woman who is working full time as an accountant. She has no children. She has been HIV seropositive for eight years. Her CD4 cell count is 225 cells/mm^3 and her HIV viral load is 40 000 copies/ml. She is clinically asymptomatic.

Over the past 6 months, she reports that she has been struggling with her work, and her mind is less sharp. She feels less efficient and less focused. She complains that her memory and her attention span for tasks seem to be worse. She also feels more irritable and down. She is worried about her work performance. She is anxious about the situation and is not sleeping well. She is concerned that she may be developing "dementia" but her friends tell her that she is just depressed.

What are the characteristics of HIV-associated minor cognitive motor disorder (MCMD)?

In HIV-associated minor cognitive motor disorder (MCMD), the cognitive impairment is mild and more subtle in nature, but may result in significant morbidity. Patients with MCMD often present with complaints of forgetfulness, decreased concentration, word-finding difficulties, and cognitive inefficiency. They often experience a loss of self-confidence in the workplace and may question their ability to work effectively. MCMD is a concern for patients who wonder why their brain is not working optimally and fear that this mild decline will progress to a more severe dementia. In contrast to HADC, this milder cognitive syndrome continues to be prevalent even with the widespread availability of HAART (Table 2.1).

What is the course of illness?

Most patients with MCMD will show some fluctuation in cognitive symptoms but are generally stable over a 2-year period. There may be no progressive deterioration or only mild, transient worsening of symptoms during periods of systemic illness. Rapid progression appears to be related to the patient's overall systemic

Table 2.1. Criteria for HIV-Associated Minor Cognitive Motor Disorder (MCMD).

Criteria	Defined by

1. Cognitive/motor/behavioral abnormalities. Must have at least two of the following (present for ≥ 1 month):
    impaired attention and concentration
    mental slowing
    impaired memory
    slowed movements
    incoordination
    personality change, irritability or emotional lability
	Abnormalities verified by both a reliable history (when possible from an informant) and by clinical neurologic examination or neuropsychological tests

2. Mild impairment of work or activities of daily living	Impairments verified objectively or by report of a key informant
3. Does not meet criteria for HIV dementia or HIV myelopathy	
4. No other etiology present. Alternative etiologies include active CNS opportunistic infection or malignancy, severe systemic illness, active alcohol or substance use, acute or chronic substance withdrawal, adjustment disorder, or other psychiatric disorder	Alternative etiologies excluded through appropriate history, physical examination, and laboratory and radiologic investigation (e.g., lumbar puncture, neuroimaging)

Note: For a probable diagnosis, a patient must meet all four criteria. A possible diagnosis of minor cognitive motor disorder can be made if criteria 1–3 are present and either an alternative etiology is present and the cause of number 1 is not certain, or the etiology of criterion 1 cannot be determined because of an incomplete evaluation.
Adapted from the American Academy of Neurology AIDS Task Force 1991.

health and immune function. Patients who are most immunocompromised and systemically unwell are at the highest risk of rapid progression.

According to the DANA Consortium on Therapy for HIV Dementia and Related Cognitive Disorders (1996), it remains unclear whether MCMD and HADC are two distinct entities or a single continuous entity differentiated only by severity (Marder *et al.*, 1998).

Any abrupt changes in mental status (e.g., rapid deterioration, new-onset focal neurologic findings, seizures, psychosis, or mania) should be investigated for causes other than or in addition to HACM.

What is the morbidity associated with HIV-related neurocognitive impairment?

HIV-related neurocognitive impairment has been associated with decreased survival, poorer quality of life, poorer medication adherence, more unemployment, and a subjective sense of diminished work performance (Heaton *et al.*, 1994,1996; Kaplan *et al.*, 1995; Albert *et al.*, 1995,1999; Ellis *et al.*, 1997; Marder *et al.*, 1998).

Patients display a wide range of reactions to cognitive losses, and the functional impact of these losses varies considerably. Intervention is focused on both biologically limiting progression and maximizing the patient's functioning and adaptation.

What is the relationship between cognitive complaints and depression?

It is often difficult to differentiate HACM from a major depressive disorder. The disorders frequently coexist. The presence of apathy, amotivation, and anergia, along with cognitive deficits consistent with HACM, and the absence of a qualitative subjective sense of sadness, are more suggestive of HACM (or consequences of advanced systemic HIV disease) than a major depressive episode. Practitioners should rule out an organic etiology in patients living with advanced HIV disease before attributing the symptom complex to major depression alone.

Subjective neurocognitive complaints can often be associated with depressed mood, but not necessarily with a decrease in objective neuropsychiatric performance (Rourke *et al.*, 1999a). While many depressed people with HIV may complain of cognitive problems, this is not necessarily reflective of their actual cognitive ability. The psychiatrist can counsel the patient that as their mood symptoms improve, they may experience a subjective improvement in their cognitive symptoms. Anxiety symptoms occurring in the context of cognitive problems have not been studied in HIV disease, but clinicians suspect that the relationship is similar to that between cognitive problems and depression. By contrast, individuals who are impaired in frontal-executive functioning may underestimate the extent of their cognitive impairment because they are not able to accurately assess their skills (Rourke *et al.*, 1999b).

Depressed patients also have more difficulty adhering to HAART (Catz *et al.*, 2000), which may lead to less than optimal treatment of their HIV disease, including HACM (Paterson *et al.*, 2000). The psychiatrist can play an important role in identifying and treating depression, and assessing the impact on the patient's adherence to HAART. The psychiatrist can also liaise with the patient's HIV/AIDS physician to help determine if a delay in starting HAART or a HAART holiday might be advisable, rather than risking the patient's ongoing non-adherence in the face of depression.

What is the treatment approach when patients have symptoms of depression and MCMD?

When clinicians identify both cognitive symptoms and symptoms of depression in an individual, it is essential that both systemic HIV disease and depression be identified as potential causes of the complaints, and each be optimally treated. If systemic medical factors (physical symptoms, CD4 count, viral load) indicate that HIV disease needs treatment, HAART should be initiated or optimized to aim for full suppression of viral replication. Similarly, if a major depression is identified, antidepressant treatment should be initiated, aimed at full remission of depressive symptoms.

Neuropsychological testing, when available, can be used to differentiate those cognitive symptoms associated with depression versus those associated with HIV disease.

In some people, MCMD can be clearly diagnosed even in the context of depression. In these cases, the clinician should treat both conditions: the patient should receive HAART for optimal treatment of their systemic disease, and an antidepressant or psychotherapy for the treatment of depression.

Studies indicate that adding HAART to the management of people with MCMD primarily improves overall psychomotor efficiency. The benefits to other specific functions (attention, working memory, learning ability) are less clear (Sacktor *et al.*, 1999; Tozzi *et al.*, 1999; Cohen *et al.*, 2001).

A psychiatrist can be instrumental in helping identify the presence and cause of both cognitive and depressive symptoms and advising the HIV/AIDS physician on the timing of HAART initiation.

When should a psychiatrist consider neuropsychological testing?

Neuropsychological testing provides objective data in the evaluation of cognitive complaints, and helps elucidate early and less obvious neurologic impairment. When used on a single occasion it can provide a cross-sectional snapshot of performance as compared to age and education-matched controls. This can help define areas of performance deficit. When used longitudinally, neuropsychological testing can be more helpful because it provides objective data at two or more points in time, which can be used to monitor both progression of deficits and response to treatments.

Examples of beneficial cross-sectional neuropsychological assessment include:
- a patient has subjective concerns about cognitive performance and wants to make important work-related decisions, e.g., return to school, change in job status/demands, decision to go on disability
- a patient is reluctant to begin HAART because of systemic/immunologic factors but may be persuaded to do so if there are objective findings of cognitive decline
- a clinician wants to differentiate between depression and HACM

Epilogue

Clair is assessed by a psychiatrist who determines that she is not depressed. Although her mood is consistently irritable, she only feels sad when she thinks about her difficulties at work. Her appetite and energy are both good, and she maintains a sense of optimism about herself and the prospect of some improvement in her symptoms.

Clair agrees to undergo neuropsychological testing, which shows deficits in attention, psychomotor speed, and working memory. She works with her psychiatrist and an occupational therapist to develop compensatory strategies that help her at home and at work. She also makes the decision to start antiretroviral therapy to treat her systemic HIV disease and improve the cognitive symptoms.

One year later, repeat neuropsychological testing shows improvement in some aspects of Clair's cognitive status, particularly psychomotor efficiency.

Case study: HIV-associated dementia complex

Ravi is a 50-year-old gay male currently employed as a vice-president of a large company. Over a 3-month period, his employer has noticed a decline in his work performance. Ravi is no longer able to remember appointments and agendas as he once did. He acknowledges that his memory has been less sharp over the past year. He says he is unable to concentrate in meetings and feels two steps behind his usual mental pace. He is having difficulty learning a new computer software package and remembering the plot of the latest book he is reading.

Ravi reports that he is frequently fatigued, has less energy, and is unenthused about his work or other activities. He has lost 3.6 kg in the past year and has a difficult time falling asleep. He is less interested in socializing with friends. His partner says that he is uninvolved in home chores, irritable, and indecisive. When pushed by his partner, Ravi can take pleasure in activities but is reluctant to participate in most things he enjoyed in the past. His partner complains that he is slower and frequently clumsy. Ravi reports feeling frustrated rather than sad. He has been drinking more alcohol at night and using over-the-counter sleep preparations without relief. He has no suicidal ideation or intent. He has no personal or family psychiatric history.

He had one episode of *Pneumocystis carinii* pneumonia (PCP) 2 years earlier, but is currently systemically well, with only mild oral candidiasis. His antiretroviral treatment includes efavirenz 600 mg qhs, zidovudine 300 mg bid, and lamivudine 150 mg bid. His CD4 cell count is 90 cells/mm^3, his nadir CD4 cell count was 25 cells/mm^3, and his HIV viral load is 50 000 copies/ml.

What are the characteristics of HIV-associated dementia complex (HADC)?

HIV-associated dementia complex (HADC) is characterized by progressive decline in cognitive function accompanied by changes in affective, behavioral, and motor function, which results in a significant decrease in a person's capacity to attend to activities of daily living. Behaviorally, many patients with HADC will experience amotivation, anergia, fatigue, social withdrawal, or irritability (Table 2.2). In addition, the most common affective disorder that accompanies HACM is depression. Mania, hypomania, or disinhibition syndromes are less common than depression, but occur most often in advanced stages of HIV disease. Since the introduction of HAART, HIV dementia is now seen less frequently.

The DSM–IV–TR diagnosis (American Psychiatric Association, 2000) for this condition is Dementia due to HIV disease.

What are the risk factors for HADC?

Risk factors that correlate with HACM in adults include:

- older age
- lower educational achievement
- anemia
- multiple head injuries
- more constitutional symptoms before the onset of clinically defined AIDS
- not currently taking HAART.

Lower CD4 cell counts are associated with higher rates of cognitive impairment (Chang et al., 1999), but the relationship between plasma HIV viral load and cognitive impairment is more equivocal (McArthur et al., 1997; Stankoff et al., 1999) The impact of substance abuse as a risk factor for HACM is unclear; however, high levels of chronic substance use are known to cause cognitive changes, and this must be considered as a comorbidity in some individuals.

Which elements in this history are important in establishing the diagnosis?

Systemic clinical disease staging, HIV viral load, and CD4 cell count are markers of disease severity, and have implications when establishing a differential diagnosis. In the case of Ravi, the patient has had an AIDS-defining clinical condition, is significantly immunosuppressed, and has insufficient suppression of viral replication.

Other important diagnostic elements in this patient are:

- cognitive, affective, and motor complaints in the midst of significant immune suppression
- a pattern of cognitive deficits consistent with a slowly progressive decline in memory, concentration, new learning, and speed of processing
- behavior that is apathetic, amotivated, withdrawn, and at times irritable
- slow and, at times, clumsy motor functions but no focal neurologic symptoms
- A decrease in ability to function in usual day-to-day activities.

Table 2.2. Criteria for HIV-associated dementia complex (HADC)

Criteria	Defined by

1. Acquired abnormality in at least two of the following cognitive abilities (present for ≥ 1 month):
  attention/concentration
  speed of processing
  abstraction/reasoning
  visuospatial skills
  memory/learning
  speech/language
	Cognitive decline verified by history and mental status examination. When possible, history should be obtained from an informant and examination should be supplemented by neuropsychological testing. The cognitive dysfunction must cause impairment of work or in activities of daily living, with impairment not attributable solely to severe systemic illness

2. At least one of the following:
  (a) Acquired abnormality in motor function or performance, including:
    slowed rapid movement
    abnormal gait
    limb incoordination
    hyperreflexia
    hypertonia
    weakness
	Abnormality verified by physical examination, neuropsychological tests (e.g., fine motor speed, manual dexterity, perceptual motor skills), or both

(b) Decline in motivation or emotional control or change in social behavior	Change characterized by any of the following: apathy, inertia, irritability, emotional lability, or new-onset impaired judgment characterized by socially inappropriate behavior or disinhibition
3. Absence of clouding of consciousness during a period long enough to establish the presence of criterion 1	
4. Exclusion of another etiology. Alternate possible etiologies include active central nervous system opportunistic infections or malignancy, psychiatric disorders (e.g., depressive disorders), active substance abuse, or acute or chronic substance withdrawal	Alternative etiologies excluded by history, physical and psychiatric examination, and appropriate laboratory and radiologic tests

Adapted from the American Academy of Neurology AIDS Task Force 1991.

By history, the presentation is very typical of HACM. As this patient has significant immune suppression (CD4 < 200 cells/mm^3, low nadir CD4 lymphocyte count), other causes of cognitive dysfunction must also be considered, including secondary AIDS-related opportunistic conditions affecting the central nervous system.

Table 2.3. Differential diagnosis of neuropsychiatric impairment in HIV disease.

Factor	Conditions
Central nervous system	CNS opportunistic infections associated with advanced HIV disease such as toxoplasmosis, cryptococcal meningitis, progressive multifocal leukoencephalopathy (PML), cytomegalovirus (CMV) encephalitis, neurosyphillis and tuberculous meningitis CNS tumors associated with advanced HIV disease, such as primary cerebral lymphoma and metastatic Kaposi's sarcoma. Other neuropsychiatric disorders
Systemic conditions	Metabolic disorders (anemia, malnutrition), endocrinopathies (hypothyroidism, hypogonadism), and vitamin deficiencies (B12 deficiency) may present with some overlapping symptoms such as fatigue, decreased concentration, and apathy. Systemic conditions that cause a delirium may present with acute mental status changes
Psychiatric disorders	Major depression may present with similar symptoms of apathy, fatigue, and decreased concentration. Major depression may coexist with HACM
Substance related disorders	Drug intoxication and withdrawal states and chronic dependence/usage may present with cognitive signs and symptoms similar to those found in HACM
Medication side effects	Some medications commonly used in the treatment of HIV/ AIDS are associated with neuropsychiatric symptoms. See medical overview

What is the differential diagnosis and how can the physician narrow it?

The clinical history is helpful in determining the diagnosis (Table 2.3). No single piece of information or investigation can lead to a diagnosis of HACM. Instead, the practitioner must consider data from systemic, neurologic, and psychiatric examination, as well as ancillary investigations.

When the patient's CD4 cell count is below 200 cells/mm^3, the practitioner must consider the possibility of secondary opportunistic infections and tumors. These rarely present with neurocognitive findings alone however. Most often they present with focal neurologic findings and evidence of systemic illness. In Ravi's case, the course of illness has developed over several months, which is more consistent with HACM, endocrinopathy or metabolic disturbance, vitamin deficiencies, psychiatric disorder, or substance abuse disorder, than with a secondary infection.

- Toxoplasmosis, lymphoma, CMV, PML, cryptococcal meningitis, and tubercular meningitis are usually acute in their onset and progress rapidly, although they can take a more indolent course.
- Toxoplasmosis, cryptococcal meningitis, and CMV are generally accompanied by signs of systemic illness, such as headache, fever, and decreased level of consciousness.
- Cryptococcus generally presents with some meningeal signs and symptoms, although in some cases, the only symptom is headache.
- CMV encephalitis is rare in people with CD4 counts >100 cells/mm^3 and is also rare in the absence of other sites (retina, colon) of CMV infection.
- Focal signs on neurologic examination are most commonly seen in toxoplasmosis, lymphoma, and PML.

Ravi's neurologic examination reveals brisk reflexes bilaterally, mild extrapyramidal signs, generalized psychomotor slowing and clumsiness, but no focal signs. Psychiatric examination reveals an absence of personal and family psychiatric history but a pattern of substance use, including alcohol and hypnotics, which may affect cognitive function.

What other investigations are necessary to establish a diagnosis?

Hematological and biochemical investigations, anatomic brain imaging, cerebrospinal fluid (CSF) examination, and neuropsychological testing will help support the clinical examination findings and exclude other causes of central nervous system (CNS) dysfunction. The physician should use anatomic brain imaging techniques to detect other causes of CNS dysfunction, including space-occupying lesions due to toxoplasmic encephalitis, lymphoma, or stroke, which may complicate the course of HIV disease. Brain imaging should always be done for patients with focal neurologic signs or with rapidly progressive deterioration, decreased level of alertness, or new-onset mental status change such as seizure, mania, or psychosis in the course of HIV disease. (In Ravi's case, where there were no focal findings and a clinical picture consistent with HACM, anatomic brain imaging is less necessary.) Brain imaging techniques do not reliably detect early changes of HACM, nor do they show a high degree of specificity in clinical staging. Magnetic resonance imaging (MRI) is more specific and sensitive than computerized tomography (CT). The most common finding on both is cerebral atrophy and ventricular enlargement, with a pattern of combined central and cortical atrophy. MRI may also detect patchy T2-weighted white matter lesions and is more sensitive than CT in detecting regional atrophic changes, particularly in the subcortical structures.

The CT done on Ravi confirms the absence of focal brain pathology and shows moderate atrophy and ventricular dilatation.

The physician should use a CSF examination primarily to exclude other central conditions that may lead to mental status changes, including opportunistic infections (CMV, cryptococcus), tumors, and syphilis. In HACM alone, a CSF examination may show pleocytosis, elevated immunoglobulin-G, oligoclonal bands, and increased protein. All are nonspecific and do not correlate well with clinical severity. Research investigations, including measures of immune activation, such as increased CSF β2-microglobulin or quinolinic acid levels and measures of increased levels of CSF viral load, have been shown to correlate with clinical severity of cognitive decline but remain primarily research tools.

With Ravi's history highly suggestive of HACM, no history of syphilis, a negative serum VDRL and FTA-antibodies, no focal neurologic signs, and a negative serum cryptococcal serum antigen, the physician feels a lumbar puncture would add little to the diagnostic investigations, so it is not performed.

An electro-encephalogram, which may show mild, nonspecific slowing, contributes little to the diagnostic evaluation unless the clinician suspects a seizure disorder. Functional neuroimaging with single photon emission computed tomography (SPECT), positron emission tomography (PET), or magnetic resonance spectroscopy (MRS) are primarily research tools.

Laboratory blood work that may reveal systemic conditions that contribute to a delirium include: hemoglobin, glucose, electrolytes, liver function tests, calcium, albumin, magnesium, vitamin B12, thyroid-stimulating hormone and free testosterone. The decision to order these tests should be guided by the clinical examination.

Investigations and a detailed clinical history will help exclude substance-related disorders. If the clinician suspects either chronic or acute intoxication, he or she should measure levels of psychoactive drugs, including anticonvulsants, sedatives, narcotics, antidepressants, as well as alcohol.

Could the patient's symptoms be caused by major depression?

As noted earlier, it is often difficult to differentiate HACM from a major depressive disorder, and the two disorders often coexist.

In Ravi's case, the absence of personal or family history of depression and his insistence that he does not feel sad suggest that the symptoms are caused by HACM. His symptom profile, however, including loss of interest, sleep disturbance, diminished energy, diminished concentration, decreased weight and appetite, and psychomotor slowing, does meet the criteria for a major depressive episode, so both disorders (HADC and major depression due to a medical condition) are considered in the diagnosis.

Could the symptoms be caused by the substances that the patient is using?

Alcohol, benzodiazepines, hypnotics, and narcotics can all diminish concentration, attention, learning efficiency, and processing speed, can exacerbate cognitive decline.

In Ravi's case, it is possible that alcohol and hypnotics are affecting his cognitive function, but as his condition continues to deteriorate despite stable substance use, it is unlikely that the substances account for all his symptoms. It is possible that his sleep disorder is related to either HADC, major depression, or antiretroviral use (i.e. efavirenz).

What mental status screening and assessment tools should be used?

The physician should conduct office-based mental status screening tests on all patients to document their mental status.

The Folstein Mini-Mental State Examination (MMSE), which measures functions rarely impaired until advanced stages of HACM, is not sensitive to mild dysfunction and is therefore not useful. The MMSE was developed for use in screening cortical dementias and is relatively insensitive to subcortical processes.

Psychiatrists use a mental status screening examination to obtain a global clinical impression of cognitive function. Screening should incorporate tests of attention, short-term memory, frontal executive function, and psychomotor speed that may be more useful in identifying patients with mild cognitive decline. Typically, screening includes tests of orientation to person, place, time, digit span, four-word immediate registration and five-minute recall, serial sevens, Luria repetitive hand sequence maneuvers, and Trail Making Tests (A and B). The Trail Making Test (A and B) is a general screening instrument that involves the following functions: attention, concentration, speed of information processing, abstraction, cognitive flexibility, and executive skills. The Luria repetitive hand sequence maneuvers is a screening tool for frontal lobe functioning, in which the patient is taught a sequence of 3 maneuvers to complete with each hand and is then asked to repeat this sequence. The psychiatrist observes for accuracy and fluidity in repeating the sequence. These tests are used by neurologists and psychologists, with whom psychiatrists interested in these tools can confer regarding their correct use. The psychiatrist notes the accuracy of the tasks, the speed of performance, and the qualitative manner with which the tasks are performed. This group of tests is used clinically as a screen, but as it has not been validated as a cognitive screening measure for HACM, it is not possible to include cut-off numbers for the evaluation. Functional assessment of the impact of cognitive deficits is best evaluated by an occupational therapist skilled in the assessment of activities of daily living.

A screening scale which has been validated is the HIV Dementia Scale (HDS). It screens domains of memory, attention, psychomotor speed, and construction, and has been developed as a rapid screening examination. According to Power *et al.* (1995), a validation analysis using an HDS score > 10 to detect HIV-associated dementia was found to have a sensitivity of 80%, a specificity of 91%, and a positive predictive value of 78%. This validation study was conducted prior to the advent of HAART. A validation study conducted in the HAART era, which showed a sensitivity of 39% and a specificity of 85% (Smith *et al.*, 2003), is less encouraging. Although this screening scale has received the most widespread attention to date, its clinical utility is not certain.

What other staging system can be used to describe the cognitive changes in HIV disease?

The Memorial Sloan–Kettering clinical staging system for Aids Dementia Complex can also be used to describe the quality and severity of cognitive changes in HIV disease (Price and Brew, 1992). Individuals with a Memorial Sloan–Kettering of 0 are not considered to have HACM. Individuals with a Memorial Sloan–Kettering rating of 0.5 are considered equivocal and may or may not have MCMD. A Memorial Sloan–Kettering rating of 1 usually corresponds to a diagnosis of MCMD, while ratings between 2 and 4 are generally consistent with HADC (Table 2.4).

Mental status examination conducted on Ravi reveals that he is fully oriented with a normal level of alertness. He registers four of four words immediately, but can recall only two of four words after five minutes. He can remember a digit span of five forward and three backward. He makes only one error on serial sevens, but he is remarkably slow in his performance. He is clumsy with both hands in performing the Luria repetitive hand-sequence maneuvers and has difficulty repeating a complex sequential task. Using age- and education-adjusted norms, he scores in the bottom 10th percentile on the Trail Making Test (Part A) and in the bottom 5th percentile on the Trail Making Test (Part B) – again displaying markedly slow performance suggestive of diminished cognitive flexibility. This profile is consistent with HADC, with a Memorial Sloan–Kettering stage 2, and it establishes a baseline for future examinations.

Are there specific treatments for HACM?

Treatment decisions should be considered by the patient's treating internist/family physician in concert with psychiatrist/neurologist, and if available, the neuropsychologist. As HIV is believed to be the primary factor driving HACM progression, antiretroviral agents are considered first-line therapy. The benefits of antiretrovirals in HACM can be divided into two main categories:
- the potential benefit in treating cognitive decline (that is, reversing and/or halting the progression of deficits) once deficits have emerged
- the benefit of early intervention with antiretrovirals as a means to prevent the emergence of HACM.

Recent studies support the use of HAART in the treatment of HACM. The most common combination includes two or more nucleoside reverse transcriptase inhibitors (NRTIs) in combination with at least one protease inhibitor (PI) or one

Table 2.4. Memorial Sloan-Kettering clinical staging system for AIDS dementia complex

Stage	Degree of severity	Characteristics
0	Normal	Normal mental and motor function
0.5	Equivocal	Either minimal or equivocal symptoms of cognitive or motor dysfunction characteristic of HIV-associated cognitive–motor disorder, or mild signs (snout response, slowed extremity movements), but without impairment of work or capacity to perform activities of daily living (ADLs). Gait and strength are normal
1	Mild	Unequivocal evidence (symptoms, signs, neuropsychological test performance) of functional intellectual or motor impairment characteristic of HIV-associated cognitive–motor disorder, but able to perform all but the more demanding aspects of work or ADLs. Can walk without assistance
2	Moderate	Cannot work or perform the more demanding ADLs, but able to perform basic self-care ADLs. Ambulatory, but may require a single prop
3	Severe	Major intellectual incapacity (cannot follow news or personal events, cannot sustain complex conversations, considerable slowing of all output) or motor disability (cannot walk unassisted, requiring walker or personal support, usually with slowing and clumsiness of arms as well)
4	End Stage	Nearly vegetative. Intellectual and social comprehension and output are at a rudimentary level. Nearly or absolutely mute. Paraparetic or paraplegic with double incontinence (urinary and bowel)

ADL = activity of daily living. Adapted from Price and Brew, 1992.

non-nucleoside reverse transcriptase inhibitor (NNRTI). Several studies show significantly better neuropsychological performance in cohorts of patients taking HAART. Longitudinal studies also show improvements in abnormal baseline neuropsychiatric performance in patients taking HAART (Ferrando *et al.*, 1998; Filippi *et al.*, 1998;

Galgani *et al.*, 1998; Letendre *et al.*, 1998; Martin *et al.*, 1998; Aweeka *et al.*, 1999; Sacktor *et al.*, 1999).

As individual agents, only two antiretrovirals have been examined in randomized, placebo-controlled trials:

- zidovudine (AZT) as monotherapy has been shown to be efficacious in improving neuropsychological performance at high doses, but improvements were not durable for greater than 12 months, and the doses resulted in high levels of toxicity, and far exceed currently recommended doses (Schmitt *et al.*, 1988; Sidtis *et al.*, 1993)
- abacavir was not shown to be efficacious for neuropsychological performance when tested as an add-on medication to a patient's existing antiretroviral regimen (Brew *et al.*, 1998).

In the pre-HAART era, AZT was considered the first line of treatment to halt the progression of neurocognitive impairment. Recommendations at that time were to start AZT (600–800 mg/day) as a part of the patient's antiretroviral combination, or to increase the dose of AZT in patients who were already taking it. This strategy leads to considerable toxicity, promotes antiretroviral resistance, and does not have any durable antiviral effect. Strategies of adding a single antiretroviral agent to a failing regimen should not be used to treat either systemic HIV disease or HACM. Principles for successful use of HAART in treatment of systemic HIV disease apply to the treatment of HACM as well.

Reseachers initially hypothesized that the antiretroviral had to penetrate the CNS to improve or prevent HIV-related neurocognitive impairment. Although this is theoretically plausible, evidence does not yet support the notion that the use of brain-penetrating agents is more effective than nonbrain-penetrating agents. Clinicians should choose medications most likely to ensure systemic viral load suppression. Other factors to consider in selecting antiretrovirals include:

- the patient's antiretroviral resistance profile
- tolerability of the medication
- potential for optimal medication adherence.

There may be a relationship between CSF viral load and neuropsychological impairment in persons with AIDS, but the strength of this relationship is not clear (McArthur *et al.*, 1997; Stankoff *et al.*, 1999; Ellis *et al.*, 2002). This has led researchers to investigate the use of other medications that may limit neurologic injury, minimize the inflammatory cascade, or confer neuroprotection. These agents include nimodipine, peptide T, lexipafant, selegiline, memantine, and donepezil, but none are currently clinically indicated for the treatment of HACM.

What can be done for the fatigue and apathy?

Fatigue, apathy, anergia, amotivation, and dysphoria are particularly troublesome symptoms that have a significant impact on a person's quality of life. Even in the absence of major depression, people living with HACM and late-stage HIV disease may experience these symptoms.

Low-dose psychostimulants can be used to treat these symptoms. Methylphenidate or dextroamphetamine may be started at 5 mg each morning and titrated upwards based on response and side effects in 5-mg increments every 48 hours to a daily maximum of 60 mg daily . Mean daily dosage is usually between 10 and 20 mg, and some patients benefit from a booster dose at noon to carry the effect of the morning dose through the afternoon. Others prefer the sustained release formulation given once per day. Doses after 13:00 hours should be avoided because they may interfere with nighttime sleep. Patients should be told that stimulants can be addictive, and clinicians should prescribe them judiciously to mitigate any possible abuse or misuse. This concern, however, should not prevent psychiatrists from prescribing psychostimulants when appropriate. Patients who are in recovery from substance dependence disorder may be reluctant to take a stimulant for fear of retriggering feelings associated with the addiction. Clinicians should also be aware that methylphenidate has been demonstrated to be effective for fatigue in one randomized, double blind, placebo-controlled trial (Breitbart *et al.*, 2001). However, fatigue in the context of HIV disease and HACM, are not FDA approved indications for the use of psychostimulants.

Epilogue

Ravi wants his HADC managed aggressively. The psychiatrist and Ravi discuss that optimal management of his systemic HIV disease with HAART is also the first step in treatment of HADC. In consultation with his HIV specialist, Ravi decides to start on three antiretrovirals that he has never been on before (d4t, ddI, and lopinavir), in hopes of fully suppressing viral replication. His clinicians emphasize strategies to promote optimal adherence to the antiviral medications.

Follow-up neuropsychological assessment is planned for 6-month intervals to help the clinical team document objective evidence of improvement in neuropsychological function, which would help guide treatment decisions.

The psychiatrist advises Ravi to decrease his alcohol intake and prescribes a non-benzodiazepine hypnotic to replace the over-the-counter hypnotic Ravi was using to manage his sleep problems. They also discuss a trial of low-dose trazodone (50 mg at bedtime) as a hypnotic alternative to benzodiazepines. The psychiatrist decides to monitor Ravi's mood symptoms for a period of time before initiating antidepressant treatment.

Case study: Dementia with behavioral complications

Carlo is a 37-year-old man with AIDS, an HIV viral load of 110 000 copies/ml, and a CD4 cell count of 10 cells/mm^3. Four months before he was assessed, he was in his usual state of health. At that time, he began to complain of memory difficulties and inattention. This was followed by a steady decrease in cognitive capacities and an increase in intrusive, argumentative, impulsive, and bizarre behavior. Systemically, he had several HIV-associated symptomatic conditions including candidiasis infection and wasting.

When he is examined, he has no insight into the inappropriateness of his behavior and is highly concrete in his interpretation of his situation. He reports that he stopped his antiretroviral medications 6 months ago because he felt he had been cured of HIV disease. He is emotionally labile and at times argumentative, but denies having a sense of euphoria or grandiosity.

He is fully oriented in all spheres and scores 25/30 on a Folstein MMSE, with deficits in serial sevens and sequential task performance. He is unable to perform the Luria hand sequence maneuvers, is markedly inaccurate and concrete in his clock drawing, and is unable to perform complex tasks requiring planning, organizing, and sequencing.

He has no personal or family history of psychiatric problems. He denies alcohol and drug use and is taking no new medications. He displays no focal neurologic findings other than cognitive, behavioral, and personality changes, suggesting a frontal lobe syndrome.

An occupational therapy assessment confirms that he is unable to perform basic activities of self-care required for independent living, and a home visit reveals that his apartment has become unsafe.

An MRI reveals patchy T2-weighted white matter lesions in the frontal region with diffuse cortical and central atrophy and enlarged ventricles. Two sleep-deprived electro-encephalograms show diffuse slow-wave activity but no focal discharges.

Carlo appears to have an organic mental condition secondary to HIV disease.

Opportunistic conditions described earlier in this chapter are ruled out.

Carlo does not have the capacity to make treatment decisions due to his inability to understand and appreciate that he has HIV disease and needs ongoing treatment. Because of his behavior, he is found to be at risk of imminent harm to himself through lack of self-care; he is admitted involuntarily to a psychiatric inpatient unit under regional mental health legislation.

What impact does HADC have on behavior?

HADC may involve affective and behavioral symptoms that require psychiatric care. Apathy and amotivation are the more common affective problems of HADC, but HADC may also be complicated by behavioral disinhibition syndromes including hypomania and frontal lobe impairment, resulting in impulsivity, disinhibition, mood instability, and poor judgment.

How should behavioral symptoms associated with HADC be treated?

The first step in managing behavioral symptoms associated with HADC is to treat the underlying HADC with HAART, while using psychiatric interventions to stabilize the affective and behavioral symptoms.

Apathy and amotivation can be treated by low-dose psychostimulants, in a manner similar to that suggested earlier. However, clinicians should consider depression in the differential diagnosis, as psychostimulants are not effective as a sole agent in treating major depression.

There are limited outcome data on treatments for frontal lobe executive deficit symptoms and manic symptoms in HIV disease. Treatment is based on the limited data and clinical experience accrued from similar populations. (For more information on treating manic syndromes, See Chapter 4 on Mood Disorders.) The strategies employed to manage frontal lobe and executive deficit symptoms include mood stabilizers or antipsychotics.

- Divalproex sodium is often chosen as a mood stabilizer as it is thought to be well tolerated in persons with HIV disease. It must be used with some caution as recent in vitro data suggest that it causes an increase in HIV replication (Simon *et al.*, 1994; Moog *et al.*, 1996; Witvrouw *et al.*, 1997). Retrospective clinical data suggest that in the presence of adequate antiretroviral therapy, HIV viral load may not be increased in response to divalproex sodium; sample sizes in these studies were small however, so monitoring of HIV viral load is still recommended as a precaution (Maggi and Halman, 2001). Dosing usually begins at 250 mg bid and is titrated against symptoms.
- Olanzapine and risperidone are also used at low doses for control of impulsivity, agitation, disinhibition, and mood instability associated with the later stages of HACM. Typical doses include 2.5–5 mg/day of olanzapine or 0.5–1 mg bid of risperidone.

It is important to remember that patients with HADC are vulnerable to the side effects of several medications, including the antipsychotic agents that block dopamine (D2) receptors. As Hriso *et al.* (1991) note, psychiatrists should use lower doses of these agents to treat delirium and behavioral disorders in people living with HIV (i.e., use doses comparable to those used with geriatric patients).

Are there nonpharmacological interventions that should be considered in the management of HADC?

The psychiatrist can play an important role in helping to coordinate psychosocial support for the patient. Psycho-education can help the patient and family learn about the nature of HADC and management strategies.

In the early stages of HADC, people can often adjust to their cognitive losses and continue to function somewhat normally. They can use an adaptation strategy to reinforce their remaining cognitive abilities and compensate for their limitations. Patients are encouraged to:

- keep a written record of appointments and important dates using a daytimer
- slow down and undertake only one task at a time
- keep mentally active (e.g., play games such as Scrabble, cards, and video games, and do crosswords and jigsaw puzzles, and ensure the activities are challenging but not frustrating)
- get plenty of rest
- schedule appointments at times when they are less likely to be fatigued
- improve their ability to concentrate and focus by problem-solving out loud
- avoid stressful situations and environments such as busy shopping malls
- use stress reduction and relaxation techniques
- avoid tasks they once did easily but now find frustrating (e.g., balancing a cheque book)
- exercise regularly
- use a pill box to manage their own medications as long as possible, and work with someone to ensure correct medication management (e.g., a caregiver, friend, registered nurse, occupational therapist).

As HADC progresses, cognitive problems become more marked, and patients have more difficulty adapting to them. At that stage, caregivers can use environmental engineering to provide an external structure that makes the world less confusing for the patient. The more structured the environment, the easier it is for people to understand and process what is happening around them. Depending on the severity of the cognitive impairment, this may include:

- frequently orienting the person to the year, month, date, time, and place
- keeping calendars and clocks in view
- posting the day's date and the person's schedule for the day on a wall or blackboard
- using nightlights, particularly for people who become disoriented in the dark
- ensuring that familiar objects and pictures are placed in the person's room (especially if the person is in a hospital or other setting away from home)
- keeping furniture, personal objects, and daily living utensils in the same place
- having the same home-care attendant assigned to the patient
- putting up large, clear signs to label different rooms
- ensuring the person carries an identification card with the names, addresses, and phone numbers of caregivers on it
- presenting information slowly, one step at a time, and asking the person to repeat instructions to make sure he or she has understood them

- encouraging the person to talk about familiar places, interests, and past experiences
- assessing the person's ability to manage stimulation and adjusting the amount of stimulation in the environment accordingly (e.g., keeping the space uncluttered, setting a maximum number of people to visit at one time)
- removing anything from the environment that seems to trigger anxiety
- simplifying tasks and allowing the person to do them at his or her own pace.

The most important intervention is consultation with a knowledgeable occupational therapist, psychologist, or rehabilitation counselor who can design an individualized care plan or strategy and help the patient implement this strategy.

In practice, these strategies only minimally address the difficult nature of this problem. With increasing severity of cognitive deficits, the functional limitations become extremely cumbersome. After maximizing medical treatment with HAART, there is little else that has been proven effective. Researchers are currently examining the use of cognitive rehabilitation in the treatment of HADC, as better strategies are urgently needed.

What is the prognosis for a person presenting with HADC?

It is unclear how much recovery may occur in patients with HADC. Use of HAART to achieve full viral suppression results in significant improvement in some patients, including halting disease progression and in some cases improvement in psychomotor efficiency. Usually there is little change seen in symptoms such as learning and working memory. To maintain the improvements, it appears to be necessary to maintain full viral suppression with HAART. In some patients, brain disease is too advanced and no significant recovery occurs.

A treatment plan is designed by Carlo's internist and authorized by Carlo's partner who is his substitute decision maker. Carlo is started on abacavir, AZT, 3TC and lopinavir in an attempt to reduce his systemic and brain viral load. The psychiatrist is involved in assisting to manage the behavioral disturbance. A trial of haloperidol 1 mg at bedtime results in problematic extrapyramidal symptoms, but Carlo's behavioral symptoms improve somewhat on risperidone 0.5 mg twice a day. Mood lability and disinhibition remain a concern. Divalproex sodium is added, and titrated up to 1000 mg at bedtime with good results.

Within the first 2 weeks of treatment, Carlo's systematic health improves. After 2 months, his viral load decreases to 12 000 copies/ml and his CD4 cell count increases to 150 cells/mm^3.

There is mild improvement in his psychomotor efficiency over the 2-month period. Despite HAART therapy, working memory and complex tasks such as organization remain a significant problem for Carlo. He continues to have marked difficulties in some of his self-care activities. Ultimately, he accepts a transfer to a supportive housing facility with 24- hour staff to assist with activities of daily living and nursing care.

Conclusion

In diagnosing and managing cognitive disorders associated with HIV disease, the psychiatrist should work closely with the treating internist, primary care physician, neurologist, and neuropsychologist where available. Psycho-pharmacological management must involve treating both the symptomatic condition and the underlying disease process.

REFERENCES

Albert, S. M., Marder, K., Dooneief, G. *et al.* Neuropsychologic impairment in early HIV infection: A risk factor for work disability. *Archives of Neurology,* **52**(5) (1995): 525–30.

Albert, S. M., Weber, C., Todak, G. *et al.* An observed performance test of medication management ability in HIV: relation to neuropsychological status and medication adherence outcomes. *Aids and Behavior,* **3**(2)(1999): 121–8.

American Academy of Neurology AIDS Task Force. Nomenclature and research case definitions for neurologic manifestations of human immunodeficiency virus type-1 (HIV-1) infection. *Neurology,* **41**(6)(1991): 778–85.

American Psychiatric Association. *Diagnostic and Statistical Manual of Mental Disorder. 4th edn text revised.* Washington, DC: American Psychiatric Association, 2000.

Aweeka, F., Jayewardene, A., Staprans, S. *et al.* Failure to detect nelfinavir in the cerebrospinal fluid of HIV-1-infected patients with and without AIDS dementia complex. *Journal of Acquired Immune Deficiency Syndrome and Human Retrovirology,* **20** (1999): 39–43.

Breitbart, W., Rosenfeld, B., Kaim, M. and Funesti-Esch, J. A randomized, double-blind, placebo-controlled trial of psychostimulants for the treatment of fatigue in ambulatory patients with human immunodeficiency virus disease. *Archives of Internal Medicine,* **161**(3)(2001): 411–20.

Brew, B. J., Brown, S. J., Catalan, J.*et al.,* Safety and efficacy of abacavir (ABC, 1592) in AIDS dementia complex (study CNAB 3001) (abstract no. 32192). 12th World AIDS Conference, Geneva, Switzerland, 1998.

Catz, S. L., Kelly, J. A., Bogart, L. M. *et al.* Patterns, correlates, and barriers to medication adherence among persons prescribed new treatment for HIV disease. *Health Psychology,* **19**(2) (2000): 124–133.

Chang, L., Ernst, T., Leonido-Yee, M. *et al.* Cerebral metabolite abnormalities correlate with clinical severity of HIV-1 cognitive motor complex. *Neurology,* **52**(1) (1999): 100–8.

Cohen, R. A., Boland, R., Paul, R. *et al.* Neurocognitive performance enhanced by highly active antiretroviral therapy in HIV-infected women. *AIDS,* **15**(3) (2001): 341–5.

Cummings, J. L. *Subcortical Dementia.* New York: Oxford University Press, 1990.

Dore, G. J., Correll, P. K., Li, Y. *et al.* Changes in AIDS dementia complex in the era of highly active antiretroviral therapy. *AIDS,* **13**(1999): 1249–53.

Ellis, R. J., Deutsch, R., Heaton, R. K. *et al.* Neurocognitive impairment is an independent risk factor for death in HIV infection. *Archives of Neurology*, **54** (1997): 416–24.

Ellis, R. J., Moore, D. J., Childers, M. E. *et al.* Progression to neuropsychological impairment in human immunodeficiency virus infection predicted by elevated cerebrospinal fluid levels of human immunodeficiency virus RNA. *Archives of Neurology*, **59**(6) (2002): 923–8.

Ferrando, S., van Gorp, W., McElhiney, M. *et al.* Highly active antiretroviral treatment in HIV infection: benefits for neuropsychological function. *AIDS*, **12**(8) (1998): F65–70.

Filippi, C. G., Sze, G., Farber, S. J. *et al.* Regression of HIV encephalopathy and basal ganglia signal intensity abnormality at MR imaging in patients with AIDS after the initiation of protease inhibitor therapy. *Radiology*, **206** (1998): 491–8.

Galgani,S., Balestra, P., Tozzi, V. *et al.* Comparison of efficacy of different antiretroviral regimens on neuropsychological performance in HIV-1 patients (abstract). *Journal of NeuroVirology*, **4**(1998): 350.

Grant, I. and Adams, K. M. (eds.) *Neuropsychological Assessment of Neuropsychiatric Disorders.* New York: Oxford University Press, 1996.

Grant, I. and Martin, A. *Neuropsychology of HIV infection.* New York: Oxford University Press, 1994.

Heaton, R. K. and Grant, I. *Neurobehavioral Progress Report/Preliminary Studies (research plan presented to NIMH, Office on AIDS)*, Grant, I., ed. San Diego, CA: HIV Neurobehavioral Research Center, 1995.

Heaton, R. K., Marcotte, T. D., White, D. A. *et al.* Nature and vocational significance or neuropsychological impairment associated with HIV infection. *Clinical Neuropsychologist*, **10** (1996): 1–14.

Heaton, R. K., Velin, R. A., McCutchan, J. A. *et al.* Neuropsychological impairment in human immunodeficiency virus-infection: implications for employment. HNRC Group, HIV Neurobehavioral Research Center. *Psychosomatic Medicine*, **56**(1)(1994): 8–17.

Hriso, E., Kuhn, T., Masdeu, J. C. and Grundman, M. Extrapyramidal symptoms due to dopamine-blocking agents in patients with AIDS encephalopathy. *American Journal of Psychiatry*, **148** (11)(1991): 1558–61.

Kaplan, R. M., Anderson, J. P., Patterson, T. L. *et al.* Validity of the quality of well-being scale for persons with human immunodeficiency virus infection. HNRC Group, HIV Neurobehavioral Research Center. *Psychosomatic Medicine*, **57**(2) (1995): 138–47.

Letendre, S., Ellis, R., Heaton, R. K. *et al.* Change in CSF RNA level correlates with the effects of antiretroviral therapy on HIV-1 associated neurocognitive disorder (abstract no. 32198). *Journal of NeuroVirology*, **4** (1998): 357.

Maggi, J. D. and Halman, M. H. The effect of divalproex sodium on viral load: a retrospective review of HIV-positive patients with manic syndromes. *Canadian Journal of Psychiatry*, **46**(4) (2001): 359–62.

Marder, K., Albert, S. M., McDermott, M. and the DANA Consortium on therapy for HIV dementia and related disorders. Prospective study of neurocognitive impairment in HIV (DANA cohort): dementia and mortality outcomes. *Journal of NeuroVirology*, **4** (1998): 358.

Martin, E. M., Pitrak, D. L., Pursell, K. J. *et al.* Information processing and antiretroviral therapy in HIV-1 infection. *Journal of the International Neuropsychological Society*, **4** (1998): 329–35.

Masliah, E., Heaton, R.K., Marcotte, T. D. *et al*. Dendritic injury is a pathological substrate for human immunodeficiency virus-related cognitive disorders. *Annals of Neurology*, **42** (1997): 963–72.

McArthur, J. C., Hoover, D. R., Bacellar, H. *et al*. Dementia in AIDS patients: incidence and risk factors. Multicenter AIDS Cohort Study. *Neurology*, **43**(11) (1993): 2245–52.

McArthur, J. C., McClernon, D. R., Cronin, M. F. *et al*. Relationship between human immunodeficiency virus-associated dementia and viral load in cerebrospinal fluid and brain. *Annals of Neurology*, **42**(5) (1997): 689–98

Moog, C., Kuntz-Simon, G., Caussin-Schwemling, C. and Obert, G. Sodium valproate, an anticonvulsant drug, stimulates human immunodeficiency virus type 1 replication independently of glutathione levels. *Journal of General Virology*, **77** (1996): 1993–9.

Neuenburg, J. K., Brodt, H. R., Herndier, B. G. *et al*. HIV-related neuropathology, 1985 to 1999: rising prevalence of HIV encephalopathy in the era of highly active antiretroviral therapy. *Journal of Acquired Immune Deficiency Syndromes*, **31**(2) (2002): 171–7.

Parks, R. W., Zec, R. F. and Wilson, R. S. (eds.). *Neuropsychology of Alzheimer's Disease and Other Dementias*. New York: Oxford University Press, 1993.

Paterson, D. L., Swindells, S., Mohr, J. and Brester, M. Adherence to protease inhibitor therapy and outcomes in patients with HIV infection. *Annals of Internal Medicine*, **133**(1) (2000): 21–30.

Power, C., Selnes, O. A., Grim, J. A., and McArthur, J. C. HIV Dementia Scale: a rapid screening test. *Journal of Acquired Immune Deficiency Syndrome and Human Retrovirology*, **8**(3) (1995): 273–8.

Price, R. W. and Brew, B. J. The AIDS dementia complex. *Journal of Infectious Diseases*, **158** (1992): 1079–83.

Rourke, S. B., Bassel, C. and Halman, M. H. Neurocognitive complaints in HIV-infection and their relationship to depressive symptoms and neuropsychological functioning. *Journal of Clinical and Experimental Neuropsychology*, **21** (1999a): 737–56.

Rourke, S. B., Bassel, C. and Halman, M. H. Neuropsychiatric correlates of memory-metamemory dissociations in HIV-1 infection. *Journal of Clinical and Experimental Neuropsychology*, **21** (1999b): 757–68.

Sacktor, N. C., Lyles, R. H., Skolasky, R. L. *et al*. Combination antiretroviral therapy improves psychomotor speed performance in HIV-seropositive homosexual men. Multicenter AIDS Cohort Study (MACS). *Neurology*, **52**(8) (1999): 1640–7.

Schmitt, F. A., Bigley, J. W., McKinnis, R. *et al*. Neuropsychological outcome of zidovudine (AZT) treatment of patients with AIDS and AIDS-related complex. *New England Journal of Medicine*, **319**(24) (1988): 1573–8.

Sidtis, J. J., Gatsonis, C., Price, R. W. *et al*. Zidovudine treatment of the AIDS dementia complex: results of a placebo-controlled trial. AIDS Clinical Trials Group. *Annals of Neurology*, **33**(4)(1993): 343–9.

Simon, G., Moog, C. and Obert, G.. Valproic acid reduces the intracellular level of glutathione and stimulates human immunodeficiency virus. *Chemico-Biological Interactions*, **91** (1994): 111–21.

Smith, C. A., van Gorp W. G., Ryan, E. R. *et al*. (2003). Screening subtle HIV-related cognitive dysfunction: the clinical utility of the HIV Dementia Scale. *Journal of AIDS*, **33**(1) (2003): 116–18.

Stankoff, B., Calves, V., Suarez, S. *et al*. Plasma and cerebrospinal fluid human immunodeficiency virus type-1 (HIV-1) RNA levels in HIV-related cognitive impairment. *European Journal of Neurology*, **6**(6) (1999): 669–75.

Tan, S. V. and Guiloff, R. J. Hypothesis on the pathogenesis of vacuolar myelopathy, dementia, and peripheral neuropathy in AIDS [comment]. *Journal of Neurology, Neurosurgery and Psychiatry*, **65**(1) (1998): 23–8.

Tozzi, V., Balestra, P., Galgani, S. *et al.* Positive and sustained effects of highly active antiretroviral therapy on HIV-1-associated neurocognitive impairment. *AIDS*, **13**(14) (1999): 1889–97.

Tyor, W. R., Wesselingh, S. L., Griffin, J. W. *et al.* Unifying hypothesis for the pathogenesis of HIV-associated dementia complex, vacuolar myelopathy, and sensory neuropathy. *Journal of Acquired Immune Deficiency Syndrome and Human Retrovirology*, **9** (1995): 379–88.

Wesselingh, S. L., Glass, J., McArthur, J. C. *et al.* Cytokine dysregulation in HIV-associated neurological disease. *Advances in Neuroimmunology*, **4**(3) (1994): 199–206.

White, J. L., Darko, D. F., Brown, S. J. *et al.* Early central nervous system response to HIV infection: sleep distortion and cognitive-motor decrements. *AIDS*, **9**(9) (1995): 1043–50.

Witvrouw, M., Schmit, J. C., Van Remoortel, B. *et al.* Cell type-dependent effect of sodium valproate on human immunodeficiency virus type 1 replication in vitro. *AIDS Research and Human Retroviruses*, **13** (1997): 187–92.

3

General principles of pharmacotherapy for the patient with HIV infection

Sanjay M. Sharma, M.D., M.B.A.[1], J. Stephen McDaniel, M.D.[2] and Nancy L. Sheehan, B.Pharm, M.Sc.[3]

[1] Assistant Professor, Department of Psychiatry and Behavioral Sciences, Emory University School of Medicine, Atlanta, GA
[2] Professor, Department of Psychiatry and Behavioral Sciences, Emory University School of Medicine, Atlanta, GA
[3] HIV Pharmacotherapy Specialist, McGill University Health Centre, Montréal, Canada

Introduction

Over the past several years, highly active antiretroviral therapy (HAART) has become the pharmacological mainstay in the ongoing management of HIV infection and AIDS. This treatment regimen comprises a combination of antiretroviral medications which fall into four major classes including nucleoside/nucleotide reverse transcriptase inhibitors (NRTIs), non-nucleoside reverse transcriptase inhibitors (NNRTIs), protease inhibitors (PIs), and entry inhibitors (Table 3.1). Each medication within its respective class acts to inhibit the replication process of HIV at a distinct point in its viral life cycle. When used in combination therapy, these medications form a highly effective and powerful tool in the treatment of HIV infection and AIDS.

However, as effective and beneficial as these combination antiretroviral treatments are, the ongoing management of HIV infection may be complicated by potential side effects and drug–drug interactions.

In addition to being concerned about the impact of antiretrovirals on psychotropic medications, the clinician has to ensure that the psychopharmacological agents do not compromise HIV treatment or lead to the development of resistant strains of the virus. This chapter:

- describes the various potential drug–drug interactions and neuropsychiatric side effects that may occur when psychotropic medications, narcotics, recreationally used/abused drugs, and alternative agents are utilized concomitantly with antiretroviral treatment
- offers practical recommendations on choosing psychotropic medications for a variety of psychiatric illnesses while respecting issues of safety and not compromising HIV care.

HIV and Psychiatry. A Training and Resource Manual, Second Edition, ed. Kenneth Citron, Marie-Josée Brouillette, and Alexandra Beckett. Published by Cambridge University Press. © Cambridge University Press 2005.

Table 3.1. Currently available antiretroviral agents

Nucleoside/nucleotide reverse transcriptase inhibitors (NRTIs)
    Abacavir sulfate (Ziagen[R])
    Didanosine (Videx[TM]/Videx EC[TM])
    Emtricitabine (Emtriva[TM])
    Lamivudine (Epivir[R])
    Stavudine (Zerit[TM]/Zerit XR[R])
    Tenofovir disoproxil fumarate (Viread[R]) – nucleotide
    Zalcitabine (Hivid[R])
    Zidovudine (Retrovir[R])
    Abacavir sulfate–lamivudine–zidovudine (Trizivir[TM])
    Lamivudine–zidovudine (Combivir[R])
Non-nucleoside reverse transcriptase inhibitors (NNRTIs)
    Delavirdine mesylate (Rescriptor[R])
    Efavirenz (Sustiva[R])
    Nevirapine (Viramune[R])
Protease inhibitors (PIs)
    Amprenavir (Agenerase[TM])
    Atazanavir (Reyataz[R])
    Fosamprenavir (Lexiva[TM])
    Indinavir sulfate (Crixivan[R])
    Lopinavir–ritonavir (Kaletra[TM])
    Nelfinavir mesylate (Viracept[R])
    Ritonavir (Norvir[R] SEC)
    Saquinavir – soft gel capsules (Fortovase[R])
    Saquinavir mesylate – hard gel capsules (Invirase[R])
Entry inhibitors
    Enfuvirtide (Fuzeon[R])

Case study: A woman with bipolar disorder and HIV infection

Fani is a 35-year-old woman with a long history of bipolar disorder. For the past several years, she has been well maintained on a stable dose of valproic acid. Diagnosed HIV seropositive 4 years ago, she had not required any antiretroviral medication until 3 weeks ago, when she was started on a regimen of lopinavir–ritonavir and lamivudine–zidovudine.

Today, she presents to the emergency room with symptoms of decreased sleep, increased energy, racing thoughts and increased libido, which she recognizes as indications of incipient mania. A check of her valproic acid serum level reveals that it has decreased by one-third since the previous one measured 2 months ago. Fani insists that she has been fully adherent to her psychiatric medication.

What is the main mechanism responsible for interactions between antiretrovirals and psychotropic medications, narcotics, recreationally used/abused substances, and alternative products?

The mechanisms of drug–drug interactions may be divided into two major categories:

- Pharmacodynamic interactions, which occur when two medications have additive, synergistic, or antagonistic pharmacologic properties. For example, clozapine and zidovudine may interact with each other as they can both cause bone marrow suppression.
- Pharmacokinetic interactions, which occur when a medication interferes with another's absorption, distribution, metabolism, and elimination. Both the interference with phase I metabolism (oxidation, reduction, hydrolysis) and with phase II metabolism (conjugation to sulfate or glucuronide moieties) may be at the origin of clinically significant drug interactions (Boroujerdi, 2002).

This chapter will focus mainly on metabolic pharmacokinetic interaction as this is the principal mechanism behind interactions between antiretrovirals and psychotropic drugs, narcotics, recreationally used/abused drugs, and herbal medicines.

The liver, primarily through the cytochrome P450 (CYP) microsomal oxidases, serves as the major site in the body for the metabolism of many medications, alternative compounds such as herbal preparations, and recreationally used/abused drugs. The CYP enzyme system is a large family of related isoenzymes found mainly in the liver and intestine that are specifically involved in the formation of metabolites through oxidative biotransformation of numerous substances (Dresser *et al.*, 2000). The metabolites can then be eliminated by the kidneys or be conjugated to compounds that will make them hydrophilic and stable prior to renal or fecal elimination (Boroujerdi, 2002).

In terms of drug–drug interactions between psychotropic medications, narcotics, herbal medicines, recreationally used/abused drugs and antiretrovirals, the clinically relevant CYP isoenzyme subfamilies include CYP2D6, 3A4, 1A2, 2B6, 2C9, and 2C19.

Significant drug–drug interactions occurring in the liver are usually caused by either inhibition or induction of the CYP isoenzymes and of the transferase (conjugation) enzyme systems (Krishnan *et al.*, 1996; Boroujerdi, 2002).

- Enzyme inhibition occurs when one drug decreases the metabolic activity and functioning of a CYP isoenzyme or a transferase, thereby decreasing the metabolism of other drugs that are substrates of this enzyme.
- Enzyme induction occurs when one drug stimulates the metabolic activity and functioning of a CYP isoenzyme or a transferase, thereby increasing the metabolism of drugs that are substrates of this enzyme.

How are antiretrovirals metabolized and how can they influence the bioavailability of psychotropic medications?

The NRTIs predominantly undergo renal elimination with or without prior hepatic transformation. The enzymes involved in the metabolism of the NRTIs are for the most part not CYP isoenzymes but rather UDP-glucuronosyltransferase (for zidovudine and abacavir), alcohol dehydrogenase (for abacavir), and xanthine oxidase (for didanosine) (Tseng *et al.*, 2002). For this reason, few pharmacokinetic interactions exist between the NRTIs and the psychotropic drugs.

The NNRTIs are all substrates of the CYP3A4 isoenzyme. They are also substrates of other CYP isoenzymes but to a minor extent. While it is clear that delavirdine is a CYP3A4 inhibitor and nevirapine a CYP3A4 inducer, efavirenz can both inhibit and induce various isoenzymes (Tseng *et al.*, 2002).

The PIs are also extensively metabolized by CYP3A4. Within the PI family, ritonavir is the most potent CYP3A4 enzyme inhibitor, followed by indinavir, amprenavir, lopinavir, nelfinavir, and saquinavir (Eagling *et al.*, 1997; Von Moltke *et al.*, 1998; Cozza and Armstrong, 2001; Tseng *et al.*, 2002). Preliminary studies also suggest that atazanavir inhibits the metabolism of medications that are substrates of CYP3A4 (O'Mara *et al.*, 2000). Though CYP3A4 is the primary enzyme involved, the PIs can also inhibit and induce other isoenzymes. The enzymes that metabolize the NNRTIs and the PIs as well as the capacity of these antiretrovirals to inhibit or induce various isoenzymes are shown in Table 3.2.

The newly developed entry inhibitor, enfuvirtide, is thought to be partly eliminated by the liver, however the exact isoenzyme involved is unclear. Clinically significant interactions are not expected between enfuvirtide and medications metabolized by CYP isoenzymes (Fletcher, 2003).

What are the clinical implications of these pharmacokinetic interactions?

- 3A4: As the PIs, delavirdine and at times efavirenz have an inhibitory effect upon the CYP3A4 system. Psychotropic agents that are primarily metabolized by CYP3A4 (e.g., benzodiazepines) may therefore encounter a decrease in their metabolism and an increase in their plasma levels when co-administered with these antiretrovirals, potentially leading to toxicity. On the other hand, as nevirapine and efavirenz induce CYP3A4, benzodiazepines may be metabolized more rapidly with a resultant decrease in their plasma levels when co-administered with these antiretrovirals. Clinically, this may translate into an individual who may have previously been stable on a benzodiazepine regimen experiencing the signs and symptoms of benzodiazepine withdrawal syndrome as the level of this medication falls.
- 2D6: Regimens containing ritonavir, with its inhibitory effect on CYP2D6, may increase the levels and side effect profile of psychotropic drugs that are primarily

Table 3.2. Metabolism of non-nucleoside reverse transcriptase inhibitors and protease inhibitors

Antiretroviral	Substrate of following enzymes	Enzymes inhibited	Enzymes induced
Non-nucleoside reverse transcriptase inhibitors (NNRTIs)			
Delavirdine	3A4 > 2D6	3A4, 2C9, 2C19	
Efavirenz	3A4 > 2B6, UDP-GT	3A4, 2C9, 2C19, 2B6	3A4
Nevirapine	3A4 > 2B6		3A4
Protease inhibitors (PIs)			
Amprenavir	3A4	3A4 (moderate), 2C19	3A4?
Atazanavir	3A4	3A4, UDP-GT	
Indinavir	3A4	3A4 (moderate)	
Lopinavir*	3A4	3A4 (weak)	3A4?
Nelfinavir	3A4 >> 2C19, 2D6, 2C9	3A4 (moderate), 2B6	UDP-GT
Ritonavir	3A4 > 2D6	3A4 (potent) > 2D6 > 2C9 > 2C19 > 2B6, 2A6, 2E1	1A2, 2C9, 2C19, UDP-GT, 3A4 auto-induction
Saquinavir	3A4	3A4 (weak)	

*As lopinavir is formulated with low dose ritonavir in Kaletra™, the CYP3A4 inhibition capacity is increased.
UDP – GT: Uridine diphosphate glucuronosyltransferase.
Sources: Tseng and Foisy, 1999; O'Mara *et al.*, 2000; Tseng *et al.*, 2002; Park-Wyllie and Antoniou, 2003.

metabolized by CYP2D6 (e.g., tricyclic and selective serotonin reuptake inhibitor antidepressants, typical and atypical antipsychotic agents).

- 2B6: Ritonavir-containing regimens, which inhibit CYP2B6, may significantly increase bupropion levels, which may increase the risk of seizures and other bupropion-related toxicities. In fact, high-dose ritonavir (400–600 mg twice daily) is contraindicated with bupropion and clinicians should prescribe reduced doses of bupropion with regimens that contain low doses of ritonavir (100 mg twice daily), such as Kaletra™ (Park-Wyllie and Antoniou, 2003).

- The induction or inhibition of isoenzymes other than CYP3A4 and 2D6 by the antiretrovirals may also be responsible for clinically significant interactions with psychotropic drugs. For example, as ritonavir and nelfinavir induce UDP-glucuronosyltransferase (glucuronidation), plasma levels of mood stabilizers such as lamotrigine and valproic acid that are eliminated by this route may significantly decrease leading to suboptimal plasma levels. Clinicians may have to adjust the doses of these mood stabilizers after introducing one of these antiretroviral agents.

For the most part, few pharmacokinetic studies have been conducted to evaluate interactions between psychotropic drugs and antiretrovirals. Clinicians should anticipate potential interactions based on the metabolism of the various drugs taken concomitantly. The documented or theoretical impact of the various NNRTIs and PIs on psychotropic drugs is shown in Table 3.3.

What medications used in HIV care (other than antiretrovirals) can have an impact on the metabolism of psychotropic medications?

In addition to the potential drug–drug interactions between psychotropic medications and antiretrovirals noted in Table 3.3, other medications can also affect the metabolism of psychotropic medications.

In terms of hepatic CYP enzyme inhibition, macrolide antibiotics (notably erythromycin and clarithromycin) as well as azole antifungal medications (i.e., ketoconazole and itraconazole) are potent inhibitors of CYP3A4 (Cozza *et al.*, 2001). These agents can potentially increase the blood levels of psychotropic medications metabolized by this enzyme system, leading to increased side effects and possible toxicities.

In terms of hepatic CYP enzyme induction, antimycobacterial/antitubercular agents (i.e., rifampin, rifabutin, and rifapentine) are inducers of CYP3A4 (Cozza and Armstrong, 2001). These agents can potentially decrease the blood levels of psychotropic medications metabolized by this enzyme system, leading to decreased efficacy.

Clinicians who treat patients with HIV should be mindful of the potential interactions and subsequent effects that may occur when psychotropic medications are used concomitantly with other medications and prepared to adjust psychotropic medication dosages accordingly.

The clinician increases Fani's dose of valproic acid in order to reach the previous serum level at which she had been stable, and temporarily adds a benzodiazepine. The symptoms of hypomania resolve. In terms of HIV care, Fani responds well to the antiretroviral regimen and her viral load becomes undetectable.

Several months later, following a series of setbacks, she develops depressive symptoms including crying spells, anhedonia, decreased motivation, and fatigue. Fani has always resisted taking antidepressants. On the recommendation of a friend, she decides to start St. John's Wort because it is natural. However, she decides not to mention it to her physicians for fear they will disapprove. At her next visit with her HIV specialist, she learns her viral load has increased to 800 copies/ml.

Table 3.3. Documented and potential impact of antiretrovirals on the plasma levels of psychotropic drugs

Psychotropic drug	Nevirapine, efavirenz		Delavirdine, indinavir, saquinavir, amprenavir, atazanavir, nelfinavir, at times efavirenz		Lopinavir + low dose ritonavir (Kaletra™), low dose ritonavir 100 mg twice daily		High dose ritonavir (400–600 mg twice daily)	
	Effect on psychotropic	Effect on antiretroviral	Effect on psychotropic	Effect on antiretroviral	Effect on psychotropic	Effect on antiretroviral	Effect on psychotropic	Effect on antiretroviral
Antidepressants								
Amitriptyline	↓	↓	↑		↑↑		↑↑↑	
Bupropion	↓		↑		↑↑		↑↑↑(1)	
Citalopram	↓		↑	↓	↑	↓	↑↑	↓
Clomipramine	↓		↑		↑↑		↑↑↑	
Desipramine					↑		↑↑	
Doxepin	?	?	?	?	?	?	?	?
Fluoxetine	↓	↓		↓	↑↑(2)	↑	↑↑↑(2)	↓
Fluvoxamine		↑?		↓	↑↑	↓	↑↑	↓
Imipramine	↓		↑		↑↑		↑↑↑	
Mirtazapine	↓		↑		↑↑		↑↑↑	
Moclobemide					↑		↑↑	
Nefazodone	↓	↓	↑	↓	↑↑	↓	↑↑↑	↓
Nortriptyline					↑		↑↑	
Paroxetine					↑		↑↑	
Phenelzine								
Sertraline	↓		↑		↑↑		↑↑↑	

Tranylcypromine	↓?		↑?		↑↑?
Trazodone	→		↑↑	↑	↑↑↑
Trimipramine	↑↓?		↑	↑?	↑↑
Venlafaxine	→		↑↑	↑	↑↑↑
Antipsychotics					
Chlorpromazine			↑	↑	↑↑	↑
Clozapine			↑↑		↑↑↑(1)
Fluphenazine			↑	↑	↑↑	↑
Haloperidol	↑↓?		↑	↑?	↑↑
Loxapine	→		↑	↑	↑↑
Methotrimeprazine			↑	↑	↑↑	↑
Olanzapine			→	↑	↓↓	↑
Perphenazine			↑	↑	↑↑	↑
Pimozide	→	↑(3)	↑↑(1)		↑↑↑(1)
Quetiapine	→		↑↑	↑	↑↑↑
Risperidone			↑	↑	↑↑
Thioridazine	→		↑↑	↑	↑↑
Ziprasidone	→		↑		↑↑↑	↑
Zuclopenthixol				↑	↑↑
Sedatives/anxiolytics					
Alprazolam	→		↑↑(3)	↑	↑↑(3)
Bromazepam	→		↑↑	↑	↑↑↑
Buspirone	→		↑↑	↑	↑↑↑
Chloral hydrate					
Clonazepam	↓?		↑↑?		↑↑?
Clorazepate	→		↑↑(1)	↑	↑↑↑(1)
Diazepam	→		↑↑	↑	↑↑↑
Flurazepam	↓?		↑↑?(3)		↑↑↑?(1)
Lorazepam	↓(4)				↓↓
Midazolam	→	↑(1)	↑↑(1)		↑↑↑(1)

Table 3.3. (cont.)

Psychotropic drug	Nevirapine, efavirenz		Delavirdine, indinavir, saquinavir, amprenavir, atazanavir, nelfinavir, at times efavirenz		Lopinavir + low dose ritonavir (Kaletra™), low dose ritonavir 100 mg twice daily		High dose ritonavir (400–600 mg twice daily)	
	Effect on psychotropic	Effect on antiretroviral	Effect on psychotropic	Effect on antiretroviral	Effect on psychotropic	Effect on antiretroviral	Effect on psychotropic	Effect on antiretroviral
Nitrazepam	↓?		↑?		↑↑?		↑↑↑?	
Oxazepam	→		↓ (4)		→		↓↑	
Temazepam	→		↓ (4)		→		↓↑	
Triazolam	→		↑ (1)		↑↑ (1)		↑↑↑ (1)	
Zaleplon	→		↑		↑↑		↑↑↑	
Zolpidem	→		↑		↑↑ (1)		↑↑↑ (1)	
Zopiclone	→		↑		↑↑		↑↑↑	
Mood stabilizers								
Carbamazepine	→	↓↑	↑	↓↑	↑	↓↑	↑	↓↑
Gabapentin								
Lamotrigine			↓ (4)		→		↓↑	
Lithium								
Valproic acid			↓ (4)		→		↓↑	
Stimulants								
Dextroamphetamine					↑		↑↑	

| Methylphenidate | ↓? | ↑ | ↑ | ↑? | ↑ | ↑? |
| Modafinil | ↓ | → | ↓ | ↑ | → | ↑↑ |

(1) Contraindicated
(2) Caution
(3) Avoid
(4) With nelfinavir

Sources: Bertz and Granneman,1997; Bezchlibnyk-Butler *et al.*, 1997; Tseng and Foisy, 1999; Brosen and Naranjo, 2001; Organon, 2000; Penzak *et al.*, 2002; Prior and Baker, 2003; Montplaisir *et al.*, 2003; Robertson and Hellriegel, 2003.

How can psychotropic medications have an impact on the bioavailability of antiretroviral agents and what are the clinical implications?

The potential impact of psychotropic medications on the bioavailability of antiretroviral agents is extremely important. To avoid developing resistant strains of the virus, patients on antiretroviral therapy must adhere to 95% or more of the doses (Paterson *et al.*, 2000). A drop in bioavailability of antiretrovirals caused by psychotropic medications could compromise the immune response and foster resistance. On the other hand, an increase in plasma levels may lead to increased side effects associated with the use of these agents, which can lead to nonadherence.

Some psychotropic medications may have an effect on the plasma levels of various antiretrovirals through pharmacokinetic interactions. For example:

- The antidepressant nefazadone is a potent inhibitor of the CYP system at the CYP3A4 site (Bertz and Granneman, 1997). When used concomitantly with antiretrovirals metabolized by CYP3A4 (PIs and NNRTIs), nefazadone may decrease the overall metabolism of these antiretrovirals and increase their plasma levels. Under these conditions an increase in the physiological and neuropsychiatric side effects of the antiretrovirals may occur. It has been demonstrated that higher efavirenz plasma levels correlate with an increased prevalence of efavirenz-related neuropsychiatric side effects (Marzolini *et al.*, 2001). These intolerable side effects may ultimately translate into treatment nonadherence and the development of viral resistance.

- The mood stabilizer, carbamazepine, is a potent inducer of CYP3A4, which means the metabolism of the PIs and NNRTIs will be accelerated, leading to subtherapeutic antiretroviral plasma levels (Tseng and Foisy, 1999). This almost always results in the development of viral resistance and the permanent loss of effectiveness of the antiretroviral taken. Cross-resistance within an antiretroviral class may rapidly occur, leading to a significant decrease in treatment options. Potent inducers of CYP3A4 such as carbamazepine, phenobarbital, phenytoin, and rifampicin should be avoided in patients receiving PIs or NNRTIs.

Are there significant interactions between antiretrovirals and alternative products (herbal medicines)?

Significant interactions may occur between alternative agents such as herbal preparations and antiretrovirals. This can be seen in people with HIV who are using St. John's Wort (*Hypericum perforatum*), an inducer of the CYP3A4 isoenzyme, and the PI, indinavir. In this scenario, St. John's Wort, through its induction of indinavir's metabolism, may significantly lower the plasma levels and effectiveness of indinavir. Presumably, other CYP3A4 substrates (including other PIs and NNRTIs) may be similarly affected (Piscitelli *et al.*, 2000a; de Maat *et al.*, 2001). Studies have also shown that milk thistle and garlic supplements can induce the metabolism of antiretrovirals (Piscitelli *et al.*, 2002a,b). From a clinical standpoint, this type of interaction may increase the risks of developing resistance to the antiretroviral and cross-resistance to the antiretrovirals in the same pharmacological class, potentially compromising the treatment and ongoing management of an individual infected with HIV. The use of milk thistle, garlic supplements, and St. John's Wort should be avoided in patients taking a PI or an NNRTI.

When the clinician explores with Fani possible explanations for the increase in the viral load, she reveals that she started taking St. John's Wort for depression. The clinician instructs Fani to discontinue her use of it and measures the trough level of lopinavir–ritonavir, which is subtherapeutic and explains the virologic failure. Three weeks later, a repeat measure of the lopinavir–ritonavir trough level shows that it is now back in the therapeutic range. Over the next few weeks, Fani's viral load once again becomes undetectable (less than 50 copies/ml). The clinician uses this incident to clarify with Fani the importance of honest communication in reaching their common goal of treating her HIV infection.

> ## Case study: HIV seropositive man on methadone maintenance therapy
>
> Sam is a 35-year-old HIV-seropositive man with a significant past history of intravenous heroin use who has been on chronic methadone maintenance therapy for the past 10 years. He has been on a stable dose of 80 milligrams per day during this time, with a serum methadone level at 0.75 µg/ml. He has been maintained on an antiretroviral regimen consisting of abacavir sulfate and zidovudine. Because of a significant increase in viral load, the regimen has to be changed. The clinician initiates a new antiretroviral regimen consisting of lamivudine, didanosine, and nevirapine. Approximately 10 days after starting his new antiretroviral regimen, Sam begins experiencing symptoms consistent with opiate withdrawal, including myalgias, nausea, diarrhea, abdominal pain, increased lacrimation, rhinorrhea, piloerection, and diaphoresis.

How can antiretrovirals interact with opiate medications?

Some opiate analgesic medications, such as codeine and hydrocodone, must be converted into active metabolites in order to produce their analgesic effects. This conversion process can be impaired by agents (such as the protease inhibitors) that inhibit the CYP3A4 and 2D6 isoenzyme systems, thereby causing an accumulation of unmetabolized drug products and decreasing the level of pain control. This interaction increases the risk of adverse reactions due to the build-up of unmetabolized drug products, and may also trigger recurrence of pain that may have been previously well controlled, prompting an appropriate adjustment in the pain medication regimen (American Psychiatric Association, 2000a).

In contrast, ritonavir is thought to induce meperidine metabolism leading to opiate withdrawal and an increase in the normeperidine metabolite (Piscitelli *et al.*, 2000b). This metabolite is responsible for significant CNS toxicity (e.g., seizures).

As morphine and hydromorphone are eliminated by glucuronidation, antiretrovirals that induce UDP-glucuronosyltransferase such as ritonavir and nelfinavir may increase the opiate's metabolism leading to a need for increased doses of these analgesics (Bertz and Granneman, 1997). This interaction is less relevant for morphine as the morphine-6-glucuronide metabolite produces some analgesic effect (Osborne *et al.*, 1988).

Interactions between fentanyl and the PIs and NNRTIs may also occur. As fentanyl is metabolized by CYP3A4, PIs and delavirdine are expected to decrease its elimination and increase the risk of opiate toxicity, whereas the NNRTIs efavirenz and nevirapine are expected to induce its elimination and cause suboptimal analgesia and withdrawal symptoms (Bertz and Granneman, 1997).

The clinical consequences of enzyme induction can also be seen when methadone (mainly metabolized by 3A4 and glucuronidation) is taken together with certain antiretrovirals. For example, methadone levels may be decreased secondary to the induction of its metabolism by the PIs ritonavir, nelfinavir, amprenavir, and lopinavir–ritonavir, or by the NNRTIs nevirapine and efavirenz. Methadone metabolism induction can also be seen secondary to the antimycobacterial/anti-tubercular drug rifampicin (Altice *et al.*, 1999; American Psychiatric Association, 2000a; Gourevitch and Friedland, 2000; Gourevitch, 2001; Hendrix *et al.*, 2000; Clarke *et al.*, 2002). Interactions such as these can precipitate an opiate withdrawal syndrome or loss of pain control in people who had previously been stable on methadone.

Another example of interactions between opiate medications and antiretrovirals is that which occurs between methadone and the NRTIs, didanosine, zalcitabine, and stavudine (Thiemann and Lalazeri, 1999; Rainey *et al.*, 2000). By delaying gastric motility, methadone decreases the oral bioavailability of these antiretrovirals (Gourevitch and Friedland, 2000). Clinically, this may reduce the effectiveness of these antiretrovirals in treating the HIV infection and increase the risk of viral resistance. This clinical scenario may prompt clinicians to increase the dosage of these antiretrovirals or change to other antiretrovirals that may not have significant drug–drug interactions with methadone. Methadone may also substantially increase the plasma levels of zidovudine by inhibiting UDP-glucuronosyltransferase (glucuronidation) (Schwartz *et al.*, 1992; Gourevitch and Friedland, 2000), which may increase the development of zidovudine toxicity (e.g., bone marrow toxicity, myopathy, and gastrointestinal upset).

Sam's serum methadone level has dropped from 0.75 mg/ml to 0.15 mg/ml. The clinician increases the dose of methadone from 80 mg per day to 100 mg per day, and Sam's withdrawal symptoms resolve. One week later, the serum methadone level is 0.50 mg/ml. As the full impact of nevirapine induction takes approximately 2 weeks to appear, the clinician steadily increases Sam's dose of methadone over the next several weeks to 130 mg per day. He does quite well at this dose and experiences no further symptoms of opiate withdrawal.

Are there significant interactions between antiretrovirals and recreationally used/abused substances?

Clinicians should be aware of the numerous significant interactions that may occur between antiretrovirals and recreationally used/abused substances. Potentially clinically significant drug interactions may occur between antiretrovirals and amphetamines, gamma-hydroxybutyrate (GHB), ketamine, phencyclidine (PCP), lysergic acid diethylamide (LSD), cocaine, heroin, tetrahydrocannabinol (THC), and ethanol (Antoniou and Tseng, 2002). Table 3.4 presents the possible interactions and complications related to the concomitant use of these recreational drugs and antiretrovirals.

Alcohol, especially if consumed on a regular basis, can increase the risk of developing pancreatitis when combined with NRTIs, such as didanosine, zalcitabine, stavudine, and lamivudine, or with the protease inhibitor, ritonavir (Thiemann and Lalazeri, 1999). Furthermore, alcohol can increase abacavir levels as it competes for the same metabolic pathway, alcohol dehydrogenase (McDowell et al., 2000). The clinical significance of this interaction, however, appears limited and dose adjustments of abacavir are not necessary.

In other instances, the protease inhibitor, ritonavir, by inhibiting CYP2D6, 2B6 and 3A4, may increase the blood levels and therefore the likelihood of possible intoxication and overdose of methylenedioxymethamphetamine (MDMA, ecstasy), methamphetamine (crystal meth, speed), GHB, ketamine, PCP, and THC (the active ingredient in marijuana) (Henry and Hill, 1998; Thiemann and Lalazeri, 1999; Antoniou and Tseng, 2002). Death related to the concomitant use of ritonavir and MDMA has been reported. In one such case, the MDMA level was close to ten times the expected level (Henry and Hill, 1998). Caution should also be used with the other antiretrovirals that inhibit CYP3A4 or 2B6 (PIs, delavirdine, and efavirenz). If HIV-infected patients insist on taking rave drugs, they should be counseled to reduce their intake significantly (take approximately a quarter of the usual dose), remain well hydrated by avoiding alcohol and drinking plenty of water, and take breaks from dancing (Antoniou and Tseng, 2002).

A similar interaction may be encountered between the PI indinavir and barbiturates, yielding an increase in the blood levels of the barbiturates, thereby increasing the likelihood of potential barbiturate intoxication and overdose (Thiemann and Lalazeri, 1999).

Table 3.4. Potential interactions between antiretrovirals and recreationally used/abused substances

Recreational drug	Other names	Metabolism	Interactions with antiretrovirals		Comments
			PIs / Delavirdine Efavirenz	Nevirapine Efavirenz	
Cocaine (Ladona et al., 2000)	Coke, crack	Spontaneous hydrolysis, cholinesterases, N-demethylation (CYP3A4) < 10 %	May cause ↓ norcocaine metabolite, less hepatotoxicity expected	May cause ↑ norcocaine metabolite, monitor for hepatotoxicity	Interaction theoretical, clinical relevance unknown
Ethanol (McDowell et al., 2000)	Alcohol	Alcohol dehydrogenase, aldehyde dehydrogenase	Increased risk of pancreatitis with ritonavir	Unlikely	Interaction with the NRTI, abacavir (clinically nonsignificant increase in abacavir levels). Increased risk of pancreatitis with NRTIs
γ-hydroxybutyrate (Harrington et al., 1999)	GHB, G, Grievous bodily harm	First-pass metabolism (CYP?), expired as CO_2	Possible risk ↑ GHB toxicity (ritonavir +++)	Possible risk ↓ GHB effect	Life-threatening reaction documented in a patient receiving ritonavir (bradycardia, cardiac arrest)
Heroin (Bertz and Granneman, 1997)		Deacetylase (formation 6-monoacetyl –morphine), then glucuronidation	Nelfinavir and ritonavir expected to increase elimination of active metabolite, may cause opiate withdrawal	Unlikely	Monitor for signs and symptoms of opiate withdrawal (rhinorrhea, diaphoresis, piloerection, lacrimation, anxiety, agitation, insomnia, hallucinations, psychosis, dilated pupils, nausea, vomiting, abdominal cramps)
Ketamine (Yanagihara et al., 2001)	Kit Kat, Special K	CYP2B6 > 3A4, 2C9	Efavirenz, nelfinavir and ritonavir expected to increase ketamine effect	Efavirenz expected to increase ketamine effect	Monitor for signs and symptoms of ketamine toxicity (respiratory depression, cardiac arrythmias, tremors, tonic-clonic movements)

Drug	Common names	CYP	Protease inhibitor interaction	NNRTI interaction	Comments / recommendations
Lysergic acid diethylmide	LSD, acid, blotters	CYP?	Unknown, use with caution	Unknown, use with caution	LSD effects: agitation, insomnia, hallucinations, psychosis, flashbacks
Methamphetamine (Lin et al., 1997)	Crystal meth, Speed	CYP2D6	Ritonavir expected to increase levels	Unlikely	Monitor for signs/symptoms of amphetamine toxicity, avoid combination; if taken, use reduced dose of methamphetamine (1/4), avoid alcohol, rest, ensure hydration
Methylenedioxy-methamphetamine (Lin et al., 1997; Henry and Hill, 1998; Kreth et al., 2000)	MDMA, Ecstasy, XTC, Adam, Essence	CYP2D6 > 1A2, 2B6, 3A4	Significant increase of MDMA levels (ritonavir +++, 1 death reported)	Efavirenz: possible increase or decrease in MDMA levels Nevirapine: Possible decrease	Monitor for signs / symptoms of amphetamine toxicity, avoid combination; if taken, use reduced dose of MDMA (1/4), avoid alcohol, rest, ensure hydration
Phencyclidine (Laurenzana and Owens, 1997)	PCP, rocket fuel, angel dust, killer weed	CYP3A4	Increased levels of PCP	Decreased levels of PCP	Monitor for signs and symptoms of PCP toxicity (hypertension, seizures, rhabdomyolysis, hyperthermia)
Tetrahydrocannabinol (Bornheim et al., 1992, Watanabe et al., 1995, Abrams et al., 2001) Kosel et al., 2001)	THC, Marijuana, Pot	CYP3A4, 2C9	Possible increase in THC levels, decreases in nelfinavir and indinavir levels reported	Possible decrease in THC levels	Decrease in nelfinavir and indinavir levels considered clinically nonsignificant

Sources: Antoniou and Tseng, 2002.

The potential for interactions between cocaine or heroin and antiretrovirals is unclear. Only 10% of cocaine's metabolism is related to the CYP enzyme system (CYP3A4) (Ladona *et al.*, 2000). The concomitant use of CYP3A4 inhibitors (PIs, delavirdine, efavirenz) or inducers (nevirapine, efavirenz) may have little impact on cocaine levels since other metabolic pathways play a more determinant role in the elimination of this drug. However, it should be noted that since CYP3A4 metabolism transforms cocaine into norcocaine, a hepatotoxic metabolite, CYP3A4 inhibitors may decrease the risk of hepatotoxicity while CYP3A4 inducers may increase this type of toxicity (Antoniou and Tseng, 2002). Heroin levels may also be reduced when used concomitantly with the PI ritonavir, possibly precipitating a heroin (opiate) withdrawal syndrome in someone who is dependent upon heroin (Thiemann and Lalazeri, 1999; Antoniou and Tseng, 2002).

The use of smoked THC or its synthetic oral analogues is very common among patients with HIV. Other than recreational uses, THC can be taken for medical reasons such as to control pain and nausea, and to stimulate appetite in wasting patients. THC has been shown to decrease nelfinavir and indinavir 'area under the curves' by 17% and 24%, respectively (Kosel *et al.*, 2001). As no changes in viral suppression and immune restoration have been documented, this is not considered clinically significant (Abrams *et al.*, 2001) (Table 3.4).

Case study: Medication-induced neuropsychiatric side effects

Deborah is a 40-year-old HIV-seropositive female with no prior psychiatric history who begins experiencing symptoms of mania, paranoia, and hallucinations approximately 2 weeks after initiating her antiretroviral regimen of didanosine, lopinavir–ritonavir, and efavirenz. Her initial symptoms include insomnia, vivid "lifelike" dreams, and irritability. Her symptoms progress to agitation, feeling "hyper", rapid and pressured speech, racing thoughts with difficulty in concentration and ability to remain focused, and ongoing sleeplessness. Deborah begins experiencing psychotic symptoms of paranoia with associated thoughts that she is being poisoned by her medication and that people are out to get her. She also has auditory and visual hallucinations that frighten her. The clinician develops a plan to temporarily discontinue her antiretroviral medications and initiate a low dose of risperidone to alleviate her symptoms. Shortly thereafter, her psychosis begins to improve and the risperidone is eventually discontinued without a recurrence of symptoms. She is later restarted on an antiretroviral regimen consisting of didanosine, lopinavir–ritonavir, and nevirapine without any difficulty or reemergence of her psychiatric symptomatology.

What types of neuropsychiatric side effects have been associated with the use of antiretrovirals and other agents used in HIV infection?

A wide spectrum of neuropsychiatric side effects may be associated with the use of antiretrovirals and other HIV therapeutic agents. These side effects may include mood disturbances such as depression and mania, anxiety, irritability, agitation, fatigue, sleep disturbances, headache, neuropathic pain syndromes, confusion and disorientation. Patients taking antiretrovirals as well as other therapeutic agents to treat HIV infection or related complications may also experience psychotic symptoms, including delusions, paranoia, and hallucinations.

The strength of evidence for a causal relationship between the antiretrovirals and the psychiatric adverse reactions is weak. Most of these adverse reactions were noted in the antiretroviral clinical trials. During these trials, there may not have been a systematic inquiry into the symptoms of psychiatric disorders (possibly leading to under-reporting) and no attempt to diagnose according to DSM criteria. On the other hand, when a psychiatric symptom was reported, no attempt was made to rule out other possible causes of that symptom (possibly leading to over-reporting). For example, if a patient reported insomnia, there was no exploration of other potential causes of insomnia. This is particularly significant in view of the fact that HIV infection is often accompanied by important psychosocial stress and patients are on several medications.

Another source of information on the neuropsychiatric side effects of antiretrovirals is case reports. While attempts are made to clarify causality, no agent is associated with enough case reports to clearly demonstrate the relationship between the neuropsychiatric effect and the HIV medication, with two notable exceptions: NRTI-related peripheral neuropathy and efavirenz-related neuropsychiatric symptoms.

Approximately 50% of HIV-infected patients who receive efavirenz will develop neuropsychiatric symptoms, including: dizziness, headache, impaired concentration, confusion, insomnia, nervousness, anxiety, vivid dreams or nightmares, daytime somnolence, morning hangover feelings, abnormal thinking, amnesia, depersonalization, euphoria, depression, and hallucinations. The symptomatology usually begins after the first few days of therapy and gradually diminishes over 1–4 months of treatment (Halman, 2001). Most patients will develop only a few of these symptoms. According to different clinical studies, the efavirenz discontinuation rate related to the neuropsychiatric adverse events varies between 2.6% and 16% (Halman, 2001).

How does one choose a psychopharmacological agent for a patient with HIV infection?

Potential drug–drug interactions and side effects can have a significant impact and should be important considerations when deciding to prescribe a particular medication or medication regimen for a patient with HIV infection. The following summary provides the rationale for considering various medications to manage psychiatric conditions.

Major depressive disorders

- Selective serotonin reuptake inhibitors (SSRIs) are good choices in treating both depressive and anxiety symptoms. Of this group, fluoxetine has the longest elimination half-life, while sertraline and citalopram (as well as its isomeric formulation, escitalopram) have an overall decreased incidence of drug–drug interactions as compared with fluoxetine and paroxetine. With respect to the concomitant use of antiretrovirals, significant interactions with paroxetine and fluoxetine are expected with regimens containing ritonavir. In fact, a case series of serotonin syndromes has been reported with the concomitant use of fluoxetine and ritonavir (DeSilva *et al.*, 2001). In HIV-infected patients receiving a PI, clinicians should start SSRIs with half the usual initial dose and titrate the dose slowly.

- Venlafaxine XR is a good medication choice in individuals who have concomitant depressive and anxiety symptoms. Blood pressure should be monitored when using venlafaxine XR at higher doses (greater than 300 mg/day) because of the possibility of worsening hypertension. Individuals taking venlafaxine XR may experience nervousness, agitation, and/or insomnia because of its possible "activating effect" and may also experience headaches while taking the medication. Significant drug–drug interactions are possible between venlafaxine XR and regimens containing ritonavir, as venlafaxine is metabolized by CYP2D6 and ritonavir inhibits this isoenzyme (Tseng and Foisy, 1999). Interactions with the other PIs or with NNRTIs are less likely. Patients taking ritonavir should begin with lower doses of venlafaxine XR and their blood pressure should be monitored closely as increased venlafaxine plasma levels may result from the interaction.

- Bupropion SR may be used in individuals with depression who are experiencing sexual dysfunction caused by other antidepressant agents. It should not be administered in doses exceeding 400 mg/day (in twice daily divided doses) due to an increased risk of seizures (particularly in those individuals who have a history of seizures, head injury, and/or CNS compromise). As bupropion is metabolized primarily by CYP2B6, and ritonavir, nelfinavir, and efavirenz inhibit this isoenzyme, caution should be used when giving bupropion SR to HIV-infected patients taking these antiretrovirals (Tseng *et al.*, 2002; Park-Wyllie and Antoniou, 2003). Increased plasma levels of bupropion with an increased risk of seizures may be anticipated (Park-Wyllie and Antoniou, 2003). The concomitant use of bupropion with ritonavir 400–600 mg twice daily is contraindicated, whereas smaller doses of bupropion (i.e., 150 mg daily) can be used with caution with the other PIs, including ritonavir 100 mg twice daily.

- Mirtazapine may be a particularly useful antidepressant choice when insomnia is a significant symptom of depression because of its sedating side effect (hence, it should be dosed at bedtime). It may also be used in depressed individuals who are experiencing sexual dysfunction caused by other antidepressant agents. While taking mirtazapine, individuals may experience an increase in appetite and weight gain (which may be a wanted effect in the context of decreased appetite and weight loss associated with depression and/or HIV/AIDS). As mirtazapine is metabolized by CYP2D6, 1A2 and 3A4, all PIs (in particular ritonavir) as well as delavirdine (and at times efavirenz), may increase mirtazapine concentrations (Organon, 2001). Clinicians should use lower doses of mirtazapine when starting this antidepressant in an HIV-infected patient taking ritonavir. On the contrary, nevirapine and efavirenz may induce mirtazapine metabolism resulting in the need for higher doses.

- Nefazadone has been found to cause liver dysfunction and life-threatening liver failure in some cases, prompting the US Food and Drug Administration to issue a so-called "black box" warning to caution clinicians of the possibility of a serious or life-threatening adverse event. It should not be used in treating individuals with HIV/AIDS and/or in individuals with impaired liver function (i.e., hepatitis infection). Nefazadone also has significant effects upon the hepatic CYP enzyme system (it inhibits CYP3A4) and can affect the metabolism of various other medications/drugs.

- Tricyclic antidepressants can be used to treat a variety of disorders including depression, insomnia, and neuropathic pain. Tricyclic antidepressants undergo metabolism via the CYP2D6 enzyme system; therefore medications such as ritonavir, fluoxetine, and paroxetine that are inhibitors of this enzyme system will invariably raise the blood levels of tricyclic antidepressants. For more information on the use of tricyclic antidepressants in this population, see Chapter 4 on Mood Disorders. If tricyclic antidepressants are used as a pharmacological treatment modality, clinicians should carefully monitor therapeutic blood levels, keeping in mind that these medications have narrow therapeutic windows that can be surpassed through drug–drug interactions. The use of tricyclic antidepressants as first-line agents for the treatment of depression for people with HIV (who may be on a complex regimen of medications and are susceptible to drug–drug interactions and side effects) is not recommended, particularly as other pharmacological treatment options exist.

- Psychostimulants such as methylphenidate, dextroamphetamine, and modafinil may be used as a treatment for secondary depression (depression in the context of a medical illness, such as HIV infection), particularly in individuals in whom apathy and anergia is a primary component of their depression. These agents may also be used as adjuncts to augment current antidepressant therapy. These agents, by virtue of their stimulant effects, can be used in the treatment of fatigue, which is commonly encountered in individuals with HIV/AIDS.

Nervousness, agitation, tremulousness, and insomnia are some of the most common side effects that may be experienced during psychostimulant use. Cardiovascular effects may also occur (with the exception of modafinil, which has no/minimal significant cardiovascular effects) and can include increased blood pressure and heart rate, heart palpitations, and cardiac dysrhythmias. Psychostimulants have a strong abuse potential and individuals taking these agents must be counseled and monitored for the emergence of tolerance, abuse, and dependency. Care must be taken in prescribing psychostimulants to patients with a past or current history of mania, psychosis, seizures, hypertension, and/or substance use as these agents may trigger or exacerbate these conditions.

With regard to interactions with antiretrovirals, regimens containing ritonavir may increase dextroamphetamine levels and increase the risk of amphetamine toxicity (Bezchlibnyk–Butler et al., 1997), and methylphenidate can theoretically increase the PI and NNRTI levels (Tseng and Foisy, 1999). Patients should be closely monitored for the presence of increased antiretroviral toxicity. Modafinil's metabolism may be slightly affected by medications that either induce (such as nevirapine, efavirenz, and carbamazepine) or inhibit (such as the PIs and ketoconazole) the CYP3A4 enzyme system. In these cases, it may be necessary to adjust the dosage of modafinil to account for these potential interactions (Physicians' Desk Reference, 2003). Modafinil also induces CYP3A4 and therefore may decrease the plasma concentrations of CYP3A4 substrates, such as the NNRTIs and PIs (Robertson and Hellriegel, 2003). This can lead to the development of permanent viral resistance to the antiretroviral as well as cross-resistance to the antiretrovirals in the same pharmacological class. Whenever possible, therapeutic drug monitoring of the NNRTIs and PIs should be done if modafinil is added, to ensure that the plasma levels of the antiretrovirals remain therapeutic. Dose adjustments of the antiretrovirals may be required.

Bipolar disorders

- Lithium carbonate is not metabolized and is excreted through urine virtually unchanged. Since it is cleared from the body via the kidneys, clinicians must pay careful attention to an individual's renal function prior to starting the medication and throughout the course of treatment, making dosage adjustments in the context of renal impairment. Its therapeutic index is low and toxic side effects may arise rapidly. Lithium can have numerous interactions with other medications including antibiotics (such as tetracycline and metronidazole), nonsteroidal anti-inflammatory drugs (NSAIDs, such as ibuprofen), angiotensin converting enzyme (ACE) inhibitors (such as lisinopril), and thiazide diuretics (such as hydrochlorothiazide) that can elevate lithium levels within the body and produce toxicity. Dehydration, which may be encountered secondary to vomiting and/or diarrhea, can also elevate lithium levels within the body, so the use of lithium in people with advanced HIV disease can be problematic. There have been a number of cases of lithium neurotoxicity at therapeutic levels in people with AIDS (Tanquary, 1993).

- Valproic acid is metabolized hepatically through both CYP enzyme and glucuronic acid conjugation pathways. Since it is metabolized by the liver and can potentially be hepatotoxic, it carries a US Food and Drug Administration black box warning (Physicians' Desk Reference, 2003). Clinicians must pay careful attention to an individual's hepatic function prior to starting the medication and throughout the course of treatment, adjusting the dosage or discontinuing the medication if hepatic impairment occurs.

   Valproic acid inhibits UDP-glucuronosyltransferase (glucuronic acid conjugation pathway) and may therefore increase the serum concentrations of other agents that are substrates of this enzyme. Clinically significant interactions between valproic acid and ritonavir or nelfinavir may also occur as these PIs can induce valproic acid's metabolism and lower valproic acid concentrations (Tseng and Foisy, 1999). A loss of efficacy may be noted and valproic acid dose increases may be required. Valproic acid plasma levels should be measured before starting nelfinavir or ritonavir and once again 3 weeks after the start of the PI.

   In addition to its effects on the liver, valproic acid can also affect platelet function and cause thrombocytopenia. As such, clinicians should monitor platelet counts closely. Valproic acid also carries US Food and Drug Administration black box warnings for teratogenicity (in association with neural tube defects) and potentially life-threatening pancreatitis (Physicians' Desk Reference, 2003). It must be used with some caution as recent data suggest that it may cause an increase in HIV replication (Maggi and Halman, 2001).

- Carbamazepine is metabolized via the hepatic CYP enzyme system, so clinicians should pay careful attention to the patient's hepatic function prior to starting the medication and throughout the course of treatment, adjusting the dosage or discontinuing the medication if hepatic impairment occurs. Carbamazepine has an auto-inductive and inductive effect upon the hepatic CYP enzyme system and can decrease the serum concentrations of other agents whose metabolism is via these isoenzymes. In particular, carbamazepine should be avoided in HIV-infected patients receiving NNRTIs and/or PIs, as the carbamazepine-related CYP3A4 induction will produce a clinically significant decrease in antiretroviral plasma concentrations, a loss of virologic suppression, and an acceleration of the development of viral resistance and cross-resistance (Tseng and Foisy, 1999). In addition to its effects on the liver, carbamazepine can also affect hematologic function causing bone marrow suppression, aplastic anemia, and agranulocytosis. Carbamazepine carries a US Food and Drug Administration black box warning for its association with aplastic anemia and agranulocytosis (Physicians' Desk Reference, 2003), so complete blood counts should be closely monitored.

- Lamotrigine has been found to be an effective agent for treating bipolar depression (the depressive pole of bipolar disorder) (Calabrese *et al.*, 2002). Lamotrigine is metabolized hepatically primarily via glucuronic acid conjugation reactions and its clearance can be significantly decreased in the context of hepatic or renal impairment. Lamotrigine can have a significant, potentially life-threatening interaction with valproic acid, which when coadministered with lamotrigine can increase the elimination half-life and therefore decrease the clearance of lamotrigine from the body (Keck and McElroy, 2002). The reaction, which has led to a black box warning on lamotrigine by the US Food and Drug Administration, can range from a severe skin rash to Stevens–Johnson syndrome involving multiorgan failure. The appearance of a rash in the context of lamotrigine treatment is an indication for immediate discontinuation of treatment (Physicians' Desk Reference, 2003). Similar to the interaction between ritonavir or nelfinavir and valproic acid, these PIs can accelerate lamotrigine's metabolism and cause a decrease in lamotrigine plasma levels and efficacy (Tseng and Foisy, 1999). Therapeutic drug monitoring of lamotrigine is recommended before and 3 weeks after starting nelfinavir or ritonavir.

- Gabapentin is not metabolized and is excreted by the kidneys essentially unchanged. Since it is cleared from the body via the kidneys, clinicians must pay careful attention to the patient's renal function before starting the medication and throughout the course of treatment, adjusting the dosage in the context of renal impairment. Gabapentin has a good safety and tolerability profile with no significant drug–drug interactions. Gabapentin has been used effectively to treat neuropathic pain, insomnia, and certain anxiety states (such as social phobia, panic, and generalized anxiety disorder) (Freeman *et al.*, 2002). Although gabapentin showed early promise in various case reports as a potential mood-stabilizing agent, it has more recently been shown to be ineffective in the treatment of bipolar spectrum disorders (Pande *et al.*, 2000).

- Atypical antipsychotic medications such as risperidone, olanzapine, quetiapine, and ziprasidone can also be used effectively in lieu of the mood-stabilizing agents mentioned above for the treatment of mood and affective lability and instability. These medications offer a better safety profile and do not have the potentially deleterious effects of the other agents. For further discussion of these medications, see below.

In the management of a patient with bipolar disorder, the goal is to maximize mood-stabilizing treatments as quickly as possible. In terms of pharmacotherapy, both lithium carbonate and valproic acid are recommended first-line agents that are effective in treating and stabilizing acute manic episodes in bipolar disorder. The recommended first-line treatment for bipolar depression is either lithium or lamo-trigine. More complex bipolar disorder types, such as mixed and rapid cycling states, may be more responsive to valproic acid, lamotrigine, and/or atypical antipsy-chotic medication treatment. Both lithium and valproic acid have been shown to be effective in the maintenance phase treatment of bipolar disorders (American Psychiatric Association, 2000b; Moller and Nasrallah, 2003; Goldberg and Irving, 2003; Keck *et al.*, 2004).

However, in certain cases, such as that of an acute manic episode with agitation and/or psychosis, an atypical neuroleptic agent such as olanzapine may need to be administered immediately to rapidly and acutely control the symptoms and prevent injury to the patient or others. This can then be followed by the addition of a mood-stabilizing agent. Given the necessity of regular hematological monitoring as well as the potential for significant drug–drug interactions and toxicities that may be encountered when using mood-stabilizing agents such as lithium carbonate, val-proic acid, carbamazepine, and lamotrigine, clinicians must remain vigilant when prescribing these medications for the treatment of mood and affective lability and instability states, such as those encountered in bipolar disorders.

Anxiety disorders

- Benzodiazepines. Clinicians should choose relatively longer acting agents as well as agents without major pharmacologically active metabolites such as loraze-pam, oxazepam, and temazepam (thereby decreasing the overall burden on the liver). These three benzodiazepines undergo metabolism within the liver via glucuronic acid conjugation reactions and are much less susceptible to the inhibitory/inductive drug–drug interaction effects that are encountered in oxidative metabolism involving the hepatic CYP enzyme system. As a result, they are ideal choices in patients with significant hepatic impairment (e.g., secondary to hepatic disease), and in patients who are on complex medication regimens where drug–drug interactions are of concern.

Benzodiazepines should be used only as short-term treatment for the acute manage-ment of anxiety disorders because of tolerance, abuse, and dependency issues that may be of special concern to individuals with an active or past history of addiction. Antidepressant agents such as the SSRIs and venlafaxine should be used in the longer-term management of anxiety disorders (see above section on major depres-sive disorders). When treating someone with an anxiety disorder, a useful strategy may be to start both a low-dose benzodiazepine and an antidepressant concomi-tantly, then titrate the antidepressant until therapeutic effects are seen (antidepres-sant dosages to treat anxiety symptoms are generally lower than those needed to treat depressive symptoms), and finally maintain the antidepressant at the thera-peutic dose while gradually tapering and discontinuing the benzodiazepine (to avoid possible withdrawal symptoms). Benzodiazepines can lead to behavioral disinhibition and delirium with symptoms including confusion, disorientation, memory impairment, mood lability, and agitation (particularly in the elderly and in those with CNS compromise such as AIDS dementia).

Potential drug–drug interactions may occur between benzodiazepines and other medications that inhibit benzodiazepine metabolism, thereby yielding elevated benzodiazepine levels within the body and possibly causing respiratory suppression and death. For example, PIs and delavirdine (and at times efavirenz) are expected to increase plasma concentrations of benzodiazepines that are metabolized by CYP3A4, whereas nevirapine and efavirenz are expected to decrease the plasma concentrations. Plasma concentrations of benzodiazepines that are eliminated by glucuronidation (lorazepam, oxazepam, temazepam) may be decreased by nelfinavir and ritonavir via UDP-glucuronosyltransferase induction (Antoniou and Tseng, 2002).

- Buspirone is a non-benzodiazepine anxiolytic agent that is indicated for the treatment of generalized anxiety disorder. Common side effects of buspirone may include light-headedness and dizziness. Buspirone has a low abuse potential, but clinicians should be cautious about potential drug–drug interactions. As buspirone is extensively metabolized by CYP3A4, numerous clinically significant interactions with CYP3A4 inhibitors (itraconazole, erythromycin, nefazodone, fluvoxamine) and inducers (rifampicin) are possible (Bezchlibnyk-Butler *et al.*, 1997). PIs and NNRTIs (efavirenz and nevirapine) are expected to inhibit and induce, respectively, buspirone's metabolism.

- Antihistaminergic agents such as hydroxyzine may also be used to manage anxiety symptoms. They can have anticholinergic side effects and cause problems as such.

Psychotic disorders

- Atypical antipsychotic medications, such as risperidone, olanzapine, quetiapine, and ziprasidone, offer a better safety profile than the older, typical neuroleptic medications (such as haloperidol, fluphenazine, and chlorpromazine) in terms of the risks of side effects such as anticholinergic effects, extra-pyramidal symptoms, and tardive dyskinesia. These newer medications are relatively safe in terms of hepatic function, have minimal drug–drug interactions, and are effective in the treatment of agitated states, delirium, psychotic disorders, and mood and affective lability and instability. Of the atypical antipsychotic agents mentioned above, risperidone, quetiapine, and olanzapine may cause weight gain, whereas ziprasidone is weight neutral. Weight gain may be beneficial in patients suffering with severe cachexia (HIV wasting). Of the atypical neuroleptic agents discussed above, olanzapine has been noted to precipitate or exacerbate diabetes in susceptible patients through an unclear mechanism. In susceptible patients, the onset of hyperglycemia can occur relatively soon after the initiation of olanzapine therapy, with the spectrum of symptoms ranging from mild hyperglycemia to diabetic ketoacidosis and coma (deaths have also been reported). Glycemic control can improve when olanzapine treatment is either discontinued or its dosage decreased (Koller and Doraiswamy, 2002). The implication of this altered glycemic control in the context of olanzapine treatment, particularly in a clinical setting where the use of PIs can also favor the development of diabetes, is that both patients and clinicians must be vigilant, monitor blood glucose levels regularly, and be prepared to adjust treatment in the face of symptoms such as hyperglycemia, weight loss, polyuria, polydipsia, and altered mental status that may indicate abnormal glucose metabolism. Interactions between atypical antipsychotic medications and antiretrovirals may occur. The concomitant use of high-dose ritonavir and clozapine is contraindicated as ritonavir may substantially increase clozapine levels by inhibiting CYP2D6 and C3A4. However, at the same time, ritonavir may induce clozapine CYP1A2 metabolism and glucuronidation (Tseng and Foisy, 1999). Low-dose ritonavir (100 mg twice daily) can be used with caution with clozapine. Similarly, by inducing CYP1A2 and UDP-glucuronosyl-transferases, ritonavir can induce olanzapine's metabolism fostering the need to increase olanzapine dosage to obtain the desired effect (Penzak *et al.*, 2002). PIs and NNRTIs (efavirenz and nevirapine) are expected to inhibit and induce, respectively, quetiapine's and ziprasidone's metabolism. Regimens containing ritonavir are also expected to increase risperidone plasma levels and favor the development of adverse drug reactions.

Sleep disorders

Insomnia is widespread in individuals infected with HIV and is especially prevalent among those with neurocognitive impairments (Rubinstein and Selwyn, 1998). Insomnia in people with HIV can have multiple etiologies, including ongoing medical issues, pain syndromes, neurocognitive impairments, psychosocial stress, medication effects, active substance abuse/dependence, and concomitant psychiatric illness (such as depression, anxiety, hypomania/mania, and psychosis). As a result, the evaluation of insomnia should first focus on obtaining a thorough sleep history in order to properly identify the underlying cause of the problem.

Treatment should not only focus on the potential causative condition, but also on addressing the insomnia itself. The treatment of insomnia may be addressed nonpharmacologically as well as pharmacologically (Lippman *et al.*, 2001). Nonpharmacological techniques include education about good sleep hygiene (such as maintaining a regular bedtime and avoiding naps), behavioral modifica-tions (such as exercising, avoiding caffeine/alcohol after the late afternoons/early evenings, and having early evening dinners), and stress relaxation activities before bedtime (such as yoga and meditation). Pharmacologically, insomnia may be addressed with various options including antihistamine agents (such as diphenhydramine and hydroxyzine), benzodiazepines (such as temazepam, lorazepam, and oxazepam), tricyclic antidepressants, antidepressants such as the SSRIs and mirtazapine, gabapentin and nonbenzodiazepine sedative-hypnotic agents such as zolpidem, zaleplon, and zopiclone. These latter three medications have relatively short elimination half-lives and may be used for the short-term treatment of insomnia. Long-term use is not recommended due to concerns of habituation and the potential for abuse/dependency (Lippman *et al.*, 2001). As in other cases, proper attention must be paid to potential drug–drug interactions (see Table 3.3) and side effects that may occur when using pharmacological means to treat insomnia.

What precautions should a clinician take in order to safely prescribe medications in an HIV-infected individual?

- Always take a complete and thorough medication/substance use history from the patient, paying attention to the prescribed medications, over-the-counter (OTC) medications, herbal/alternative supplements, and recreational drugs. Taking a careful initial history can make the clinician mindful of any potential negative drug–drug interactions and side effects that may arise and have an adverse impact on the patient. The use of investigational medications in HIV-infected individuals is common. Because information about their interactions and neuropsychiatric side effects is limited, the clinician should use extra caution when starting an additional medication.

- In prescribing medications, always start with a low dose and gradually titrate the dose over time, following up with the patient especially closely during the early stages. Once a patient is successfully started on a medication, find the lowest effective maintenance dose.

- To lessen the overall pill burden for the patient and reduce the risk of medication errors, adverse drug reactions, and any potential negative drug–drug interactions, avoid polypharmacy as much as possible. Limiting pill burden and the development of adverse reactions can significantly improve patient adherence to his/her psychotropic drugs and antiretrovirals, and lead to better control of the psychiatric illness, better virologic suppression, and a decreased risk of viral resistance.

- To avoid any potential negative drug–drug interactions, be aware of the hepatic CYP enzyme system responsible for the metabolism of many substances (e.g., prescribed and OTC medications, alternative compounds, recreationally used/ abused drugs) that enter the body. Know which substances can induce and/or inhibit this enzyme system and avoid agents that are metabolized solely by a single enzymatic pathway (i.e., clinicians should choose agents that have multiple metabolic pathways through the hepatic CYP enzyme system so that, if one pathway is altered or impaired, the agent may still be metabolized via others).

- Advise patients to be aware and knowledgeable about their medications and any potential side effects and interactions that may occur. Encourage them to be vigilant about the emergence of possible new side effects or interactions that may occur when new medications are added to their regimen and/or if they begin consuming alternative products or recreational drugs. Encourage them to consult a physician or pharmacist before starting any new prescribed or OTC medication, alternative agent, or recreational drug to ensure that there are no adverse drug interactions.
- Be aware that the side effects of certain psychotropic medications may actually negatively affect an individual's medical condition.
- If in doubt about a particular medication or substance, a potential side effect, or a possible drug–drug interaction, consult a pharmacist, website, or resource manual/text (see suggested reading).
- Stress the importance to the patient of obtaining all medications from the same pharmacy if possible in order to maintain consistency, to give the clinician and patient a single resource for future medication questions/concerns, and to avoid potential confusion from receiving multiple medications from multiple different sources.
- Emphasize and encourage strict adherence with a given medication regimen and educate the patient not to change and/or discontinue his or her medications in spite of "feeling better" because of the potential for a recurrence of symptoms and the development of viral resistance.
- Foster an environment where information about medications, alternative agents, and recreational drug use/abuse can be freely and easily exchanged between the clinician and the patient, and encourage open communication. Allow patients to be active participants in the treatment planning process.

Conclusion

Psychopharmacological interventions and management can be used appropriately and effectively in patients with HIV, but care must be taken when using these medications concomitantly with antiretroviral agents. The clinician must have a working knowledge and understanding of the potential drug–drug interactions that may occur when antiretrovirals and other HIV therapeutic agents are used with other medications. To complement the efforts of the clinician, the patient should also be knowledgeable about his or her medications, the possible side effects that may occur, and the risk for interactions. Open communication between the clinician and patient is vital to ensure the success of the overall treatment process.

REFERENCES

Abrams, D., Leiser, R., Shade, S. *et al.* Short-term safety of cannabinoids in HIV patients [Abstract 744]. *8th Conference on Retroviruses and Opportunistic Infections*, Chicago, USA, February 4–8, 2001.

Altice, F. L., Friedland, G. H. and Cooney, E. L. Nevirapine induced opiate withdrawal among injection drug users with HIV infection receiving methadone. *AIDS*, **13** (1999): 957–62.

American Psychiatric Association. *Practice Guideline for the Treatment of Patients with HIV/ AIDS*. Washington, DC: American Psychiatric Association, 2000a.

American Psychiatric Association. Treatment recommendations for patients with bipolar disorder. In *Practice Guidelines for the Treatment of Psychiatric Disorders* (compendium), pp. 555–6. Washington, DC: American Psychiatric Association, 2000b.

Antoniou, T. and Tseng, A. L. Interactions between recreational drugs and antiretroviral agents. *Annals of Pharmacotherapy*, **36** (2002): 1598–613.

Armstrong, S. C. The Cytochrome P450 system drug interaction principles for medical practice. Washington, DC: American Psychiatric Publishing, Inc., 2001.

Bertz, R. J. and Granneman, R. Use of *in vitro* and *in vivo* data to estimate the likelihood of metabolic pharmacokinetic interactions. *Clinical Pharmacokinetics*, **32** (1997): 210–58.

Bezchlibnyk-Butler, K. Z. and Jeffries, J. J. *Clinical Handbook of Psychotropic Drugs*, eds. 7th edn. Seattle, WA: Hogrefe and Huber Publishers, 1997.

Boroujerdi, M. *Pharmacokinetics: Principles and Applications*. New York: McGraw-Hill Companies, 2002.

Bornheim, L. M., Lasker, J. M. and Raucy, J. L. Human hepatic microsomal metabolism of delta l-tetrahydrocannabinol. *Drug Metabolism and Disposition*, **20** (1992): 241–6.

Brosen, K. and Naranjo, C. A. Review of pharmacokinetic and pharmacodynamic interaction studies with citalopram. *European Neuropsychopharmacology*, **11** (2001): 275–83.

Calabrese, J. R., Shelton, M. D., Rapport, D. J. *et al.* Long-term treatment of bipolar disorder with lamotrigine. *Journal of Clinical Psychiatry*, **63** (Suppl. 10) (2002):18–22.

Clarke, S., Mulcahy, F., Bergin, C. *et al.* Absence of opioid withdrawal symptoms in patients receiving methadone and the protease inhibitors lopinavir–ritonavir. *Clinical Infectious Diseases*, **34** (2002): 1143–5.

Cozza, K. L. and Armstrong, S. C. *The Cytochrome P450 System Drug Interaction Principles for Medical Practice*. Washington, DC: American Psychiatric Publishing, 2001.

De Maat, M. M. R., Hoetelmans, R. M. W., Mathot, R. A. A. *et al.* Drug interaction between St. John's wort and nevirapine. *AIDS*, **15** (2001): 420–1.

DeSilva, K. E., LeFlore, D. B., Marston, B. J. and Rimland, D. Serotonin syndrome in HIV-infected individuals receiving antiretroviral therapy and fluoxetine. *AIDS*, **15** (2001): 1281–5.

Dresser, G. K., Spence, J. D. and Bailey, D. G. Pharmacokinetic–pharmacodynamic consequences and clinical relevance of cytochrome P450 3A4 inhibition. *Clinical Pharmacokinetics*, **38** (2000): 41–57.

Eagling, V. A., Back, D. J. and Barry, M. G. Differential inhibition of cytochrome P450 isoforms by the protease inhibitors, ritonavir, saquinavir and indinavir. *British Journal of Clinical Pharmacology*, **44** (1997): 190–4.

Fletcher, C. V. Enfuvirtide, a new drug for HIV infection. *Lancet*, **361** (2003): 1577–8.

Freeman, M. P., Freeman, S. A. and McElroy S. L. The comorbidity of bipolar and anxiety disorders: prevalence, psychobiology, and treatment issues. *Journal of Affective Disorders*, **68** (2002): 1–23.

Goldberg, J. and Irving, K. Treatment goals of bipolar disorder. *Medscape Psychiatry and Mental Health* **8** (2003): 1–3 (Available as a living document at www.medscape.com).

Gourevitch, M. N. Interactions between HIV-related medications and methadone: an overview. *The Mount Sinai Journal of Medicine*, **68** (2001): 227–8.

Gourevitch, M. N. and Friedland, G. H. Interactions between methadone and medications used to treat HIV infection: a review. *The Mount Sinai Journal of Medicine*, **67** (2000): 429–36.

Halman, M. Management of depression and related neuropsychiatric symptoms associated with HIV/AIDS and antiretroviral therapy. *Canadian Journal of Infectious Diseases*, **12** (Suppl. C) (2001): 9–19.

Harrington, R. D., Woodward, J. A., Hooton, T. M. *et al*. Life-threatening interactions between HIV-1 protease inhibitors and the illicit drugs MDMA and gamma-hydroxybutyrate. *Archives of Internal Medicine*, **159** (1999): 2221–4.

Hendrix, C., Wakeford, J., Wire, M. B. *et al*. Pharmacokinetic and pharmacodynamic evaluation of methadone enantiomers following co-administration with amprenavir in opioid-dependent subjects [Abstract 1649]. *40th Interscience Conference on Antimicrobial Agents and Chemotherapy*, Toronto, Canada, September 17–20, 2000.

Henry, J. A. and Hill, I. R. Fatal interaction between ritonavir and MDMA [research letter]. *Lancet*, **352** (1998): 1751–2.

Keck, P. E. and McElroy, S. L. Clinical pharmacodynamics and pharmacokinetics of antimanic and mood-stabilizing medications. *Journal of Clinical Psychiatry*, **63** (Suppl. 4) (2002): 3–11.

Keck, P. E., Perlis, R. H., Otto, M. W. *et al*. The expert consensus guideline series: treatment of bipolar disorder 2004. *Postgraduate Medicine* (2004): 1–47.

Kreth, K., Kovar, K., Schwab, M. and Zanfar, U. M. Identification of the human cytochromes P450 involved in the oxidative metabolism of "Ecstasy"-related drugs. *Biochemical Pharmacology*, **15** (2000): 1563–71.

Koller, E. A. and Doraiswamy, P. M. Olanzapine-associated diabetes mellitus. *Pharmacotherapy*, **22** (2002): 841–52.

Kosel, B., Aweeka, F., Benowitz, N. *et al*. The pharmacokinetic effects of marijuana (THC) on nelfinavir and indinavir [Abstract 747]. *8th Conference on Retroviruses and Opportunistic Infections*, Chicago, USA, February 4–8, 2001.

Krishnan, R. R., Steffens, D. C. and Doraiswamy, P. M. *Psychotropic Drug Interactions*. New York: MBL Communications, Inc, (1996).

Ladona, M. G., Gonzalez, M. L., Rane, A. *et al*. Cocaine metabolism in human fetal and adult liver microsomes is related to cytochrome P450 3A expression. *Life Science*, **68** (2000): 431–3.

Laurenzana, E. M. and Owens, S. M. Metabolism of phencyclidine by human liver microsomes. *Drug Metabolism and Disposition*, **25** (1997): 557–63.

Lin, L. Y., Di Stefano, E. W., Schmitz, D. A. *et al.* (1997). Oxidation of methamphetamine and methylenedioxymethamphetamine by CYP2D6. *Drug Metabolism and Disposition*, **25** (1997): 1059–64.

Lippman, S., Mazour, I. and Shahab, H. Insomnia: therapeutic approach. *Southern Medical Journal*, **94** (2001): 866–73.

Maggi, J. D. and Halman, M. H. The effect of divalproex sodium on viral load: a retrospective review of HIV-1-positive patients with manic syndromes. *Canadian Journal of Psychiatry*, **46**(4) (2001): 359–62.

Marzolini, C., Telenti, A., Decosterd, L. A. *et al.* Efavirenz plasma levels can predict treatment failure and central nervous system side effects in HIV-1-infected patients. *AIDS*, **15** (2001): 71–5.

McDowell, J. A., Chittick, G. E., Pilati-Stevens, C. *et al.* Pharmacokinetic interaction of abacavir (1592U89) and ethanol in human immunodeficiency virus-infected adults. *Antimicrobial Agents and Chemotherapy*, **44** (2000): 1686–90.

Moller, H. J. and Nasrallah, H. A. Treatment of bipolar disorder. *Journal of Clinical Psychiatry*, **64** (Suppl. 6) (2003): 9–17.

Montplaisir, J., Hawa, R., Moller, H. *et al.* Zoplicone and zaleplon vs benzodiazepines in the treatment of insomnia: Canadian consensus statement. *Human Psychopharmacology: Clinical and Experimental*, **18** (2003): 29–38.

O'Mara, E. M., Mummaneni, V., Burchell, B. *et al.* Relationship between uridine diphosphate-glucuronosyl transferase 1A1 genotype and total bilirubin elevations in healthy subjects receiving BMS-232632 and saquinavir [Abstract 1645]. *40th Interscience Conference on Antimicrobial Agents and Chemotherapy*, Toronto, Canada, September 17–20, 2000.

O'Mara, E., Mummaneni, V., Randall, D. *et al.* BMS-232632: A summary of multiple dose pharmacokinetic, food effect and drug interaction studies in healthy subjects [Abstract 504]. *7th Conference on Retroviruses and Opportunistic Infections*, San Francisco, USA, January 3–February 2, 2000.

Organon Canada Ltd. *Remeron (mirtazapine) product monograph*. Scarborough, ON, 2001.

Osborne, R., Joel, S., Trew, D. and Slevin, M. Analgesic activity of morphine-6-glucuronide (letter). *Lancet*, **1** (1988): 828.

Pande, A. C., Crockatt, J. G., Janney, C. A. *et al.* Gabapentin in bipolar disorder: a placebo-controlled trial of adjunctive therapy [abstract]. *Bipolar Disorders*, **2** (2000): 249–55.

Park-Wyllie, L. Y. and Antoniou, T. Concurrent use of bupropion with CYP2B6 inhibitors, nelfinavir, ritonavir and efavirenz: a case series [letter]. *AIDS*, **17** (2003): 638–40.

Paterson, D. L., Swindells, S., Mohr, J. *et al.* Adherence to protease inhibitor therapy and outcomes in patients with HIV infection. *Annals of Internal Medicine*, **133** (2000): 21–30.

Penzak, S. R., Hon, Y. Y., Lawhorn, W. D. *et al.* Influence of ritonavir on olanzapine pharmacokinetics in healthy volunteers. *Journal of Clinical Psychopharmacology*, **22** (2002): 366–70.

Physicians' Desk Reference, 57th edn. Montvale, NJ: Medical Economics, (2003).

Piscitelli, S. C., Burstein, A. H., Chaitt, D. *et al.* Indinavir concentrations and St. John's Wort [research letter]. *Lancet*, **355** (2000a): 547–8.

Piscitelli, S., Rock-Kress, D., Bertz, R., Pau, A. and Davey, R. The effect of ritonavir on the pharmacokinetics of meperidine and normeperidine. *Pharmacology*, **20** (2000b): 549–53.

Piscitelli, S., Formentin, E., Burstein, A. H. *et al.* Effect of milk thistle on the pharmacokinetics of indinavir in healthy volunteers. *Pharmacotherapy*, **22** (2002a): 551–6.

Piscitelli, S. C., Burstein, A. H., Welden, N. *et al.* The effect of garlic supplements on the pharmacokinetics of saquinavir. *Clinical Infectious Diseases*, **34** (2002b): 234–8.

Prior, T. I. and Baker, G. B. Interactions between cytochrome P450 system and the second-generation antipsychotics. *Journal of Psychiatry and Neuroscience*, **28** (2003): 99–112.

Rainey, P. M., Friedland, G., McCance-Katz, E. F. *et al.* Interaction of methadone with didanosine and stavudine. *Journal of Acquired Immune Deficiency Syndrome*, **24** (2000): 241–8.

Robertson, P. and Hellriegel, E. T. Clinical pharmacokinetic profile of modafinil. *Clinical Pharmacokinetics*, **42** (2003): 123–37.

Rubinstein, M. L. and Selwyn, P. A. High prevalence of insomnia in an outpatient population with HIV infection [abstract]. *Journal of Acquired Immune Deficiency Syndromes*, **19** (1998): 260–5.

Schwartz, E. L., Brechbuhl, A. B., Kahl, P. *et al.* Pharmacokinetic interactions of zidovudine and methadone in intravenous drug-using patients with HIV infection. *Journal of Acquired Immune Deficiency Syndrome*, **5** (1992): 619–26.

Tanquary, J. Lithium neurotoxicity at therapeutic levels in an AIDS patient. *Journal of Nervous and Mental Disorders*, **181**(8)(1993): 518–19.

Thiemann, L. and Lalazeri, J. *Double Jeopardy: The HIV/HCV Co-Infection Handbook*. New York: Community Prescription Service, 1999.

Tseng, A. and Foisy, M. Significant interactions with new antiretrovirals and psychotropic drugs. *Annals of Pharmacotherapy*, **33** (1999): 461–72.

Tseng, A., Foisy, M. and Fletcher, D. *2001 Handbook of HIV Drug Therapy*. Toronto, 2002. (available as a live document at www.tthhivclinic.com/pdf/regimens01.pdf)

Von Moltke, L. L., Greenblatt, D. J., Grassi, J. M. *et al.* Protease inhibitors as inhibitors of human cytochromes P450: high risk associated with ritonavir. *Journal of Clinical Pharmacology*, **38** (1998): 106–11.

Watanabe, K., Matsunaga, T., Yamamoto, I. *et al.* Involvement of CYP2C in the metabolism of cannabinoids by human hepatic microsomes from an old woman. *Biological and Pharmaceutical Bulletin*, **18** (1995): 1138–41.

Yanagihara, Y., Kariya, S., Ohtani, M. *et al.* Involvement of CYP2B6 in n-demethylation of ketamine in human liver microsomes. *Drug Metabolism and Disposition*, **29** (2001): 887–90.

SUGGESTED READING

Further resources pertinent to this topic may be found within the American Psychiatric Association's *Practice guideline for the treatment of patients with HIV/AIDS* (2000) as well as at the following websites:

www.aidsmap.com

www.aegis.com

www.tthhivclinic.com

www.hivinsite.com/InSite.jsp?page=ar-00-02

www.hivpharmacology.com

www.drug-interactions.com

4

Mood disorders and psychosis in HIV

Andrea Stolar, M.D.[1], Glenn Catalano, M.D.[2], Sheryl M. Hakala, M.D.[3], Robert P. Bright, M.D.[4] and Francisco Fernandez, M.D.[5]

[1] Assistant Professor, Department of Psychiatry and Behavioral Medicine, University of South Florida, College of Medicine, FL, Staff Psychiatrist, Women's Program, Bay Pines Veterans Administration Medical Center, Bay Pines, FL, USA

[2] Associate Professor, University of South Florida College of Medicine, FL, Medical Director of Psychiatry, Tampa General Hospital, Tampa, FL, USA

[3] Child Fellow, Department of Psychiatry and Behavioral Medicine, University of South Florida, College of Medicine, FL, USA

[4] Assistant Professor of Psychiatry, University of North Carolina, Attending Psychiatrist, Carolinas HealthCare System, Charlotte, NC, USA

[5] Professor and Chairperson, Department of Psychiatry and Behavioral Medicine, University of South Florida, College of Medicine, Tampa, FL, USA

Introduction

Reported rates of depression among people infected with HIV vary. During the course of their disease, up to 85% of HIV-seropositive individuals report some depressive symptoms, and up to 50% experience a major depressive disorder. The variability across studies may be due to small sample size, population character-istics, and evaluation tools. However, in their meta-analysis of published studies, Ciesla and Roberts (2001) found that people with HIV were almost twice as likely as those who are HIV-seronegative to be diagnosed with major depressive dis-order, and that depression was equally prevalent in people with both symptomatic and asymptomatic HIV. In their recent analysis of rates of depression and anxiety disorders in people with HIV, Morrison et al. (2002) found a fourfold increase in the risk of current major depressive disorder in HIV-seropositive women com-pared with an HIV-seronegative group.

The data regarding the prevalence of mania in people with HIV is scant. Although less common than depression, the risk of mania is still thought to be significant, particularly as the disease progresses (Ellen et al., 1999). Mania may be the behavioral manifestation of direct central nervous system (CNS) pathology or toxicity or, if the patient has a family or personal history of bipolar disorder, mania may suggest a primary affective disorder.

HIV and Psychiatry. A Training and Resource Manual, Second Edition, ed. Kenneth Citron, Marie-Josée Brouillette, and Alexandra Beckett. Published by Cambridge University Press. © Cambridge University Press 2005.

The occurrence of psychosis is not too surprising since people with HIV experience marked disturbances in dopamine metabolism (Berger *et al.*, 1994). Early samples found frequencies ranging between less than 0.5% to 15% (Sewell *et al.*, 1994), while more recent studies indicate a prevalence rate closer to 3% for new onset psychosis (De Ronchi *et al.*, 2000; Alciati *et al.*, 2001a) with the variability due in part to differences in disease stages studied and defining criteria. The association of psychosis with prominent mood symptoms seems to be frequent: 65% and 81% in two different studies (Harris *et al.*, 1991; Sewell *et al.*, 1994).

One of the methodological difficulties in teasing out the contribution of HIV in a clinical picture of depression, mania, or psychosis is that the age of infection with HIV corresponds to the age of onset of affective and schizophrenic illnesses in the general population. The differential diagnosis is important because several medical conditions responsible for mood or psychotic symptoms are, at least in part, treatable.

Given that HIV has evolved into a chronic condition affecting a demographically diverse population, psychiatrists are more likely to encounter HIV disease as a confounding factor in the management of affective and psychotic disorders and should be aware of the relevant diagnostic and management issues.

Case study: a woman with an adjustment disorder

Sandra, a 42-year-old, divorced African-American woman, was recently diagnosed with HIV. She was tested for HIV after learning that her ex-husband had died of an AIDS-related illness. Her CD4 cell count is 430 cells/mm^3 and her viral load is 79 000 units/ml. Sandra has no prior psychiatric or substance abuse history. A single mother of three children, ages 8 to 16, she presents with complaints of depression and anxiety about her and her children's future. She has never known anyone with HIV and has told no one about her diagnosis. She holds her secret close, for fear of being socially stigmatized and rejected by her family. She has overheard remarks about people with AIDS that now take on personal significance. For example, a friend who worked in a prison was afraid to touch inmates with HIV.

Sandra is turning down dating opportunities, isolating herself, and having suicidal thoughts, although she denies intent and plan. Her sleep is disturbed. She awakens with anxiety attacks and night sweats. She is having crying spells and missing work due to fatigue. She has lost interest in food, is losing weight, and struggles with diarrhea. She expresses a belief that her death is imminent.

What is the differential diagnosis?

- Sandra's presenting symptoms may represent an adjustment disorder with mixed anxiety and depressed mood.
- Given her suicidal thoughts, anorexia with significant weight loss, and significant sleep disturbance, the clinician should consider a major depressive episode

in the initial differential diagnosis. When trying to establish a psychiatric diagnosis in medically ill patients, differentiating constitutional symptoms from psychiatric symptoms is a challenge. However, in studies that eliminate the somatic items of the Hamilton Depression Rating Scale (HAM-D) while screening for the prevalence of depression, people with HIV are still at clear risk of major depression (Cockram *et al.*, 1999).

- The panic attacks and excessive worry suggest the possibility of an anxiety disorder, including posttraumatic stress disorder, which is also suggested by the sense of foreshortened future, feelings of detachment and hyperarousal.
- Early in the course of HIV, the differential diagnosis of depressive symptoms is complicated by an appropriate grief reaction. The grief associated with the loss of loved ones, the potential loss of one's own health, and, for many with HIV, the multiple losses in families and support systems create layers of grief and multiple bereavement. When the mode of transmission of infection is through sexual contact, the patient's anger toward the sexual partner may be internalized and subsumed under grief, or it may trigger guilt and self-loathing for the patient's own choices. Grief may be justified, but it may also reflect a more psychologically acceptable expression of underlying anger or mask a deeper depression. Suicidal ideation indicates a diagnosis of a serious depressive illness and the need for timely intervention.

Complicating both diagnosis and symptom burden is Sandra's grief. Anger with her ex-husband, whose risk-taking behavior (i.e., injection drug abuse) led to his abandonment of his family and his untimely death, complicates her dysphoria and manifests in excessive guilt about her own choices. Sandra's grief and anger are directed not only at what has passed, but also to her own future and that of her children. As a single mother, the anticipated physical debilitation and the fear of being unable to care for her children is a significant psychological stress.

What are the risk factors for the development of depression and suicidality?

Individuals who are most at risk of a depressive disorder are those with:
- a prior psychiatric history, particularly a history of depressive disorders and prior suicide attempts, alcohol and substance abuse, and anxiety disorders
- female gender
- a positive family psychiatric history including a family history of suicide
- social factors including lack of social support and exposure to chronic stress
- psychological factors including passive coping style
- the presence of a medical illness that may cause affective symptoms.

Suicidality is a risk for people with a personal or family history of psychiatric illness or suicide. People with HIV are at higher risk of suicide at two stages of the illness: early in the course of HIV disease, when they are adjusting to the diagnosis, and late in the disease, when the physical burden of AIDS becomes severe. Psychological factors, including a pervasive sense of helplessness and hopelessness, increase the risk of suicide. Supportive psychological intervention, including education to teach positive coping strategies, may reduce this risk.

What impact does depression have on disease progression?

As in other chronic diseases, depression has a negative impact on quality of life and on the person's ability to function socially and in work situations. It has also been implicated in mediating cellular immunity. Studies of both men and women with HIV identify a relationship between depression and immune function. Depression is associated with lower natural killer cell activity among HIV-seropositive women (Evans *et al.*, 2002) and with HIV disease progression in general (Leserman, 2003). A longitudinal analysis from the HIV Epidemiology Research Study, which controlled for clinical, substance use, and socio-demographic characteristics, found that depressive symptoms in HIV-seropositive women were associated with disease progression (Ickovics *et al.*, 2001). Adequate psychiatric assessment and judicious management of depression may improve quality of life, reduce hospital and healthcare utilization, and slow disease progression at a cellular level and reduce HIV mortality.

What are the risks associated with untreated depression?

Polypharmacy, including potential drug–drug interactions and their impact on patients' ability to adhere to complicated medication regimes required to suppress the virus, is a concern in treating people with HIV. A conservative diagnostic approach may reduce the risk of prescribing unnecessary medication for a population already burdened by multiple, often poorly tolerated medications. However the depression itself, along with active or passive suicidal ideation or simply an attitude of fatalistic indifference, may also compromise adherence to antiretrovirals. Therefore, the risk of inadequate psychiatric intervention is increased morbidity and mortality (Tucker *et al.*, 2003)

Given the high rate of suicide and suicidal behavior in HIV-infected individuals (similar to that found in other chronically medically ill patients) and the risks of depressive comorbidity, it is important to avoid under-treatment. In evaluating depression in the context of HIV, clinicians should adopt an inclusive approach and place particular emphasis on the psychological manifestations of depression: the anhedonia, low self-esteem, excessive or inappropriate guilt, and suicidal ideation. Given the risks associated with under-treatment, the availability of well tolerated antidepressants, and the ability to identify potential drug–drug interactions, clinicians do better to err on the side of psychiatric intervention.

What is the nonpharmacological management of depressive disorders in people with HIV?

Optimal management of depressive disorders in people with HIV addresses the biopsychosocial context of the illness.

- Within supportive psychotherapy, clinicians should provide education about disease, treatment, and social service, community, and healthcare resources to help patients develop a safety net as the illness progresses. Education must include prognosis and management of HIV and comorbid conditions, as well as preventive healthcare education, including preventing transmission to future sexual partners.
- Cognitive–behavioral group therapy may reduce anxiety and depression, and provide a context for support and psycho-education.
- Interpersonal psychotherapy has demonstrated efficacy for the treatment of depression in people with HIV (Markowitz *et al.*, 1992).

Mothers of young children burdened by caregiving responsibilities have very low rates of adherence to antiretroviral regimens (Murphy *et al.*, 2002) and may need education about the benefits of complying with medication as well as interventions that promote compliance.

For a more complete discussion of psychotherapeutic issues, please see Chapter 9.

Sandra was diagnosed with an adjustment disorder with mixed anxiety and depressed mood and began taking citalopram, which the clinician prescribed because of its low risk of drug–drug interactions, single daily dosing and good coverage for both depressive and anxiety symptoms. Sandra joined an HIV support group for women through her church, and found tremendous relief in being able to admit and process her fears. Aided by her renewed spirituality, she was able to come to terms with her anger and loss. Within the group, she developed a new and important support network that encouraged her to make her own health a priority, rather than always focusing first on her children's health and welfare. A caseworker secured through her church provided the education and advocacy that allowed Sandra to successfully navigate the social service and medical resources that ultimately provided the means for her to resume her independence and restore her psychological health.

Case study: a man with cognitive decline and depression

Cesar is a 54-year-old divorced HIV-seropositive Hispanic male. He is brought to the emergency department after being found unresponsive by a passerby. Once Cesar's mental state has improved, he tells the emergency room physician that he took an intentional overdose of heroin in a suicide attempt. His urine drug screen is positive for opioids, benzodiazepines, and cocaine.

When Cesar is medically stable, he is transferred to the inpatient psychiatry unit. Previously employed as a construction worker, Cesar stopped working 4 years ago. He reports a four-month history of severely depressed mood, insomnia, and suicidal ideation. Other symptoms include a decreased appetite with an associated 45-pound weight loss, decreased energy, decreased ability to concentrate, and feelings of hopelessness and worthlessness. No manic symptoms are described.

His past psychiatric history is significant. He had two prior suicide attempts. He also has a long history of substance abuse and dependence, and continues to use. He has abused opioids, cocaine, alcohol, and benzodiazepines. He is currently involved in a methadone maintenance program, but has had multiple relapses. He has a family history of cocaine dependence, and his mother committed suicide.

Cesar was first diagnosed with HIV infection 10 years ago. Currently, his CD4 cell count is 14 cells/mm^3, and his viral load is 100 000 units/ml. He is unsure about his past usage of antiretroviral agents, and claims that he does not remember all the medications with which he has been treated but believes that there have been no recent changes. His most recent medication regimen includes zidovudine, lamivudine, and efavirenz, but his adherence has been intermittent at best. Cesar notes that this medication regimen often gives him "terrible nightmares."

During the interview, the patient is pleasant, but seems confused by some direct questioning. His mood is depressed, and his affect is blunted but mood-congruent. His thinking is logical and goal directed, but with slight tangentiality when speaking about his substance abuse. He has no obvious delusions or hallucinations, and is not attending to internal stimuli. No fluctuations in his level of consciousness are noted, and he is fully oriented. Cognitive evaluation reveals difficulty with short-term memory and serial 7 subtractions. His Mini Mental Status Examination (MMSE) is 21 out of 30.

Laboratory results reveal no major abnormality except for a low white blood cell count. A magnetic resonance imaging (MRI) scan of his head reveals subcortical atrophy. No cortical atrophy or white matter changes are noted.

What is the differential diagnosis?

It is possible that Cesar has developed a major depression over the past 4 months. The differential diagnosis of depression in HIV infection can be found in Table 4.1. All of this patient's symptoms can be explained by a diagnosis of major depression: he did have two previous suicide attempts, and the fact that the patient's mother had substance abuse disorder and committed suicide lends some genetic support to this diagnosis. However, given his prior substance abuse history and HIV infection, a diagnosis of primary affective disorder cannot be definitively made.

A mood disorder due to a general medical condition is more likely as the disease progresses. For example:

- a number of reports have associated some opportunistic infections with depression
- the development of CNS malignancies secondary to the immunocompromised state has been associated with mood symptoms (Fernandez et al., 2002)
- hypogonadism is not uncommon in advanced HIV infection and may be associated with depressive symptoms (Dobs et al., 1988).

Table 4.1. Differential diagnosis of depression in HIV infection

Primary mood disorder	Major depression
Mood disorder due to a general medical condition	Opportunistic infections (1)
	CNS malignancies
	Nutritional deficiencies (B12, folate)
	Neurosyphilis
	Hypogonadism
	HIV-related neuropathological changes
	Thyroid dysfunction
	Diabetes mellitus
	Inflammatory diseases
	Anemia
Substance-induced mood disorders	Recreational drugs
	Antiretrovirals
	Medications used to treat other medical conditions (2)
Other	Adjustment disorder with depressed mood
	Bereavement
	Grief

1. *Toxoplasma gondii*, herpes simplex virus, herpes varicella virus
2. For example, beta blockers, trimethoprim–sulfamethoxazole, quinolones.

Cesar is also at risk for nutritional deficiencies associated with his long-standing substance abuse. Deficiency in vitamin B12 or folate is associated with the development of depressive symptoms (Dommisse, 1991; Bottiglieri, 1996). It is also equally plausible that his symptoms may have been induced by either substance use/abuse or medication. He describes long-term use of multiple substances, including alcohol, cocaine, heroin, benzodiazepines, and methadone. He continued to use all these psychoactive substances, which can induce depression, up until admission. Many antiretroviral agents, including zidovudine, the protease inhibitors (PIs) and alpha-interferon, are also associated with depression. In fact, efavirenz, a medication Cesar had been taking intermittently, has been found to cause neuropsychiatric side effects, including depression, insomnia, disorientation and vivid dreams, in 50% of patients (Halman *et al.*, 2002).

Because of the multiple significant stressors in Cesar's life, it is also possible that he has developed an adjustment disorder or an episode of bereavement. However, as Cesar does not seem to have any new-onset stressors, this diagnosis is less likely. Men who have known of their HIV infection for over a year have negligible rates of adjustment disorders (Grant and Atkinson, 2000).

What is the relationship between depression and cognitive difficulties in HIV infection?

While depression and dementia are separate entities with significantly different end points, many symptoms commonly seen in major depression are also present in early HIV dementia. A patient who presents with poor concentration, irritability, psychomotor retardation, mental slowing and poor memory would likely be diagnosed with a depressive illness. However, all these symptoms could be part of the clinical picture of HIV-associated cognitive/motor disorder. People with HIV also have high rates of comorbidity between cognitive and mood symptoms. Early dementia has been known to "masquerade" as a major depression with symptoms including lethargy, apathy, and social withdrawal (Goodkin *et al.*, 2001). Symptoms such as loss of interest, anhedonia, poor concentration and mental slowing, should always be fully evaluated, even if it is early in the course of the patient's illness (Maldonado *et al.*, 2000). Given that severe depressive illness can produce a "pseudodementia" in susceptible patients (Wise and Gray, 1994), it would be relatively easy, without a rigorous neuropsychiatric evaluation, to mistake the two entities.

HIV is commonly found in the central nervous system and the virus has a direct effect on CNS structures, which can lead to the onset of new episodes of depression (Martin *et al.*, 2002). HIV is thought to invade the subcortical areas and can destroy the basal ganglia, thalamus, and temporolimbic structures. It also destroys support cells such as the astrocytes (Fernandez *et al.*, 2002; Martin *et al.*, 2002). In these cases, a careful cognitive examination and comprehensive psychiatric evaluation will be helpful in clarifying the diagnosis. For more information, see Chapter 2 on cognitive disorders in people living with HIV disease.

Which medications for HIV are associated with depression?

While the medications available to treat HIV/AIDS have greatly decreased morbidity, many have multiple cognitive and behavioral side effects:

- trimethoprim–sulfamethoxazole, efavirenz, interferon-alpha, isoniazid, steroids, vinblastine, vincristine, zidovudine, and the PIs have all been reported to cause depression (Halman *et al.*, 2002).
- abacavir, acyclovir, amphotericin B, didanosine, and ganciclovir have not been associated with depression, but have been reported to cause depressive symptoms such as tearfulness, insomnia, anorexia, and irritability (Halman *et al.*, 2002).

Which opportunistic infections may induce or mimic depression?

While opportunistic infections commonly induce episodes of delirium or cause dementia, some have been sporadically associated with depression, including:

- *Toxoplasma gondii* (Fernandez *et al.*, 2002)
- Herpes simplex virus (Andersson *et al.*, 1996)
- Herpes varicella-zoster virus (Soldatovic-Stajic and Drezgic-Vukic, 1996).

What is the initial evaluation for depression?

An initial evaluation should include:

- An in-depth psychiatric interview with special emphasis on cognitive evaluation. It is important to clarify the onset of any cognitive difficulty relative to the onset of depressive symptoms.
- A medication history. The possibility that the patient's depressive symptoms are actually side effects of antiretroviral medications should always be considered (McDaniel *et al.*, 2000).
- A substance use history.
- A comprehensive medical evaluation to identify potential organic components of the illness (Martin *et al.*, 2002).
- Laboratory testing, including thyroid function tests, free testosterone levels, arterial blood gases, toxicology screens, levels of vitamins B12 and folate, serum syphilis test and a comprehensive blood chemistry panel and liver function tests (McDaniel *et al.*, 2000; Fernandez, 2002; Martin *et al.*, 2002).
- If HIV CNS involvement is suspected, neurodiagnostic studies, including neuro-imaging, CSF analysis to rule out opportunistic infection evaluation, and EEG (Martin *et al.*, 2002).

What are some considerations in prescribing an antidepressant for people with HIV?

Medication side effects

Anticholinergic side effects are irritating and uncomfortable, and can be dangerous in people with HIV. A dry mouth can lead to a risk of oral candidiasis. Anticholinergic medications, including the tricyclic antidepressants (TCAs), paroxetine and other older antidepressants, can also worsen cognitive impairment, induce a delirium, and even cause seizures (Martin *et al.*, 2002) and should be used with caution. Although these medications are effective, they should not be first line agents. Clinicians should consider using antidepressants without significant anticholinergic activity.

Medication interactions

The great majority of antidepressants commonly used are inhibitors of the cytochrome P450 system (Nemeroff *et al.*, 1996) and are also substrates of the cytochrome P450 (Gillenwater and McDaniel, 2001). Problems may arise when other medications that inhibit or induce the cytochrome P450 system are added to a patient's medication regimen. Unfortunately, the PIs and the non-nucleoside-analogue reverse transcription inhibitors (NNRTIs) have cytochrome P450 activity (Gillenwater and McDaniel, 2001). PIs and NNRTIs can cause changes in the metabolism of antidepressants, and the antidepressants may affect blood levels of the anti-HIV medications. Adding a 3A4 isoenzyme-inhibiting antidepressant (such as nefazodone or fluvoxamine) to a stable antiretroviral regimen could increase blood levels of the antiretrovirals and thereby increase side effects (Gillenwater and McDaniel, 2001). Adding a medication that induces the 3A4 isoenzyme, such as carbamazepine, could decrease the blood levels of the PIs and NNRTIs, possibly leading to decreased efficacy and viral resistance (Gillenwater and McDaniel, 2001). See Chapter 3 for a fuller discussion of drug–drug interactions in HIV infected individuals.

Which antidepressants should be used in this population?

Choosing antidepressants to treat depression in the HIV-infected patient is a challenging task.

- The tricyclic antidepressants (TCAs) have proven to be effective for depression, neuropathic pain, and sleep disorders, but are likely not first line agents due to their side-effect profile. Clinicians who decide to use a TCA should consider using one with a low anticholinergic burden, such as nortriptyline or desipramine (Kaplan and Sadock, 1998). Cardiac toxicity is a concern, particularly in the presence of ritonavir or other medications that inhibit cytochrome P450 2D6, which is responsible for the metabolism of the TCAs.

- Clinicians would not likely initiate treatment with a monoamine oxidase inhibitor (MAOI), but patients previously on MAOIs can continue with these regimens even after antiretroviral treatment has been started (Fernandez and Levy, 1994). This combination must be monitored closely, as MAOIs are theoretically incompatible with concurrent treatment with zidovudine, possibly due to zidovudine's reported inhibition of catechol-O-methyltranferase. Patients on such a regimen are at increased risk of MAOI toxicity (Maldonado et al., 2000).

- Many newer antidepressant agents, including fluoxetine, sertraline, citalopram, and paroxetine, are effective (Fernandez, 2002). Clinicians should avoid antidepressants that significantly inhibit the 2D6 or 3A4 isoenzymes, such as nefazodone and fluvoxamine. There have been no reported adverse events noted in patients taking antiretroviral therapy and either mirtazapine or citalopram (McDaniel et al., 2000). Citalopram has minimal drug interaction potential. Mirtazapine is very helpful in patients with poor appetite and insomnia (McDaniel et al., 2000), is well tolerated and effective, and has been reported not to have hematopoietic toxicity (Maldonado et al., 2000). Bupropion is an activating agent in the majority of patients, and may be helpful in withdrawn and anergic patients. However, seizures have been noted with doses over 200 mg per day (Maldonado et al., 2000). Its use is contraindicated with full dose ritonavir, and lower doses are required in the presence of low-dose ritonavir, nelfinavir, and efavirenz. Venlafaxine has a low potential for drug–drug interactions due to its low affinity for the P450 isoenzyme system. However, a small, uncontrolled study suggested a possible decrease in indinavir concentrations in subjects on both medications concurrently (Levin *et al.*, 2001).

- The psychostimulants have also been used to treat depression in people with HIV. Methylphenidate and dextroamphetamine have both been studied, and been found to be extremely effective in the treatment of depression and cognitive impairment in HIV-seropositive patients (Fernandez, 2002). Rapid benefit has been seen within hours of beginning treatment. The symptoms that responded first were poor appetite, cognition, and psychomotor retardation (Fernandez, 2002; Martin *et al.*, 2002).

- Hypogonadism is common in this population, and testosterone for the treatment of depression has been studied. It was found to have response rates of over 80% in patients with mild depressions (Wagner *et al.*, 1996). Clinical response to testosterone in people with HIV is not correlated with serum testosterone levels at baseline (McDaniel *et al.*, 2000).

Cesar did relatively well on the inpatient psychiatric unit. He denied suicidality, but his severe depressive symptoms persisted. He had problems with withdrawal from the multiple substances he abused and often required doses of lorazepam for symptoms of alcohol withdrawal. While on the inpatient psychiatry unit, he was evaluated by the infectious disease consultation team, who recommended re-instituting antiretroviral therapy. Cesar agreed and restarted medications at that time.

After the patient was judged to no longer be a threat to himself or others, he was transferred to an inpatient substance abuse treatment program. After 28 days he was discharged and returned to the outpatient mental health clinic. At that time, the patient was still noted to have a significantly depressed mood, but was without any suicidal ideations. He still had thoughts of hopelessness, insomnia, and a poor appetite. However, his cognition was greatly improved. The patient asked to be placed on an antidepressant. Because Cesar had been restarted on saquinavir, stavudine, and didanosine to treat his HIV infection, the clinician prescribed mirtazapine.

Over the course of the next 12 months, Cesar's dose of mirtazapine was increased to 30 mg each night with good results. He reported a complete resolution of depressive symptoms and a healthy 20-pound weight gain. He began searching out his family and friends, and moved into an apartment. He has remained free of all substances, and adherent to his HIV treatment. His CD4 count increased and his health improved.

> ## Case study: A man presenting with mania
>
> Jamie is a 22-year-old gay white male who was diagnosed with HIV 2 years ago. His family bring him to the hospital complaining of increased energy and decreased need for sleep. He has dropped out of school and lost his job waiting tables.
>
> His family report that his room is piled six feet deep with garbage that he has collected from the side of the road. He says that he is going to use these items to build a great invention that will make him internationally famous. Jamie also claims that he is going to become a great chef, but his family report that he is preparing inedible combinations of disgusting foods. He has been leaving pots on the stove and forgetting about them. He has also been driving at high speeds at night without any headlights. According to the family, these behaviors started a month ago and have gradually become worse.
>
> Jamie has no previous psychiatric history, and there is no family history of psychiatric problems. However, he does have a reported history of methamphetamine use. Jamie currently has a CD4 cell count of 87 cells/mm^3 with a viral load of 45 000 units/ml. He started taking sertraline (50 mg a day) a month ago. Other medications include indinavir, stavudine, and didanosine. His adherence to these prescriptions is unknown.
>
> Mental status examination reveals a thin white disheveled male, with food-stained clothes and unzipped pants. He exhibits disorganized behavior and appears to not have any insight in to the fact that there is something wrong. There is no disturbance in consciousness. He scores 20 out of 30 in his MMSE because he is only able to register one out of three objects, he is unable to recall three objects, and he cannot follow a three-step command. He is also unable to maintain concentration to spell "world" backwards correctly.

What is the differential diagnosis of mania in HIV?

A manic episode in someone with HIV may be a primary episode (initial presentation of an underlying bipolar disorder) or a secondary episode due to a number of other etiologies (Table 4.2).

- Bipolar disorder. If the patient has a family history of bipolar disorder and is under 30 years of age, the clinician should consider bipolar disorder.
- Substance-induced mania. Manic episodes may be substance induced, either from prescription medication or illicit drug use. A number of antiretroviral agents have been implicated in the induction of mania (Brouillette *et al.*, 1994; Maxwell *et al.*, 1988).
- Mania due to general medical condition. Mania may be caused by opportunistic infection of the CNS or another CNS disease process causing structural changes (Fernandez *et al.*, 2002). Because HIV infection has been reported to increase the likelihood of a false negative serum syphilis test, neurosyphilis is also an important consideration – even with a negative serum syphilis test (Whitefield *et al.*, 1991). The manic episode may also be caused by direct pathophysiological

Table 4.2. Differential diagnosis of mania in HIV infection

Primary mood disorder	Bipolar disorder, mania
Mood disorder due to a general medical condition	Opportunistic infections of the CNS[a]
	CNS malignancies
	Neurosyphilis
	HIV-related neuropathological changes
	Cerebrovascular changes
Substance-induced mood disorder	Recreational drugs
	Antidepressants
	Antiretrovirals
	Medications used to treat other medical conditions[b]

[a] For example, cytomegalovirus encephalitis, herpes simplex virus encephalitis, toxoplasmosis cerebritis, cryptococcal meningitis, *Candida albicans* meningitis, mycobacterial tuberculosis meningitis.
[b] For example, steroids.

changes caused by HIV infection, particularly in the frontal lobes and subcortical areas (Navia *et al.*, 1986). Often this occurs in later stages of disease progression (Lyketsos and Federman, 1995).

- Hyperactive delirium. An episode of mania may sometimes be confused with hyperactive delirium. The MMSE is a useful screening tool for cognitive failure but does not distinguish between delirium and dementia (Breitbart and Strout, 2000). For more information on evaluating delirium, please see Chapter 7.

As is the case for many with HIV, Jamie is young enough for this to be the first presentation of an underlying bipolar disorder. However, there is no family history of bipolar disorder. Given his history of methamphetamine use and one-month history of antidepressant therapy, substance-induced mania should also be considered. In the context of advanced HIV infection and in the presence of cognitive difficulties, the manic symptoms may reflect HIV-related neuropathological changes. Because his symptoms developed over a period of a month rather than hours or a few days and do not fluctuate over time, Jamie does not exhibit signs or symptoms of hyperactive delirium.

Would the diagnostic considerations have been different if the patient had presented with psychosis in the absence of prominent mood symptoms?

If the patient had presented with psychosis, the clinician would consider:

- Primary psychotic disorder. There may be a family history of psychosis, particularly if the patient is under age 35 at onset.
- Substance-induced psychosis. Illicit drug use or prescribed medications, especially efavirenz, can cause psychosis, with case reports of abacavir and nevirapine

causing psychosis as well (de la Garza *et al.*, 2001; Jan Wise, 2002; Foster *et al.*, 2003; Poulsen and Lublin, 2003).

- Psychosis due to a general medical condition. Neurological conditions (seizures, vascular lesions, space-occupying lesions – infectious, or neoplasm), endocrine conditions, metabolic abnormalities, and systemic infections related to the pathophysiological changes caused by HIV infection (Navia *et al.*, 1986; Alciati *et al.*, 2001b) can trigger psychosis. In most of these cases, the patient has either demonstrable neuropsychiatric impairment at the time of onset of the psychotic symptoms or will progress to dementia within months (Busch, 1989; Alciati *et al.*, 2001b)
- Delirium. Delirium can cause psychotic symptoms.

What is the initial evaluation for mania and psychosis in HIV infection?

An initial evaluation should include:

- An in-depth psychiatric interview with special emphasis on cognitive evaluation. It is important to clarify the onset of any cognitive difficulty relative to the onset of manic symptoms.
- A medication history. Clinicians should always consider the possibility that the patient's manic symptoms are actually side effects of antiretroviral medications, and review all medication changes in the past 4 months. Didanosine has been implicated in inducing mania up to 3 months after its initiation (Brouillette *et al.*, 1994).
- A substance use history.
- A comprehensive medical evaluation to identify potential organic components of the illness (Martin *et al.*, 2002).
- Laboratory testing, including toxicology screens and serum syphilis test.
- If HIV CNS involvement is suspected, neurodiagnostic studies, including neuroimaging, and CSF analysis to rule out opportunistic infection evaluation.
- An EEG, which may provide diagnostic benefit in distinguishing a hyperactive delirium or indicating a manic episode due to drug use.

How do you treat mania and psychosis in HIV infection?

Any potentially implicating medications should be discontinued if possible. Once the manic episode resolves, restart antiretroviral agents in lower doses.

Mood stabilizers

- Valproic acid is generally used as a first-line treatment for mania among HIV patients. Valproic acid has been used to control mania associated with brain lesions in HIV disease (Halman *et al.*, 1993). The divalproex sodium preparation causes fewer gastrointestinal side effects than the sodium valproate preparation. *In vitro* studies indicate that valproic acid may increase the viral load (Moog *et al.*, 1996; Witvrouw *et al.*. 1997). However, there is only one report of increased viral load with valproic acid use in a patient who was not on an antiretroviral regimen. This was reported as part of a case review of 15 patients, 11 of whom were taking valproic acid (Maggi and Halman, 2001). The effect that valproic acid may have on viral load is likely to be negligible, but clinicians should continue to monitor viral load closely with use of this medication. Side effects of valproic acid may be more marked in the HIV-seropositive patient, including elevation of liver enzymes to three times normal. Valproic acid may also increase levels of zidovudine by decreasing its glucuronidation (Akula *et al.*, 1997; Trapnell *et al.*, 1998).

- Lithium has been useful in treating mania in HIV-seropositive patients. However, there have been a number of cases of lithium neurotoxicity at therapeutic levels in people with AIDS (Tanquary, 1993), possibly due to the fact that lithium may accumulate in abnormal neurons (Goldberger *et al.*, 1980). Lithium must be used with extreme caution, and levels and blood chemistry closely monitored, because patients may develop toxicity with dehydration due either to nausea and vomiting side effects of antiretroviral agents or infectious causes of diarrhea or dehydration (Maldonado *et al.*, 2000; Fernandez *et al.*, 2002).

- Although there are case reports of carbamazepine efficacy in HIV mania, it is theoretically contraindicated in people with HIV because of its potential hematopoietic toxicity (Maldonado *et al.*, 2000). Significant drug–drug interactions may be troublesome with antiretroviral agents due to carbamazepine's cytochrome p450 profile. There is also a case report of carbamazepine causing antiretroviral therapy to fail (Hugen *et al.*, 2000).

- Although there are no case reports in the medical literature on the use of lamotrigine for mania in an HIV patient, it has been used successfully to treat HIV neuropathy, which suggests that it may be an alternative mood stabilizer (Backonja, 2002; Simpson *et al.*, 2003). The incidence of rash was lower in people with HIV.

- Because of its low potential for drug–drug interactions, gabapentin may also play a role as an adjunctive agent in mood stabilization.

Antipsychotics

The clinician should be cautious when using neuroleptics because people with AIDS are at a greater risk of developing extrapyramidal side effects with high potency agents, including risperidone. They also are more sensitive to the anticholinergic side effects of low-potency agents and at greater risk for neuroleptic malignant syndrome. However, neuroleptics may be necessary for acute control of mania symptoms and in the treatment of psychosis. Second generation antipsychotics tend to have fewer side effects than the typical agents.

- Olanzapine, with its sedative effects, low risk of extra-pyramidal symptoms (EPS) and proven efficacy in controlling acute mania, provides benefits. When olanzapine is used in combination with ritonavir, higher doses may be necessary. There is an increased risk of hyperglycemia or glucose dysregulation associated with its use, particularly in the context of HIV care where the use of PIs can also foster the development of diabetes.

- Use risperidone in doses of 2 mg or greater with caution as there is an increased incidence of EPS at this dosage. However, a case series indicated that the drug is well tolerated and can be effective in treating HIV psychosis at a mean maximum daily dose of 3.29 mg (Singh *et al.*, 1997). Case reports indicate the inhibitory effects of antiretrovirals such as ritonavir and indinavir on the metabolism of risperidone (via cytochrome P450 CYP2D6 and CYP3A4), exacerbating EPS and precipitating toxicity (Jover *et al.*, 2002; Kelly *et al.*, 2002).

- Avoid clozapine due to the dose-related side effect of agranulocytosis in an immunocompromised patient population, but do not rule it out entirely. A pilot study indicated that this agent has benefits when used at conservative doses (mean dose 27.06 mg per day) in the context of HIV psychosis and drug-induced parkinsonism (Lera, 1999).

- Newer agents, such as aripiprazole, ziprasidone, and quetiapine, have yet to be studied in this population.

Benzodiazepines

Benzodiazepines may be a useful adjunct in the treatment of mania in the HIV patient with the caveat that they may worsen cognitive impairment.

- Clonazepam has been used with success as an adjunct in the treatment of mania in HIV patients.

- Lorazepam, oxazepam and temazepam may be of particular value as their metabolism is by direct conjugation via glucuronyl transferase, while other benzodiazepines are metabolized primarily by the cytochrome P450 isoenzyme 3A4. Ritonavir induces glucuronyl transferase activity, and coadministration with ritonavir may require higher doses of these benzodiazepines.

- Many antiretroviral agents inhibit the cytochrome P450 system, causing increased levels of benzodiazepines metabolized by this enzyme. For more information regarding the potential of drug–drug interactions using these drugs, please consult Chapter 3.

Other

- Although there are no case reports of an HIV-seropositive person receiving electroconvulsive therapy (ECT) for a manic episode, this should always be a consideration in a medically ill population unable to tolerate traditional medications. ECT has been successfully used in depressed patients with HIV and AIDS, although its use may be complicated by prolonged confusion (Schaerf *et al.*, 1989).

- Psycho-education is an important component in the management of a manic episode, particularly if the episode was iatrogenically produced. To ensure adherence to medication required for long-term survival, clinicians should reassure people with HIV about the safety of their medication regimen. Clinicians should inform patients who clearly had a medication-induced manic episode that, although there are case reports of subsequent manic and depressive episodes, mania and hypomania tend not to recur in people who do not have underlying bipolar disorder (Ellen *et al.*, 1999). However, mania does imply a poor prognosis for HIV progression. New onset mania without a family or personal history of mood disorders is more likely to be associated with dementia or cognitive slowing and to occur late in the course of the disease (el-Mallakh, 1991; Lyketsos *et al.*, 1997; Ellen *et al.*, 1999).

With new antiretroviral treatment regimens for HIV, the incidence and prognosis for mania in people with HIV may change. Highly active antiretroviral therapy (HAART) reverses brain metabolite abnormalities in mild HIV dementia (Chang *et al.*, 1999), which may result in decreased incidence of mania.

Jamie received small doses of haloperidol (0.5 mg) and lorazepam (1.0 mg) twice in the emergency room. Physical exam revealed no focal abnormalities. His medical workup was essentially negative, including CT of the head and EEG, except for a mild leukocytosis. Urine drug screen (UDS) was negative and all other laboratory values were within normal limits. Jamie was hospitalized on the psychiatry ward, and given divalproex sodium at 250 mg at bedtime, which was slowly titrated up to 500 mg twice daily. Sertraline was discontinued. The patient's manic symptoms resolved. The divalproex sodium was to be tapered and discontinued at follow-up visits. The family was educated about how to recognize the early stages of mania.

Two weeks after Jamie's discharge, he underwent neuropsychological testing as an out-patient, which showed mild frontal lobe impairment. Four weeks later, Jamie was brought to the emergency department by his family with marked confusion, which had become pro-gressively worse since his discharge from the hospital. He had hemiparesis, and hemianopia. An MRI revealed asymmetric areas of T1 hypointensity and T2 hyperintensity in the sub-cortical white matter in the parieto-occipital lobes as well as cortical gray matter involvement with a scalloped appearance. These changes were thought to be indicative of progressive multifocal leukoencephalopathy (PML). The patient continued to deteriorate and a brain biopsy could not be performed. Based on clinical symptoms suggesting PML, the clinician initiated intravenous cytarabine. Jamie's condition continued to deteriorate rapidly. Hospice made home visits and the patient died at home the following week.

Conclusion

Highly active antiretroviral therapy offers the possibility of long-term HIV sup-pression and with it, a reduction in the opportunistic infections, morbidity, and mortality associated with HIV. However, the CNS remains vulnerable to the direct and secondary effects of HIV. Despite the inadequate penetration and potentially troublesome side effects of antiretroviral therapy, the rates of affective disorders appear to be declining among people with HIV who are managed with HAART and triple combination therapy (Alciati *et al.*, 2001a; Starace *et al.*, 2002). The ability to reduce significant morbidity associated with mood disorders depends on several factors, including:

- an awareness of the signs and symptoms of affective disorders in people with HIV
- a careful review of potentially precipitating and exacerbating medical conditions and substances, and concerted efforts to manage or eliminate them
- the judicious use of mood-enhancing and stabilizing psychotropics, in conjunction with appropriate social and psychological intervention.

REFERENCES

Akula, S. K., Rege, A. B., Dreisbach, A. W. *et al.* Valproic acid increases cerebrospinal fluid zidovudine levels in a patient with AIDS. *American Journal of Medicine and Science*, **313** (1997): 244–6.

Alciati, A., Fusi, A., D'Arminio Monforte, A. *et al.* New-onset delusions and hallucinations in patients infected with HIV. *Journal of Psychiatry and Neuroscience*, **26**(3) (2001b): 229–34.

Alciati, A., Starace, F., Scaramelli, B. *et al.* Has there been a decrease in the prevalence of mood disorders in HIV-seropositive individuals since the introduction of combination therapy? *European Psychiatry*, **16**(8) (2001a): 491–6.

Andersson, E., Hansson, I. and Norlin, K. Depression caused by herpes simplex encephalitis. Atypical symptoms were misleading for diagnosis. *Lakartidningen*, **93** (1996): 1257.

Backonja, M. M. Use of anticonvulsants for treatment of neuropathic pain. *Neurology*, **59** (5 Suppl. 2) (2002): S14–17.

Berger, J. R., Kumar M. Kumar A. *et al.* Cerebrospinal fluid dopamine in HIV-1 infection. *AIDS*, **8** (1994): 67–71.

Bottiglieri, T. Folate, vitamin B12, and neuropsychiatric disorders. *Nutritional Review*, **54** (1996): 382–90.

Breitbart, W. and Strout, D. Delirium in the mentally ill. *Clinical Geriatric Medicine* **16** (2) (200): 357–72.

Brouillette, M. -J., Chouinard, G. and Lalonde, R. Didanosine-induced mania in HIV infection. *American Journal of Psychiatry*, **151** (1994): 12.

Busch, K. A. Psychotic states in human immunodeficiency virus illness. *Current Opinion in Psychiatry*, **2** (1989): 3–6.

Chang, L., Ernst, T., Leonido-Yee, M. *et al.* Highly active antiretroviral therapy reverses brain metabolite abnormalities in mild HIV-1 dementia. *Neurology*, **53**(4) (1999): 782–9.

Ciesla, J. A. and Roberts, J. E. Meta-analysis of the relationship between HIV-1 infection and risk for depressive disorders. *American Journal of Psychiatry*, **158** (2001): 725–30.

Cockram, A., Judd, F. K., Mijch, A. and Norman, T. The evaluation of depression in inpatients with HIV disease. *Australian and New Zealand Journal of Psychiatry*, **33** (1999): 344–52.

De la Garza, C. L. S., Paoletti-Duarte, S., Garcia-Martin, C. and Gutierrez-Casares, J. R. Efavirenz-induced psychosis. *AIDS*, **15**(14) (2001): 1911–12.

De Ronchi, D., Faranca, I., Forti, P. *et al.* Development of acute psychotic disorders and HIV-1 infection. *International Journal of Psychiatry in Medicine*, **30** (2000): 173–83.

Dobs, A. S., Dempsey, M. A., Ladenson, P. W. and Polk, B. F. Endocrine disorders in men infected with human immunodeficiency virus. *American Journal of Medicine*, **84** (1988): 611–16.

Dommisse, J. Subtle vitamin deficiency and psychiatry: a largely unnoticed but devastating relationship? *Medical Hypothesis*, **34** (1991): 131–40.

Ellen, S. R., Judd, F. K., Mijch, A. M. and Cockram, A. Secondary mania in patients with HIV infection. *Australian and New Zealand Journal of Psychiatry*, **33**(3) (1999): 353–60.

el-Mallakh, R. S. Mania in AIDS: clinical significance and theoretical considerations. *International Journal of Psychiatry in Medicine*, **21**(4) (1991): 383–92.

Evans, D. L., Ten Have, T. R., Douglas, S. D. *et al.* Association of depression with viral load, CD8 T lymphocytes, and natural killer cells in women with HIV-1 infection. *American Journal of Psychiatry*, **159** (2002): 1752–9.

Fernandez, F. Neuropsychiatric aspects of human immunodeficiency virus (HIV-1) infection. *Current Psychiatry Reports*, **4** (2002): 228–31.

Fernandez, F. and Levy, J. K. Psychopharmacology in HIV-1 Spectrum disorders. *Psychiatric Clinics of North America*, **17** (1994): 135–48.

Gillenwater, D. R. and McDaniel, J. S. Rational psychopharmacology for patients with HIV-1 infection and AIDS. *Psychiatric Annals*, **31** (2001): 28–34.

Goldberger, E., Clavere, J. L. and Espagno, J. Dosage de lithium intratumoral (glioblastome cerebral). *Encephale*, **6** (1980): 139–44.

Goodkin, K., Baldewicz, T. T., Wilkie, F. L. and Tyll, M. D. Cognitive-motor impairment and disorder in HIV-1 infection. *Psychiatric Annals*, **31** (2001): 37–44.

Grant, I. and Atkinson, J. H. Neuropsychiatric aspects of HIV-1 infection and AIDS. In *Kaplan and Sadock's Comprehensive Textbook of Psychiatry*, 7th edn., B. J. Sadock, and V.A. Sadock, eds. pp. 308–36. Philadelphia, PA: Lippincott Williams and Wilkins, 2000.

Halman, M. H., Bialer, P., Wort, J. L. and Rourke, S. B. HIV-1 Disease/AIDS. In *The American Psychiatric Publishing Textbook of Consultation-Liaison Psychiatry: Psychiatry in the Medically Ill*, 2nd edn., M. G. Wise, and J. R. Rundell, eds. pp. 807–51. Washington, DC: American Psychiatric Publishing, Inc, 2002.

Halman, M. H., Worth, J. L., Sanders, K. M. *et al.* Anticonvulsants use in the treatment of manic syndromes in patients with HIV-1 infection. *Journal of Neuropsychiatry and Clinical Neurosciences*, **5** (1993): 430–4.

Harris, M. J., Jeste, D. V., Gleghorn, A. and Sewell, D. D. New-onset psychosis in HIV-infected patients. *Journal of Clinical Psychiatry*, **53** (1991): 369–76.

Hugen, P. W., Burger, D. M., Brinkman, K. *et al.* Carbamazepine–indinavir interaction causes antiretroviral therapy failure. *Annals of Pharmacotherapy*, **34**(4) (2000): 465–70.

Ickovics, J. R., Hamburger, M. E., Vlahov, D. *et al.* Mortality, CD4 cell count decline, and depressive symptoms among HIV-1-seropositive women: longitudinal analysis from the HIV-1 epidemiology research study. *Journal of the American Medical Association*, **285** (2001): 1466–74.

Jan Wise, M. E. Neuropsychiatric complications of nevirapine treatment. *British Medical Journal*, **324** (2002): 879.

Jover, F., Cuadrado, J. M., Andreu, L. and Merino, J. Reversible coma caused by risperidone-ritonavir interaction. *Clinical Neuropharmacology*, **25**(5) (2002): 251–3.

Kaplan, H. I. and Sadock, B. J. *Mood Disorders*, pp. 524–80. Baltimore, MD: Williams and Wilkins, (1998).

Kelly, D. V., Beique, L. C. and Bowme, M. I. Extrapyramidal symptoms with ritonavir/indinavir plus risperidone. *Annals of Pharmacotherapy*, **36**(5) (2002): 827–30.

Lera, G. and Zirulnik, J. Pilot study with clozapine in patients with HIV-associated psychosis and drug-induced parkinsonism. *Movement Disorders*, **14**(1)(1999): 128–31.

Leserman, J. HIV disease progression: depression, stress, and possible mechanisms. *Biological Psychiatry*, **54**(3) (2003): 295–306.

Levin, G. M., Nelson, L. A., DeVane, C. L. *et al.* A pharmacokinetic drug–drug interaction study of venlafaxine and indinavir. *Psychopharmacology Bulletin*, **35**(2) (2001): 62–71.

Lyketsos, C. G. and Federman, E. B. (1995). Psychiatric disorders and HIV–infection: impact on one another. *Epidemiology Review*, **17** (1995): 152–64.

Lyketsos, C. G., Schwartz, J., Fishman, M. and Treisman, G. AIDS mania. *Journal of Neuropsychiatry and Clinical Neurosciences*, **9**(2) (1997): 277–9.

Maggi, J. D. and Halman, M. H. The effect of divalproex sodium on viral load: a retrospective review of HIV-1-positive patients with manic syndromes. *Canadian Journal of Psychiatry*, **46**(4) (2001): 359–62.

Maldonado, J. L., Fernandez, F. and Levy, J. K. Acquired immunodeficiency syndrome. In *Psychiatric Management of Neurological Disease*, E. C. Lauterbach, ed. pp. 271–95. Washington, DC: American Psychiatric Publishing, Inc, 2000.

Markowitz, J. C., Klerman, G. L. and Perry, S. Interpersonal psychotherapy of depressed HIV-seropositive outpatients. *Hospital and Community Psychiatry*, **43**(1992): 885–90.

Martin, L., Tummala, R. and Fernandez, F. Psychiatric management of HIV-1 Infection and AIDS. *Psychiatric Annals*, **32** (2002): 133–40.

Maxwell, S., Scheftner, W. A., Kessler, H. A. and Busch, K. Manic syndrome associated with zidovudine treatment. *Journal of the American Medical Association*, **259** (1988): 3406–7.

McDaniel, J. S., Chung, J. Y., Brown, L. *et al.* Practice guideline for the treatment of patients with HIV-1/AIDS. *American Journal of Psychiatry*, **157** (2000): 1–61.

Moog, C., Kuntz-Simon, G., Caussin-Schwemling, C. and Obert, G. Sodium valproate, an anticonvulsant drug, stimulates human immunodeficiency virus type 1 replication independently of glutathione levels. *Journal of General Virology*, **77** (1996): 1993–9.

Morrison, M. F., Petitto, J. M., Ten Have, T. *et al.* Depressive and anxiety disorders in women with HIV infection. *American Journal of Psychiatry*, **159** (2002): 789–96.

Murphy, D. A., Greenwell, L. and Hoffman, D. Factors associated with antiretroviral adherence-among HIV-infected women with children. Abstract X14 *International AIDS Conference*, 2002.

Navia, B. A., Cho, E. S., Petito, C. K. and Price, R. W. The AIDS dementia complex: II. Neuropathology. *Annals of Neurology*, **19** (1986): 525–35.

Nemeroff, C. B., DeVane, C. L. and Pollack, B. G. Newer antidepressants and the cytochrome P450 system. *American Journal of Psychiatry*, **153** (1996): 311–20.

Poulsen, H. D. and Lublin, H. K. Efavirenz-induced psychosis leading to involuntary detention. *AIDS*, **17**(3) (2003): 451–3.

Schaerf, F. W., Miller, R. R., Lipsey, J. R. and McPherson, R. W. ECT for major depression in four patients infected with human immunodeficiency virus. *American Journal of Psychiatry*, **146**(6) (1989): 782–4.

Sewell, D. D., Jeste, D. V., Atkinson, J. H. *et al.* HIV-associated psychosis: a study of 20 cases. *American Journal of Psychiatry*, **151** (1994): 237–42.

Simpson, D. M., McArthur, J. C., Olney, R. *et al.* Lamotrigine for HIV-associated painful sensory neuropathies: a placebo-controlled trial. *Neurology*, **60**(9) (2003): 1508–14.

Singh, A. N., Golledge, H. and Catalan, J. Treatment of HIV-related psychotic disorders with risperidone: a series of 21 cases. *Journal of Psychosomatic Research*, **42**(5) (1997): 489–93.

Soldatovic-Stajic, B. and Drezgic-Vukic, S. Case report of a female patient with post-infection depression. *Medicinski Pregled*, **49** (1996): 57–8.

Starace, F., Bartoli, L., Aloisi, M. S. *et al.* Cognitive and affective disorders associated to HIV infection in the HAART era: findings from the NeuroICONA study. *Acta Psychiatrica Scandinavica*, **106**(1) (2002): 20–6.

Tanquary, J. Lithium neurotoxicity at therapeutic levels in an AIDS patient. *Journal of Nervous and Mental Disease*, **181**(8) (1993): 518–19.

Trapnell, C. B., Klecker, R. W., Jamis-Dow, C. and Collins, J. M. Glucuronidation of 3'-azido-3'-deoxythimidine (zidovudine) by human liver microsomes: relevance to clinical pharmacokinetic interactions with atovaquone, fluconazole, methadone, and valproic acid. *Antimicrobial Agents and Chemotherapy*, **42** (1998): 1592–6.

Tucker, J. S., Burnam, A., Sherbourne, C. D., Kung, F. Y. and Gifford, A. L. (2003). Substance use and mental health correlates of nonadherence to antiretroviral medications in a sample of patients with human immunodeficiency virus infection. *American Journal of Medicine*, **114** (2003): 573–80.

Wagner, G. J., Rabkin, J. G. and Rabkin, R. A comparative analysis of standard and alternative antidepressants in the treatment of human immunodeficiency virus patients. *Comprehensive Psychiatry*, **37** (1996): 402–8.

Whitefield, S. G., Everett, A. S. and Rein, M. F. Neurosyphilis and human immunodeficiency virus infection (letter). *Journal of Infectious Diseases*, **164** (1991): 609.

Wise, M. G. and Gray, K. F. Delirium, dementia, and amnestic disorders. In *The American Psychiatric Press Textbook of Psychiatry*, 2nd edn, R. E. Hales, S. C. Yudofsky and J. A. Talbott, eds. pp. 311–53 Washington, DC:American Psychiatric Publishing, 1994.

Witvrouw, M., Schmit, J. C., Van Remoortel, B. *et al.* Cell type-dependent effect of sodium valproate on human immunodeficiency type 1 replication in vitro. *AIDS Research and Human Retroviruses*, **13** (1997): 187–92.

SUGGESTED READING

American Psychiatric Association Practice Guidelines for the Treatment of Patients with HIV/AIDS. *American Journal of Psychiatry*, **157** (Suppl. 11)(2000).

Cournos, F. and Forstein, M.(eds.)*What Mental Health Practitioners Need to Know about HIV and AIDS*, San Francisco, CA: Jossey-Bass/Wiley, 2000.

Maldonado, J. L. and Fernandez, F. Neurobehavioral complications of human immunodeficiency virus infection and acquired immunodeficiency syndrome. In *Neuropsychiatry,* 2nd edn. R. B. Schiffer, S. M. Rao and B. S. Fogel eds. pp. 1018–33. Philadelphia, PA: Lippincott Williams and Wilkins.

McDaniel, J. S., Chung, J. Y., Brown, L. *et al.* American Psychiatric Association Practice Guideline for the Treatment of Patients with HIV/AIDS. *American Journal of Psychiatry,* **157** (2000): 1–61.

Repetto, M. J., Evans, D. L., Cruess, D. G. *et al.* Neuropsychopharmacologic treatment of depression and other neuropsychiatric disorders in HIV-infected individuals. *CNS Spectrums,* **8**(1) (2003): 59–63.

5

Suicidal behavior and HIV infection

Jose Catalan, M.Sc. (Oxon), D.P.M., F.R.C. Psych.

Honorary Senior Lecturer, Imperial College School of Medicine, University of London Consultant Psychiatrist, Central North West London Mental Health NHS Trust, London, UK

Introduction

People with HIV infection, like others with serious diseases, may have thoughts about suicide. They may also engage in self-harming behaviors that have a significant suicide risk. These thoughts and actions may not be just a measure of distress or desperation, but may strongly suggest the presence of a severe depressive disorder that could benefit from specialist mental health intervention.

From the beginning of the epidemic and well into the 1990s, suicidal behavior in people with HIV infection was the subject of a good deal of research. Results indicated that people with HIV have a greater risk of suicide, deliberate self-harm and suicidal ideas than those without the infection, and clinical experience generally confirmed these findings. Since the introduction of highly active antiretroviral treatments in the mid 1990s, those involved in the care of people with HIV have noted a decline in the incidence of suicide, and few reports have appeared in the literature on the topic. It could be argued that the improvements in HIV-related mortality and morbidity resulting from the widespread use of combination therapy has contributed to a greater sense of hope for people with HIV and this, in turn, has led to positive changes in suicidal behavior.

Care providers should be able to assess suicidal ideas, recognize the presence of suicide risk and its degree, and formulate an intervention plan. Quite often, the person with HIV will hint at or disclose suicidal ideas to the frontline care provider (e.g., physician, nurse, family doctor) during a clinic appointment or home visit. It is important that these frontline professionals, who are not necessarily mental health specialists, have the skills to encourage patients to discuss suicidal ideas, evaluate their significance, and refer for specialist care if necessary. Monitoring thoughts and feelings about suicide and quality of life, which should be part of a long-term, continuous care process, requires a significant level of trust between the person with HIV and the care provider.

HIV and Psychiatry. A Training and Resource Manual, Second Edition, ed. Kenneth Citron, Marie-Josée Brouillette, and Alexandra Beckett. Published by Cambridge University Press. © Cambridge University Press 2005.

Mental health specialists should be able to put any suicidal ideas or feelings identified in people with HIV into context, recognizing the significance of HIV-related symptoms and treatment side-effects, fears about prognosis, and social difficulties. Some people with HIV infection have high levels of autonomy in wanting information about their condition and making decisions about their medical care. When discussing end-of-life medical decisions, people with HIV and their professional caregivers may experience practical and ethical conflicts related to issues such as discontinuing active treatment and euthanasia. Should a person's wish to discontinue treatment be regarded as equivalent to suicidal plans? Should suicide be prevented at all costs?

Case study: Deliberate self-harm by a pregnant woman with HIV

Ana is a 35-year-old black African married woman who took an overdose of anti-emetics and hypnotic tablets when she was 26 weeks pregnant. Alone in the house after an argument with her husband, she wanted to kill herself, but felt guilty about the baby and took herself to the hospital. She was referred to the psychiatrist.

Ana had been diagnosed with HIV when she attended the antenatal clinic at 12 weeks. She and her husband had been experiencing problems for about a year. She had discovered he was having an affair, and the pregnancy was unplanned. Ana was under pressure from her husband to terminate the pregnancy, but her religious beliefs prevented her from considering it – although neither she nor her husband wanted a child. Although Ana had not had any other sexual partners, her husband refused to be tested for HIV and was unsupportive, blaming her for the infection. In addition to her distress about his extramarital relationship and her unwanted pregnancy, Ana had to deal with the shock of an HIV diagnosis, her husband's attitude, and her concerns about the future. Over the last 3 months she has become increasingly sad and tearful, with frequent suicidal ideas and feelings of hopelessness. She has not confided in anyone about her HIV infection, and her attendance at the antenatal clinic has been erratic.

How should clinicians assess deliberate self-harm in a person with HIV infection?

The request for a mental health assessment usually occurs after the person has been treated for the consequences of the overdose or self-injury. The timing of the assessment is important because the pharmacological effects of the substances or treatment can influence the person's ability to remember events and describe the problems adequately.

The mental health assessment has several objectives:

- to explain the reasons for the act
- to clarify the degree of suicidal intent at the time of the act
- to find out if there is current risk of suicide or of further self-harm
- to establish whether the person has a psychiatric disorder
- to identify current problems
- to find out what further help might be appropriate.

Identify circumstances leading to act

The clinician should encourage the person to describe in detail events connected with the act over the preceding day or two, including the circumstances surrounding the act of self-harm and the problems faced. This will help identify key events, problems and factors, as well as contribute to an understanding of the person's intentions at the time. Because factors other than HIV infection can lead to suicidal thoughts and behaviors, it is important to elucidate how/if HIV-related issues contributed to the act.

Determine degree of suicide intent

The clinician should ask probing questions: Was the person alone at the time? Was anyone expected? Were any precautions taken against discovery? Was the act impulsive or planned? What was the expected outcome of the act? Was there a suicide note? Did the person wish to die?

Assess current risk of suicide or further self-harm

The clinicians should explore both past history and personal epidemiological indicators to clarify the person's current ideas and intentions. Does the person regret being alive? Does the person have social network or sources of support? The clinician can use the mental status examination to help assess risk.

Do mental status examination and complete history

The clinician should establish whether the person is suffering from a psychiatric disorder, such as major depression.

Identify need for further mental health intervention

The clinician should also identify any further help the person may need to deal with mental health problems and other difficulties. What kind of help is the person prepared to accept? Is psychotropic medication indicated? Should the person be admitted to a psychiatric bed? Is the person willing to go into hospital? If not, is involuntary admission to be considered?

What are the factors associated with an increased risk of deliberate self-harm in people with HIV infection?

The risk of deliberate self-harm is greater in people who have a history of self-harm before HIV diagnosis, and those who have a current or past psychiatric history, particularly of depression, substance misuse, and personality disorder.

An increased risk of deliberate self-harm has been reported at two stages:

- in the immediate aftermath of HIV diagnosis, especially if the diagnosis was unexpected or the news was given in an unsympathetic or tactless way

- in advanced HIV infection, particularly if the person is coping with serious health problems and treatment side-effects.

Clinically, any crisis point in the progression of the illness is potentially dangerous for those considering ending their lives.

HIV may be only one of many factors that contribute to the risk of self-harm. Other factors include: relationship difficulties (including break-up and separation), employment problems, difficulties adjusting to extended life expectancy, and bereavement.

Ana was diagnosed with a depressive disorder and considered to be at some risk of suicide – although she insisted she would never try to harm herself or the baby again. She had a previous history of depression responsive to medication (after the break up of her first marriage). Ana agreed to take antidepressant medication and to be seen regularly by a psychiatrist, who worked closely with her physician and gynaecologist. She started antiretroviral treatment. Her husband agreed to be tested for HIV and was found to be positive. Attempts were made to provide marital therapy for the couple but, as Ana's mood improved, she decided to leave her husband. Ana gave birth to a healthy baby by elective caesarean section. She did not breast-feed. Three months later the couple became reconciled. Ana continued on antidepressant medication for 6 months, and was coping well with HIV and with the baby.

Case study: Suicidal ideation in a long-term HIV survivor now facing serious health decline

Robert is a 48-year-old man who was diagnosed with HIV 17 years ago. He had been a successful publisher but had to stop work for health reasons. Five years ago, he recovered enough to return to part-time work but, in the last 2 years, his health has deteriorated. He has experienced marked fatigue and adverse side-effects from antiretroviral treatment, including lipodystrophy and gastrointestinal problems. Six months ago, Robert had to give up work. He has been relying to a much greater degree on his partner, Peter, who is now considering leaving work to care for Robert.

Robert attends hospital frequently these days. While having some blood taken by the nurse he became uncharacteristically angry, and accused her of deliberately causing him discomfort. He immediately regretted the remarks and apologized. During consultation with his physician, Robert expressed his regret again, but admitted to feeling generally angry and demoralized about his declining health, loss of independence, and becoming a burden to his partner. He spontaneously talked about his life not being worth living and, on close questioning, admitted that he has frequent thoughts about how to end his life if the situation deteriorates further. Robert became distraught and tearful, and required a good deal of time to compose himself.

Robert's physician became concerned about his mental status and his suicidal thinking. He wondered whether Robert might require admission to a psychiatric hospital and psychiatric treatment. His doctor asked the liaison psychiatrist to assess him in the outpatient department before leaving the clinic.

Should Robert be seen urgently and detained involuntarily under local mental health legislation?

While suicidal ideas can be a symptom of major depression and require specialist treatment, most suicidal thoughts in people with HIV are not a symptom of depression, but part of the process of adapting to an unpredictable disease. Suicidal ideas may provide a safety valve for feelings of fear and distress by giving people a breathing space between the current situation and what might happen in the future. Psychologically, they provide a sense of control or way out should things become unbearable.

Suicidal ideas should always be taken seriously and at face value. Healthcare professionals should allow patients to unburden themselves and share their concerns within the safety of the consulting room or bedside. The health professional should acknowledge the individual's predicament and explain the desirability of obtaining a specialist opinion. Because the thought of seeing a psychiatrist may frighten some patients, the issue of referral should be discussed sensitively.

Robert agreed to see the psychiatrist. When he met with her, he explained that he and his partner had often talked about suicide as a final option, but stressed he did not feel he had reached that point yet. He remained hopeful about maintaining a reasonable quality of life for some time. He recognized his ambivalence about ending his life, but agreed that such a decision would need to be taken after much thought rather than in the spur of the moment. He felt calmer and somehow relieved that his feelings had been taken seriously by his doctor, even if it had meant an urgent psychiatric assessment.

The psychiatrist did not feel that admission to psychiatric hospital was warranted but arranged to see Robert with his partner in the clinic in a week's time, and asked him to call her if he had any difficulties before the next scheduled appointment.

What are the different aspects of social support that should be explored as part of an assessment for suicidal ideas?

In assessing social support, the psychiatrist should consider the following:

- the patient's own perception of social support, rather than the actual number of people available
- changes in the patient's perception of social supports as the disease progresses
- degree of involvement and/or over-involvement of friends and relatives, and to what extent such over-involvement may lead the person to become more dependent or have less autonomy
- the quality of the communication between the person with HIV and his or her caregiver
- whether the person with HIV is receiving the help that he or she feels is needed – if not, the person may feel resentful and angry, and these feelings can be transformed into suicidal ideas

- the factors behind any concerns the patient may have about becoming a burden to family or friends (e.g., the person may fear the family will not be as supportive as they claim they will be, the person may find it difficult to be cared for, the person may be so frightened of what is to come that no one can provide effective help)
- whether the person is more comfortable accepting help from health and social services than from relatives or friends.

Over the next 3 months, Robert and his partner saw the psychiatrist regularly. During this time they were both able to talk about their fears for the future and adjust their lives. The psychiatrist helped arrange for daily home care to provide more support for Robert, so Peter was able to continue working, and their communication improved. Robert did not talk about suicide and was able to describe his newly rekindled interest in reading. Six months later, Robert was diagnosed with a lymphoma. He discussed with his physician his wish to avoid intensive and painful treatment for it. While in hospital he asked to see the psychiatrist again, and talked freely about how he felt the end was now approaching. She asked him about his earlier thoughts of suicide, and Robert asked for assistance to end his life painlessly.

What can psychiatrists do when asked to assist with suicide?

With few exceptions, most medical professional organizations and national laws are against physician assisted-suicide. Psychiatrists should explain that they are bound by law and by professional ethical codes that make it impossible to assist with suicide, but that they remain committed to helping the person cope with what is clearly a very difficult situation. This assistance will include:

- exploring the person's satisfaction with quality of life and the factors that affect it
- identifying and dealing with reversible factors that reduce quality of life (e.g., pain, nausea, isolation, difficulties coping with daily tasks, insomnia)
- exploring fears related to death (e.g., pain, mental incapacity, giving up family and friends, fear of the unknown, fear of retribution in the afterlife), and identifying possible ways to reduce or relieve those fears
- helping to develop good communication and trust between the patient, the family and healthcare professionals concerning end of life medical care, including discussing the patient's views about resuscitation, and what to do in the event the person becomes incapable of making decisions about further care
- helping members of the medical and nursing team deal with their own response to the patient's decline and decisions about care, in particular the risk of becoming over-involved in the patient's predicament or becoming detached and avoiding anxiety by distancing themselves from the patient's concerns
- examining the psychiatrist's own countertransference, and ensuring that the process of caring for the dying one is person-centred, rather than subject to the psychiatrist's own personal, ethical and moral views.

Robert decided with Peter that he wanted to die at home, and the palliative care team organized flexible support which gradually increased to 24-hour care. Symptom relief was pursued vigorously, and Robert managed to remain mentally alert and in control of his care for much of the time. He was able to have time with Peter and with his siblings, and died in his sleep.

Case study: Suicide of a man recently diagnosed with HIV infection

Kevin, a 38-year-old information technology manager, had been feeling unwell and suffering from persistent diarrhoea for several weeks. He consulted his family doctor but, when he failed to make progress, he became concerned and sought HIV testing. His CD4 count was very low and his viral load close to 1 million units/ml. Kevin was thought to have been HIV-seropositive for several years. He had thought about being tested in the past but, fearful of the results, had decided against it. He had always felt HIV was a death sentence and stated he would not be one to hang around and see himself deteriorate physically and mentally as had been the case with a few of his friends.

Kevin found the diagnosis very distressing and did not leave the house for a week, except for hospital appointments. He was unable to relax or sleep, was tearful and withdrawn, pushing his partner, Ric, away, and asking him to leave him. Ric was supportive but found it difficult to deal with Kevin's distress.

After 2 more weeks, Kevin returned to work but found it difficult to keep his previous level of performance. He was referred to a psychiatrist by a clinic nurse. When the psychiatrist saw Kevin, she found him to be tearful and hopeless about the future. His sleep and appetite were poor, and he had ill-defined suicidal ideas but no specific plans. He was drinking alcohol in the evenings to help him sleep, but with little effect. When he was 19 and his first relationship broke up, Kevin took an overdose of analgesics. At that time, he saw a psychiatrist and was prescribed antidepressants, which he had not taken.

After Kevin reassured her that he would take the antidepressants this time, the psychiatrist prescribed them. Over the next 3 months, Kevin continued to see the psychiatrist, occasionally missing appointments. He reduced his consumption of alcohol, and his mood and ability to cope with work improved. Ric continued to be supportive, but Kevin did not want to discuss his health with relatives or friends, or allow Ric to confide in anyone else. Kevin then decided to stop seeing the psychiatrist and soon after discontinued his antidepressants. The psychiatrist contacted Kevin and offered further appointments, but Kevin did not respond.

Two months later, Ric became concerned about Kevin, who had become withdrawn, had taken time off work, and was drinking excessively once more. Their relationship had deteriorated, and they were arguing constantly. Ric contacted the psychiatrist. Kevin agreed to see the psychiatrist again with Ric. Kevin was depressed and tearful, but denied any suicidal ideas. The psychiatrist restarted antidepressants and, in view of the tension in the relationship, suggested Kevin and Ric see a psychologist to explore and deal with their difficulties. They agreed, and the first session was arranged for 2 weeks later. They also made another appointment with the psychiatrist for the next week. The day before the appointment, Kevin hanged himself in the house after a violent row with Ric.

What else could the psychiatrist have done to prevent Kevin's suicide?

The suicide of a patient is one of the most distressing experiences psychiatrists have to deal with in their professional life. Preventing suicide is notoriously difficult, and mental health workers will inevitably encounter many instances of suicide in their patients. It is in the nature of the job that the failure to prevent suicide draws attention, and successful prevention is not usually recognized.

As soon as possible after the event, and regardless of any hospital-led requirements, the psychiatrist should explore the management of the case with colleagues in the team in a supportive and honest way. The review should include:

- a detailed examination of the care provided to the patient from the time of first contact, with input from all those involved in the person's care
- the risk assessment and decisions made
- a review of the records.

Sometimes it is useful to involve an external facilitator – someone not directly involved in the person's care.

The psychiatrist felt she had taken the right therapeutic approaches during her sessions with Kevin and Ric. She had been more concerned about Kevin's potential for suicidal behavior when she first met him, but was reassured by the support provided by his partner and by the positive response Kevin showed to antidepressant treatment. She had been concerned when Kevin had discontinued treatment, but felt at the time she could not do more to engage him in further therapy. When Ric had made contact and Kevin had agreed to attend, re-start medication, and receive help for their relationship problems, the psychiatrist felt that progress was being made, and the absence of suicidal ideas made her feel confident about ambulatory care. Her colleagues were supportive of her decisions and stressed the difficulties involved in predicting actual suicidal behaviour when dealing with individuals at increased risk.

What is the role of the psychiatrist in the care of partner and other relatives?

The impact of suicide on those close to the person can be very severe and persistent, and is often complicated by feelings of grief, guilt, rejection, stigma, and anger. It is important for the psychiatrist and others involved in the care of the person who has committed suicide to make themselves available to partners and relatives, to give an honest account of their involvement, and to be prepared to deal with the family's distress, anger, and mistrust. Sometimes it may be useful to give the family the opportunity to talk to psychiatrists or others not previously involved, so they can freely express their feelings.

The psychiatrist offered to see Ric, who felt very distressed and guilty. Over the next 2 months, Ric attended the outpatient department, and made contact with an organization to help relatives of people who had committed suicide.

Who cares for the caregivers?

Psychiatrists and other mental health workers are likely to be exposed to repeated suicidal events. The psychological impact on the professional caregivers can be short-term (e.g., shock, sadness, feelings of failure, loss of confidence in professional judgement), and long-term (e.g., depression, sickness, absenteeism, avoidance of emergency or potentially risky duties). In most cases, peer group support and discussion may be all that is needed but, in some cases, more formal individual or group support may also be appropriate. Junior staff, in particular, will need to be supported sensitively by senior colleagues (see also Chapter 19).

Conclusion

Suicidal ideas are common in people with HIV infection. They need to be taken seriously and evaluated carefully. In most cases, they present as a desire to end life at a certain point in the future, rather than as a short-term plan. Often by the time patients reach the point where they once thought life would not be worth living, their views have changed. However, when the person has more immediate plans, it is important to carry out a careful risk assessment, and to provide appropriate help, including the possibility of specialist psychiatric treatment.

Deliberate self-harm is not uncommon in people with HIV infection. It is important to assess carefully the circumstances and determinants of the act, including the degree to which HIV itself is a contributing factor, and to provide appropriate social and psychological interventions.

Suicidal ideas and plans in someone facing terminal illness can raise complex practical and ethical issues, and it is important for psychiatrists and others professional caregivers to be able to discuss the implications of these issues, while continuing to give the patient emotional support.

A successful suicide raises important practical and legal issues. Mental health teams should prepare for these events, and develop protocols to deal with the aftermath of suicide, including providing care for relatives and for members of the mental health team.

SUGGESTED READING

Catalan, J. Sexuality, reproductive cycle and suicidal behaviour. In *The International Handbook of Suicide and Attempted Suicide*, K. Hawton and K. v. Heeringen, eds. pp. 293–307. Chichester: John Wiley and Sons, 2000.

Clark, S. E. and Goldney, R. The impact of suicide on relatives and friends. In *The International Handbook of Suicide and Attempted Suicide*, K. Hawton and K. v. Heeringen, eds. pp. 467–84. Chichester: John Wiley and Sons, 2000.

Hawton, K. and Catalan, J. *Attempted Suicide*, 2nd edn. Oxford: Oxford University Press, 1987.

Komity, A., Judd, F. Grech, P. *et al.* Suicidal behaviour in people with HIV/AIDS: a review. *Australian and New Zealand Journal of Psychiatry*, **35** (2001): 747–57.

Marzuk, P. M., Tardiff, K., Leon, A. C. *et al.* HIV seroprevalence among suicide victims in New York City, 1991–1993. *American Journal of Psychiatry*, **154**(12) (1997): 1720–5.

Mitchell, C. Suicidal behaviour and HIV infection. In *Mental Health and HIV Infection*, J. Catalan, ed. pp. 114–31. London: UCL Press, 1999.

Stenager, E. N. and Stenager, E. Physical illness and suicidal behaviour. In *The International Handbook of Suicide and Attempted Suicide*, K. Hawton and K. v. Heeringen, eds. pp. 405–20. Chichester: John Wiley and Sons, 2000.

6

Anxiety disorders and HIV disease

Andrew C. Blalock, Ph.D.[1], Sanjay M. Sharma, M.D., M.B.A.[2]
and J. Stephen McDaniel, M.D.[3]

[1] Department of Psychology, Georgia State University, Atlanta , GA, USA
[2] Assistant Professor, Department of Psychiatry and Behavioral Sciences, Emory University School of Medicine, Atlanta, GA, USA
[3] Clinical Professor of Psychiatry and Behavioral Sciences, Department of Psychiatry and Behavioral Sciences, Emory University School of Medicine, Atlanta, GA, USA

Introduction

Anxiety disorders may occur any time in the course of HIV disease and are most likely to become manifest at pivotal points in disease progression (Elliott, 1998). Most people with HIV respond adequately to the stress of living with the disease and are able to limit the impact of disease-related anxiety on their daily functioning and quality of life. They cope with medical problems, employment changes, family struggles, relationship difficulties, financial hardship, and the uncertainty of the disease process itself. In these circumstances, anxiety is often considered a normal psychological response to stress (American Psychological Association, 1999).

For some patients, however, the anxiety is so severe and persistent that it can significantly impair their ability to function and would be diagnosed as a disorder. In the USA, prevalence rates for anxiety disorders among patients with HIV disease range from 5–40% (McDaniel and Blalock, 2000). The estimates vary widely for two reasons:

- anxiety is often part of a complex symptom picture that frequently includes concurrent mood disorders and psychoactive substance use disorders
- prevalence data often come from retrospective, cross-sectional studies that do not address whether anxiety preceded or followed HIV infection.

Despite this wide range in prevalence estimates, a pattern has emerged over the last 5 years. According to several recent studies, the point prevalence of anxiety disorders in HIV-seropositive patients is not significantly different from that of HIV-seronegative clinical comparison groups. However, lifetime prevalence rates of anxiety disorders are higher in the HIV clinical population as a whole than in the general population (Dew *et al.*, 1997; Rabkin *et al.*, 1997; Sewell *et al.*, 2000).

HIV and Psychiatry. A Training and Resource Manual, Second Edition, ed. Kenneth Citron, Marie-Josée Brouillette, and Alexandra Beckett. Published by Cambridge University Press. © Cambridge University Press 2005.

Patients with HIV, like those with other chronic medical conditions, may experience the entire spectrum of anxiety disorders as defined by the DSM–IV (American Psychiatric Association, 1994) including:

- anxiety disorder due to general medical conditions
- adjustment disorder with anxious mood
- generalized anxiety disorder
- substance-induced anxiety disorder
- panic disorder with or without agoraphobia
- specific and social phobia
- obsessive – compulsive disorder
- posttraumatic stress disorder.

Because treatment for the different disorders varies, accurate diagnosis is critical (Karasic and Dilley, 1998). Successful treatment depends on a thorough assessment of the patient's presenting symptoms, preferred coping style, and repertoire of coping skills. As with many other psychiatric conditions, treatment of anxiety disorders frequently involves both medication and psychotherapeutic intervention.

Case study: Anxiety in response to living with HIV

James, a 38-year-old heterosexual African-American male, was diagnosed with HIV infection 5 years ago. For the past 2 years, his disease progression has been largely controlled with a regimen of stavudine, lamivudine, and nevirapine. His latest laboratory reports indicated a CD4 cell count of 350 cells/mm^3 with an undetectable viral load. Other than his HIV infection, his past medical history is essentially unremarkable.

James is trying to date again and finding it quite stressful. He worries about how and when to disclose his HIV status. He reports that he becomes very anxious when sexual intimacy is initiated and is unable to maintain an erection. His physician determines that his erectile dysfunction is not related to his medical condition or medication, and refers him for psychiatric consultation.

Although James complains of anxiety, his overall symptom picture does not meet the diagnostic criteria for a specific anxiety disorder. The psychiatrist diagnoses James with male erectile disorder, and recommends short-term supportive psychotherapy and behavioral therapy. In therapy, James develops appropriate ways to disclose his HIV status to partners and learns to be less performance-focused in his sexual relationships. By being less self-critical and communicating more openly, James finds that both his anxiety and erectile dysfunction subside.

What are the benefits to a patient of distinguishing accurately between normal anxiety and an anxiety disorder?

Although there is a vast differential diagnosis for anxiety-related symptoms, including secondary to a general medical condition and medication-induced,

James' case provides an example of the kind of normal anxiety people can experience when negotiating life with HIV disease. It also illustrates the effectiveness of brief psychotherapy and behavioral interventions.

What factors should be considered in psychotherapy for patients with anxiety disorder?

Although anxiety in patients with HIV illness may be due to medical conditions or adverse medication side effects, it also frequently occurs at pivotal points in disease progression, such as being diagnosed with HIV, disclosing HIV status to significant others, starting/changing medication regimes, the onset of first or new HIV-related illnesses or opportunistic infections, and HIV-related changes in physical functioning/appearance and cognitive functioning. See Chapter 9 on psychotherapy for a more thorough discussion of psychotherapy issues.

Psychological treatment of anxiety disorders usually involves a two-phase approach: reducing acute symptoms in the short term and developing more adaptive coping skills in the long term. A variety of psychotherapeutic approaches may be used to treat anxiety, depending on the patient's presenting symptoms, level of dysfunction, and capacity for insight:

- Psychodynamic approaches provide the opportunity to understand emotional and relational patterns that underlie fear/anxiety and anxious coping styles.
- Cognitive-behavioral therapies are particularly useful because they focus directly on distorted thought patterns (cognitive schemas) and maladaptive behaviors.
- Progressive muscle relaxation and breathing exercises are often used to treat the physiological manifestations of anxiety and prevent impending panic attacks.
- For specific phobias and situationally determined panic attacks, systematic desensitization is helpful and frequently used in conjunction with relaxation techniques.
- For more generalized anxiety or anxious personality styles, techniques such as rational–emotive–behavioral therapy and cognitive restructuring are designed to identify and refute irrational, pessimistic, and self-defeating thought patterns and attributional styles (McDaniel and Blalock, 2000).
- With all types of anxiety disorders, concrete learning experiences, such as therapist modeling and therapist–patient role play, can be beneficial.

Most psychotherapeutic techniques can be incorporated into individual psychotherapy sessions, short-term psychoeducational groups, or ongoing interpersonal process therapy groups (Karasic and Dilley, 1998).

Case study: Medication-induced anxiety and agitation

Josette, a 29-year-old HIV-seropositive woman with no prior psychiatric history, begins experiencing symptoms of anxiety and agitation approximately 2 weeks after starting an antiretroviral regimen of combivir and efavirenz. Her initial symptoms include insomnia,

> vivid "lifelike" dreams, and irritability. This is followed by the development of agitation, restlessness, sleeplessness, and difficulties concentrating or remaining focused.
>
> Her physician discontinues her antiretroviral medications, and starts her on a low dose of trazodone (50 mg at bedtime as needed) to help her sleep. Her symptoms begin to improve. She is able to start a new antiretroviral regimen of didanosine, lopinavir–ritonavir, and nevirapine without any difficulty or reemergence of psychiatric symptoms.

Can antiretroviral or other medications contribute to anxiety?

Josette's case illustrates the potential neuropsychiatric side effects of antiretroviral medication. Anxiety has been associated with the use of several pharmacological agents used to treat HIV and related medical problems, although the causal relationship has often not been clearly established. Among these agents, the antiretroviral agent efavirenz has been associated with high rates of neuropsychiatric side effects, including anxiety, agitation, "lifelike" dreams and insomnia.

If there appears to be any link between a patient's anxiety symptoms and changes in medication, the care provider should consider discontinuing the medication to relieve the symptoms. If it is not possible to discontinue a given medication or medications that may be causing anxiety, consider adding other medications such as antidepressants, anxiolytic agents, sedative/hypnotic medications, or antipsychotics to the patient's overall medication regimen to relieve symptoms.

> ### Case study: Anxiety related to a medical condition
>
> Gary, a 40-year-old white male, was diagnosed with HIV infection approximately 6 months ago. Since then, he has had no significant illnesses or infections. His HIV infection is under control. With a very low viral load and a CD4 cell count of 300 cells/mm^3, Gary is not taking any antiretroviral medications. Recently, he has developed symptoms of depression, fatigue, anxiety, and restlessness. He reports feeling "nervous all the time" and describes clenching his jaws and biting his fingernails regularly. He also reports not being able to "stay focused" on tasks or activities, and not being able to remember things "like I used to."
>
> The clinician administers a mini mental state examination. Gary scores 26 out of 30. During the session, the clinician notes that Gary appears restless and fidgety. According to his blood work, Gary's chemistry panel and complete blood count are within normal limits, but his serum vitamin B12 level is extremely low. The clinician prescribes vitamin B12 supplementation, and Gary's depression, fatigue, anxiety, and cognitive impairment improve noticeably.

Can underlying medical disorders or HIV itself cause anxiety?

Unlike mood disorders in HIV, which may be caused by viral involvement in the CNS, the role of human immunodeficiency virus in the etiology of anxiety disorders is unclear and still under investigation (Sciolla *et al.*, 1998). In most cases, however, HIV is the symptomatic focus, rather than the cause, of anxiety disorders.

When evaluating psychiatric complications during the course of any chronic illness, clinicians should always consider the patient's medical condition and medications (prescribed and over-the-counter) as possible symptom etiologies. In patients with HIV, anxiety symptoms may occur in several HIV-related medical conditions and with psychoactive substance intoxication or withdrawal (American Psychiatric Association, 1998).

Once the underlying medical etiology is identified, it should be treated immediately.

Case study: Substance-related anxiety disorder and generalized anxiety disorder

Rita is a 44-year-old, bisexual, white female with a 12-year history of HIV disease. Three months ago, her viral load notably increased from a previously undetectable level, and her CD4 cell count dropped from 250 to 75 cells/mm^3. Her physician changed her antiretroviral regimen from zidovudine, didanosine, and indinavir to stavudine, lamivudine, and efavirenz. During a medical follow-up visit, Rita learns that, despite the new regime, her viral load and CD4 are unchanged. She becomes acutely agitated, claims she is a "treatment failure", and is convinced she is going to die. Her physician refers her for a crisis evaluation.

In her session with the psychiatrist, Rita describes herself as a recovered alcoholic with seven years of sobriety. She also reports a longstanding history of marijuana use. She had been smoking daily for the last 2 years, and only recently quit because she can no longer afford it. She reveals a long history (preceding her HIV diagnosis) of obsessive worrying, restlessness/irritability, sleep disturbance, and poor stress coping that are consistent with a diagnosis of generalized anxiety disorder. She also reports a history of sub-syndromal depressive symptoms and fear of being open with others about her sexual identity.

The psychiatrist determines that, although Rita abstained from alcohol, her continued use of marijuana had diminished her chronic anxiety. Once substance-free, her underlying psychiatric symptoms emerged. She diagnoses Rita with generalized anxiety disorder. The psychiatrist prescribes a combination of medication and cognitive–behavioral psychotherapy. Given Rita's history of substance dependence, the psychiatrist prefers to avoid benzodiazepines and prescribes the antidepressant mirtazepine 15 mg at bedtime to alleviate her anxious/depressive symptoms. Weekly psychotherapy sessions focus on preventing substance use relapse and strengthening Rita's problem-solving and stress-coping skills. During therapy, Rita makes progress in several important areas including: disclosing her HIV status and sexual orientation to family members, applying for disability income benefits, and finding a suitable housemate to reduce living expenses.

What factors must be considered in diagnosing anxiety disorders?

Rita's case illustrates three important issues in diagnosing anxiety disorders in people with HIV:

- anxiety disorders or anxious character styles may precede infection and affect the person's ability to cope with the stresses associated with a chronic illness
- psychoactive substances are frequently part of a complex history and symptom picture and must be considered carefully in assessment and treatment
- the psychiatrist must consider a thorough differential diagnosis, including medical and medication-induced causes, when assessing and treating anxiety-related symptoms.

What is the pharmacological management of anxiety disorders in the context of HIV infection?

Unless contraindicated by a history of psychoactive substance dependence, benzodiazepines can be used for short-term treatment of acute anxiety symptoms, and gradually tapered as the patient develops more psychologically or behaviorally based coping strategies. Antidepressants, particularly SSRIs, may also be quite effective.

However, clinicians should be aware of potential interactions between psychotropic medications and protease inhibitors.

When using benzodiazepines, choose longer-acting agents as well as agents without active metabolites, such as lorazepam, oxazepam, and temazepam. This will decrease the burden on the liver. Because of tolerance, abuse, and dependency issues, benzodiazepines should only be used for the acute management of anxiety disorders (particularly in patients with an active or past history of addiction). For longer-term management of anxiety disorders, use antidepressant agents such as the SSRIs and venlafaxine XR.

Recommended treatment strategy

i. Start both a low-dose benzodiazepine and an antidepressant concomitantly.
ii. Titrate the antidepressant until therapeutic effects are seen (antidepressant dosages to treat anxiety symptoms are generally lower than those needed to treat depressive symptoms).
iii. Maintain the antidepressant at the therapeutic dose while gradually tapering and discontinuing the benzodiazepine (to avoid possible withdrawal symptoms).

When prescribing benzodiazepines, be aware that they can lead to behavioral disinhibition and delirium with symptoms including confusion, disorientation, memory impairment, mood lability, and agitation (particularly in the elderly and in those with CNS compromise). Potential drug–drug interactions may occur between benzodiazepines and other medications that inhibit benzodiazepine metabolism, which can result in elevated benzodiazepine levels within the body, which may in turn lead to respiratory suppression and death.

Alternatively, non-benzodiazepine agents may be utilized to manage anxiety symptoms. Buspirone, a non-benzodiazepine anxiolytic agent with few known drug–drug interactions, is indicated for the treatment of generalized anxiety disorder (Dopheide and Park, 2001). Antihistamine agents such as hydroxyzine may also be used to manage anxiety symptoms.

For a more detailed discussion of potential drug–drug interactions, see Chapter 3 on psychopharmacology.

Conclusion

The spectrum of anxiety disorders in people with HIV can range from normal, transient episodes to severe, debilitating conditions that impair quality of life. While HIV is typically not the specific cause of the disorders, it is frequently the focus of symptoms and complaints. Thorough assessment of anxiety in people with HIV is important because the syndrome may be linked to concurrent HIV-related medical conditions, medications, or psychoactive substances. Fortunately, anxiety disorders generally respond favorably to a variety of pharmacological and behavioral interventions.

REFERENCES

American Psychiatric Association. *Diagnostic and Statistical Manual of Mental Disorders*, 4th edn. Washington, DC: APA, 1994.

American Psychiatric Association. Practice Guidelines for the Treatment of Patients with HIV/ AIDS. *American Journal of Psychiatry*, **157** (Suppl. 11) (2000): S2–62.

American Psychological Association. *Project HOPE: Training Materials, Module 3: Assessment Issues and Strategies.* Washington, DC, American Psychological Association, 1999.

Dew, M. A., Becker, J. T., Sanchez, J. *et al.* Prevalence and predictors of depressive, anxiety and substance use disorders in HIV-infected and uninfected men: a longitudinal evaluation. *Psychological Medicine*, **27**(2) (1997): 395–409.

Dopheide, J. and Park, S. (2001). An update on the pharmacotherapy of anxiety disorders. *California Journal of Health System Pharmacy*, **13**(1) (2001). (Available as a live document at www.cshp.org)

Elliott, A. Anxiety and HIV infection. *STEP Perspective*, **98**(1) (1998): 11–14.

Karasic, D. H. and Dilley, J. W. Anxiety and depression: mood and HIV disease. In *The USCF AIDS Health Project Guide to Counseling*, J. W. Dilley and R. Marks, eds., pp. 227–48. San Francisco: Josey-Bass Publishers, 1998.

McDaniel, S. J. and Blalock, A. C. Diagnosis and management of HIV-related mood and anxiety disorders. *New Directions in Psychiatric Services*, **87** (2000): 51–6.

Rabkin, J. G., Ferrando, S. J., Jacobsberg, L. B. and Fishman, B. Prevalence of Axis I disorders in an AIDS cohort: a cross-sectional, controlled study. *Comprehensive Psychiatry*, **38**(3) (1997): 146–54.

Sciolla, A., Atkinson, J. H. and Grant, I. Neuropsychiatric features of HIV disease. In *Practitioner's Guide to the Neuropsychiatry of HIV/AIDS*, W. G. van Gorp and S. L. Buckingham, eds., pp. 106–200. New York: Guilford Press, 1998.

Sewell, M. C., Goggin, K. J., Rabkin, J. G. *et al.* Anxiety syndromes and symptoms among men with AIDS: a longitudinal controlled study. *Psychosomatics*, **41**(4) (2000): 294–300.

7

General issues in hospital HIV psychiatry

Thomas N. Kerrihard, M.D.[1] and William Breitbart, M.D.[2]

[1] Director, Psychiatry and Mental Health Services, AIDS Healthcare Foundation, Los Angeles, CA, USA
[2] Chief, Psychiatry Service, Memorial Sloan-Kettering Cancer Center

Introduction

People with HIV disease frequently suffer comorbid depressive disorders, anxiety disorders, substance abuse disorders, and cognitive disorders (Dilley *et al.*, 1985; Bing *et al.*, 2001). People with advanced HIV disease often suffer from delirium, particularly in the last weeks of life. Prevalence rates of delirium range from 30–40% of medically hospitalized patients with AIDS (Breitbart *et al.*, 1990). In the hospital setting, it is also common to encounter patients with HIV who have sleep disorders and pain syndromes.

Pain syndromes in HIV-seropositive people are diverse in nature and etiology. The most common pain syndromes such as peripheral neuropathies remain a challenge for almost half the people with HIV, related both to the virus itself and to neuropathic toxicities of HAART (Hewitt *et al.*, 1996).

When mental conditions occur in the context of active medical illness and complicated medication regimens, they are difficult to diagnose and often go untreated. For these reasons, psychiatric consultation can enhance the care of people with HIV who are hospitalized. Psychiatrists can provide expertise in the medical management of psychiatric symptoms on the hospital wards, and they can also serve an important role as liaison between patients, families, physicians, supporting medical staff, social services, and hospital administration. The psychiatrist addressing acute or chronic pain issues in the hospital setting will benefit from knowledge of the psychological, social, and biological components of pain and its management.

> ## Case study: Psychiatric consultation requested to evaluate depression
>
> Mark, a 42-year-old male diagnosed with HIV 12 years ago, is hospitalized for disseminated lymphoma which was diagnosed a week ago. His attending physician asks for a

HIV and Psychiatry. A Training and Resource Manual, Second Edition, ed. Kenneth Citron, Marie-Josée Brouillette, and Alexandra Beckett. Published by Cambridge University Press. © Cambridge University Press 2005.

psychiatric consultation for the treatment of depression. Mark was treated for depression 12 years ago when he was first diagnosed, but has been stable off antidepressants for the past 9 years. The physician reports that Mark seems depressed and his personality has changed dramatically in the past three days. He is socially withdrawn, sleeps frequently throughout the day, and is sometimes difficult to rouse. Mark is less active and often does not want to talk or engage with the staff. He is unwilling to respond to questions and appears depressed to his family and staff. When alert, Mark often perseverates on insignificant issues. He frequently refuses to allow blood to be drawn and is eating little food. The nurses report that at times Mark accuses them of taking things from his room. Mark's family have never seen him like this before and are worried.

The current medical treatment for Mark includes IV fluids, three antiretroviral medications, steroids, and opiates for pain control. Mark is also getting sodium and potassium replacements for an electrolyte abnormality. The physicians are awaiting recommendations from the oncology consultants. The lymphoma is quite advanced and Mark is weak and cachectic. Mark's family is, nevertheless, quite optimistic. They refuse to discuss end-of-life treatment plans and are convinced that Mark will get better.

On psychiatric evaluation, Mark is initially difficult to awaken and minimally cooperative. He responds to questions but often gives inaccurate or inappropriate answers. On mental status examination, Mark is not oriented to the month, day, or year. He knows he has AIDS but does not articulate clearly the reason for his admission to the hospital. The psychiatric evaluation is difficult to complete because Mark frequently dozes off during the interview.

What is the psychiatrist's role in this case?

In the hospital setting, the psychiatrist has two primary duties:

- to gather data from the medical team, family, medical record, and the patient to develop a differential diagnosis and appropriate treatment plan for the patient's psychiatric condition
- to facilitate communication among the patient, family, and medical team, assist in alleviating confusion or dispute, and help develop an overall treatment plan that best serves the patient and his expressed treatment desires.

In the hospital setting, psychiatric consultations are often requested for specific diagnoses or symptoms. To be able to accurately assist the medical team with diagnosis and treatment, the psychiatrist will gather information first from the medical team, family, patient, and the medical history and laboratory data. In this case, it is important to go beyond the stated objective of treating depression. The psychiatrist should be willing to help bridge the gap between the perceptions of the medical team and the family regarding Mark's overall medical condition.

What is Mark's diagnosis?

In this case, the attending physician may have identified some depressive signs and symptoms but with acutely ill, hospitalized, HIV-seropositive patients, it is important to begin with a broad differential diagnosis. The psychiatrist must know Mark's baseline mental status prior to admission, and understand the time course of the changes. Mark has had a very abrupt change in mental status over a 3-day period. The waxing and waning nature of Mark's level of consciousness is also significant. The family report periods when he is engaged and upbeat yet, within the same day, Mark's alertness fades and he presents with confusion and a clouded sensorium. Mark's family and physician report that Mark has no recent history of depression or dementia. Although Mark may have other concomitant mental disorders, he is suffering from an overlying delirium, which should be the focus of initial psychiatric treatment.

What is delirium?

Delirium is a common neuropsychiatric complication that occurs often in hospitalized patients with AIDS. According to DSM–IV, three primary symptom clusters are required to diagnose delirium:

- a disturbance of consciousness with reduced ability to focus, sustain, or shift attention
- a change in cognition (such as memory deficit, disorientation, or language disturbance) or the development of a perceptual disturbance that is not accounted for by a pre-existing or evolving dementia. This can present as overt psychosis, often in the form of paranoia or delusions.
- the disturbance develops over a short period of time (usually hours to days) and tends to fluctuate over the course of the day. There is usually evidence of a medical condition with or without a laboratory abnormality, and/or a medication side effect that is judged to be etiologically related to the disturbance.

Delirium may present in either a hyperactive or hypoactive form. Hyperactive delirium is easier to identify and frequently presents with anxiety, agitation, or overt psychotic symptoms. Hypoactive delirium is more difficult to diagnose and may present with depression-like symptoms of hypersomnolence and social withdrawal. Both forms of delirium respond to psychiatric treatment.

Use of the Memorial Delirium Assessment Scale (MDAS), a 10-item delirium assessment tool, should be considered. The MDAS is a reliable tool for assessing delirium severity among patients with advanced disease. It has been validated among hospitalized inpatients with advanced cancer and AIDS. A cut-off score of 13 indicates delirium (Breitbart et al., 1997).

What is the differential etiology of the delirium?

Hospitalized medical patients with AIDS are at high risk for delirium and the etiology is often multi-factorial or unclear. The differential diagnosis is broad and may include:

- systemic infections
- drug intoxication: opiates, steroids, sedative-hypnotics, anticholinergics, drug and alcohol intoxication or withdrawal, antibiotics (Wood and Oats, 1991; Shuster and Stern, 1999; Salkind, 2000), anticonvulsants, and/or antineoplastics
- endocrine disorders and vitamin deficiencies: Addison's disease, thyroid disease, vitamin B12 insufficiency
- head trauma or intracranial neoplasms, infections, or hydrocephalus
- hypotension
- metabolic encephalopathies: hyper or hyponatremia, uremia, hypocalcemia, hypomagnesemia, hypoxia, hypoglycemia, acidosis, alkalosis, dehydration, hepatic insufficiency, adrenal insufficiency, or pancreatic insufficiency
- hematological disorders: severe anemia, coagulopathy, elevated white blood cell count
- seizure disorders.

In Mark's case the etiology could be multifold and include the impact of the virus itself on the CNS, his electrolyte abnormalities, his medications (including opioids), and his advancing tumor with the potential of neurotoxin release or CNS involvement.

What is the treatment for delirium?

The primary goals in treating delirium are to:
- Identify and treat the underlying etiology. This may involve reviewing and exploring the primary active medical conditions, including opportunistic infections, the list of current medications, laboratory blood tests, anatomical brain imaging, and clinical examination. It is important to cooperate closely with the medical team in working up the underlying abnormality.
- Manage the symptoms associated with delirium, including the possible agitation, confusion, or psychotic thought content or process.

Important nonspecific interventions include instituting psychosocial and environmental approaches, such as frequently orienting the patient, arranging visits by family members, providing a clock, and giving brief, simple commands.

The mainstay of symptomatic treatment of delirium involves the use of pharmacotherapies including antipsychotic drugs, benzodiazepines, and other sedatives. Patients generally respond to daily doses of antipsychotic drugs equivalent to 0.5–5.0 mg/day of haloperidol. To avoid extrapyramidal side effects, clinicians should use the lowest effective dose. Anticholinergic agents may worsen delirium. Benzodiazepines can be used in conjunction with antipsychotic agents when hyperactive delirium is present. In this situation, shorter-acting benzodiazepines are preferred. Benzodiazepines used alone frequently result in paradoxical reactions in patients with delirium and underlying CNS pathology.

Haloperidol is probably the antipsychotic most commonly used and studied to treat agitated delirium in the hospital setting. Its effects on blood pressure, pulmonary artery pressure, heart rate, and respirations are milder than those of the benzodiazepines, making it a good choice for severely ill patients with impaired cardiorespiratory function. Although haloperidol can be administered orally or parenterally, acute delirium with extreme agitation is best treated with parenteral medication. Intravenous administration is preferable to intramuscular injection. The initial bolus of haloperidol varies from 0.5–2.0 mg.

Recommended doses are usually 0.5 mg for an elderly person, 2 mg for mild agitation, 5 mg for moderate agitation, and 10 mg for severe agitation. If one dose does not calm an agitated patient after 30 minutes, a higher dose should be administered. Once the patient is stable, clinicians can prescribe lower doses on a qhs, bid, or tid scheduling, depending on the clinical response.

Chlorpromazine is another agent commonly used to treat delirium, but its alpha-blocking properties can cause a precipitous fall in cardiac output (Cassem and Murray, 1997). More recently, the newer antipsychotic medications including olanzapine, risperidone, quetiapine, and ziprasidone have been used successfully to treat delirium. Although less well studied, these agents are increasingly used as first-line agents in many medical settings. For example, olanzapine can be used at a low dose of 2.5 mg for elderly or mildly delirious patients, or 5–10 mg for more severe agitation. Although the newer atypical antipsychotics are limited by their nonparenteral formulations, they are often preferred for their lower incidence of extrapyramidal side effects.

Prior to prescribing any psychotropic agent, the clinician should review the list of medications, paying particular attention to the presence of antiretroviral agents that could lead to problematic drug–drug interactions. For more information on interactions, see Chapter 3 on Pharmacotherapy.

Mark is started on haloperidol 0.5 mg p.o. tid and responds remarkably. He is less confused and more engaged. Physicians also make corrections to his electrolytes and lower his pain medications. Within three days of these interventions, Mark is no longer delirious. His level of consciousness is stable and he is fully oriented. Mark now communicates his strong anxiety about his illness and the fear he has of cancer. He is not sleeping at night. It takes him up to 2 hours to fall asleep and he wakes frequently throughout the night.

How are sleep problems addressed in the hospital setting?

Sleep disturbances are common on in-patient units. Not only are the surroundings unfamiliar, but hospital procedures, such as checking vital signs and drawing blood, can disturb patients throughout the night. The necessity for these medical interventions must always be weighed against the benefits of adequate sleep. Lack of sleep can have adverse effects on mood, daytime function, and overall recovery. When possible, nighttime interruptions should be limited to necessary procedures only. For patients who are relatively stable, orders can be written to check vital signs and do bloodwork at times when the patient is likely to be awake.

Pharmacologic interventions are commonly used to treat sleep disturbances in the hospital setting. When prescribing medications, clinicians should consider the patient's current medical status, history of previous responses to sedatives/hypnotics, and the patient's prior medical and psychiatric history which may be contributing to the sleep disturbance. Consulting psychiatrists should be knowledgeable about medications that can precipitate insomnia and the many underlying psychiatric illnesses that often present with sleep disturbances. A review of psychiatric symptoms should be a part of any sleep assessment. Depression, anxiety disorders, and delirium can present with nighttime insomnia. In a patient diagnosed with delirium, increasing the bedtime dose of a sedating antipsychotic can significantly improve sleep. However, clinicians should be cautious when prescribing sedatives with high anticholinergic properties, such as diphenhydramine or some tricyclic antidepressants. Anticholinergic agents can exacerbate cognitive problems and cause confusion or induce delirium, especially in patients who have dementia, other mild cognitive impairments, or organic brain disease.

Non-benzodiazepine sedatives with low anticholinergic properties, such as zaleplon or zolpidem, can be quite useful in treating sleep problems. Trazodone can also be helpful and, with its highly sedating properties, it can be administered at much lower doses than those used to treat depression (i.e., 50–100 mg is sufficient to induce sleep, whereas 150–600 mg is recommended to treat depression). Because these medications are generally considered nonhabit forming, they are often preferred for those who require sleep agents for extended periods.

When the patient has other psychiatric diagnoses, it may be useful to use sedating psychotropics for dual action (e.g., using mirtazapine to treat depression and insomnia, increasing the bedtime dose of divalproex sodium to treat patients with bipolar disorder). Recently, gabapentin in bedtime doses ranging from 300–2400 mg has been used safely and effectively to treat insomnia (Norman *et al.*, 1990).

Shorter acting benzodiazepines without active metabolites, such as temazepam or lorazepam, are often useful in patients with anxiety or racing thoughts associated with the sleep disturbance, but they are recommended for short-term use only. These medications are generally not recommended for patients with substance abuse disorders. They should also be used cautiously with patients with organic brain disease or delirium because of the potential for paradoxical reactions. In these patients, benzodiazepines can cause agitation, restlessness, and can magnify the sleep disturbances.

Case reports suggest atypical antipsychotics may be useful in treating resistant insomnia. For example, quetiapine (in doses from 25–100 mg at bedtime) and olanzapine (in doses from 2.5–5 mg at bedtime) have been used safely and effectively for insomnia.

Mark's lymphoma progresses and is associated with severe pain in his abdomen and pain in his right hip. Radiological testing reveals extensive disease throughout his peritoneum with metastases to his bone. Chemotherapy is initiated but Mark, along with his family, decides to stop chemotherapy and choose hospice care. At first, his medical team is hesitant to shift from their treatment and cure oriented approach. The family's understanding of this decision was reviewed in a case conference with Mark, his family, the medical team, the social worker, and the psychiatrist. After ensuring that Mark's current expressed desire was consistent with his previously stated wishes for quality of life, the team agrees to respect Mark's decision. The goal of his treatment shifts to palliative care.

How should Mark's pain be managed?

Patients with HIV often fear pain and suffering (Lenderking *et al.*, 1994), yet their pain is often inadequately acknowledged, assessed, or treated in a hospital setting. Many physicians have not been adequately trained in pain management, and myths about addiction often lead to suboptimal pain treatment on medical wards. The problem of pain management is often compounded in patients with known comorbid substance abuse or personality disorders.

Any report of pain should be taken seriously and assessed. Special attention should be given to those who have difficulty communicating with clinicians, including patients who speak different languages, have different cultural backgrounds, or are developmentally delayed, cognitively impaired, or severely emotionally disturbed (Singer, 1998; Todd *et al.*, 1993).

A thorough pain assessment should include:

- a detailed history of the patient's pain
- a physical examination
- a psychosocial assessment
- the pain characteristics, such as quality, location, intensity, duration
- aggravating or relieving factors.

Clinicians should also take into account the patient's past responses and experiences with pain medications, including negative and positive responses and experiences of side effects. Because pain can be amplified by psychological states such as anxiety, depression, and anger (Bouckoms, 1999), the presence of any of these conditions should be taken into account during the assessment. When designing a treatment plan, every effort should be made to differentiate between chronic and acute pain, and between nociceptive and neuropathic pain.

The World Health Organization (WHO) analgesic ladder for cancer pain management can be used to treat pain in patients with HIV (World Health Organization, 1990):

- for mild to moderate pain, non-opioid drugs such as acetylsalicylic acid (ASA), acetaminophen or NSAIDs
- for moderate to severe pain, non-opioid medications can be combined with low-dose opioid preparations such as codeine, oxycodone, or hydrocodone
- severe pain requires the addition of higher potency opioid analgesic preparations to the non-opioid, such as morphine, hydromorphone, oxycodone, methadone, or fentanyl.

Chronic pain should be treated with extended release forms of the pain medication, while intermittent pain or breakthrough pain can be treated with shorter acting preparations. Patient controlled analgesia (PCA) has become popular in some settings. Many feel it is superior to regular dosing of narcotic analgesics. For information on the potential interactions between antiretroviral agents and opioid medications, see Chapter 3 on pharmacotherapy.

A number of analgesic adjuvants, such as tricyclic antidepressants, antihistamines, benzodiazepines, steroids, stimulants, and anticonvulsants, may enhance the effect of opioids or non-opioid medications, have independent analgesic activity in certain situations, or counteract side effects. Peripheral neuropathies are common in HIV patients and may respond to tricyclic antidepressants and anticonvulsants. However, the tricyclic antidepressants should be prescribed at much lower doses to treat pain than to treat depression. For example, amitriptyline, imipramine, nortriptyline, or desipramine can often can be started at 10–25 mg at bedtime and then increased slowly, as tolerated. Gabapentin, topiramate, and carbamazepine can all be initiated at lower doses than those used to treat seizure or mood disorders.

When starting pain treatment for patients with HIV, clinicians should have clear goals and consider using pain-rating scales to evaluate the effectiveness of an intervention. When treating patients with a drug addiction or substance abuse disorder, many clinicians find it helpful to use a pain contract, which spells out the limitations of safe narcotic prescribing practices and ensures patients are informed about the behaviors that could result in their pain treatment being tapered or terminated (e.g., the use of any illegal controlled substance, the sharing or selling of medications, the repeated loss of medications, the use of multiple prescribing physicians, poor attendance at regular follow-up appointments).

When a patient's pain management is complicated by uncertain etiologies, unrelenting pain, and pain that may require high-technology approaches (e.g., patient-controlled analgesia, intraspinal administration, or surgical intervention), clinicians should consider referring the patient to a pain specialist.

Conclusion

In the role of both medical consultant and liaison, the psychiatrist can have a profound impact on the quality of care provided to hospitalized patients with HIV. In fact, the psychiatrist's ability to act as liaison between the patient and the medical team is critical to improving quality of care and maximizing the benefits of a multidisciplinary approach. Physicians with psychiatric training often identify miscommunications between patients, families, treating teams, supporting medical staff, social services, and hospital administration. Facilitating communication is a key role for the consulting psychiatrist in inpatient settings.

High quality psychiatric care for hospitalized patients with HIV depends on the psychiatrist's knowledge of the psychological, social, and medical dimensions of HIV. The ability to understand and identify common psychiatric syndromes, such as depressive disorders, anxiety disorders, cognitive disorders, substance abuse disorders, delirium, pain syndromes, and sleep disorders, are essential to inpatient HIV medical care. The psychiatrist treating the hospitalized HIV-positive patient should also be aware of the array of treatment modalities and options available for each diagnosis.

REFERENCES

Bouckoms, A. J. Chronic pain: neuropsychopharmacology and adjunctive psychiatric treatment. In *Essentials of Consultation-Liaison Psychiatry*, 1st edn, J. R. Rundell and M. G. Wise, eds., pp. 555–76. Washington, DC: American Psychiatric Press, 1999.

Breitbart, W., Marotta, R. Platt, M. and Corbera, K. Pharmacologic management of delirium in medically hospitalized AIDS patients. Abstracts of the 37th Annual Meeting of Academy of Psychosomatic Medicine, Chicago, 1990.

Breitbart, W. Rosenfeld, B., Roth, A. *et al.* The Memorial Delirium Assessment Scale. *Journal of Pain Symptom Management*, **13** (1997): 128–37.

Bing, E. G., Burnam, A., Longshore, D. *et al.* Psychiatric disorders and drug use among human immunodeficiency virus-infected adults in the United States. *Archives of General Psychiatry*, **58** (2001): 721–8.

Cassem, N. H. and Murray, G. B. Delirious patients. In *Massachusetts General Hospital Handbook of General Hospital Psychiatry*, 4th edn. N. H. Cassem, T. A. Stern, J. F. Rosenbaum and M. S. Jellinek, eds., pp. 101–22. St. Louis: Mosby-Year Book, Inc, 1997.

Dilley, J. W., Ochitill, H. N., Perl, M. and Volberding, P. A. Findings in psychiatric consultations with patients with acquired immune deficiency syndrome. *American Journal of Psychiatry*, **142**(1) (1985): 82–6.

Hewitt, D., McDonald, M., Portenoy, R. *et al.* Pain syndromes and etiologies in ambulatory AIDS patients. *Pain*, **70** (1996): 117–23.

Lenderking, W. R., Gelber, R. D., Cotton, D. J. *et al.* Evaluation of the quality of life associated with zidovudine treatment in asymptomatic human immunodeficiency virus infection. *New England Journal of Medicine*, **330** (1994): 738–43.

Norman, S. E., Chediak, A. D., Kiel, M. and Cohn, M. A. Sleep disturbance in HIV-infected homosexual men. *AIDS*, **4** (1990): 775–81.

Salkind, A. R. Acute delirium induced by intravenous trimethoprim-sulfamethoxazole therapy in a patient with the acquired immunodeficiency syndrome. *Human and Experimental Toxicology*, **19** (2) (2000): 149–51.

Shuster, J. L. and Stern, T. A. Intensive care units. In *Essentials of Consultation-Liaison Psychiatry*, J. R. Rundell and M. G. Wise, eds., pp. 419–23, Washington, DC: American Psychiatric Press, 1999.

Singer, E. J. Advances in managing terminal pain in AIDS. *Annals of Long-Term Care*, **6** (13) (1998): 1–8.

Todd, K. H., Samaroo, N. and Hoffman, J. R. Ethnicity as a risk factor for inadequate emergency department analgesia. *Journal of the American Medical Association*, **269** (1993): 1537–9.

Wood, A. J. J. and Oats, J. A. (1991). Adverse reactions to drugs. In *Harrison's Principles of Internal Medicine*, J. D. Wilson, E. Braunwald, K. J. Isselbacher, R. G. Petersdorf, J. B. Martin, A. S. Fauci, and R. K. Root, eds., pp. 373–9. New York: McGraw Hill, 1991.

World Health Organization. *Cancer Pain Relief and Palliative Care. Report of a WHO Expert Committee* (World Health Organization Technical Report Series, 804). Geneva, Switzerland: World Health Organization, 1990.

8

HIV and people with serious and persistent mental illness

Karen McKinnon, M. A.[1], Francine Cournos, M. D.[2],
Richard Herman, M. A.[3] and Stephanie Le Melle, M. D.[4]

[1] Director, Columbia University HIV Mental Health Training Project,
   Research Scientist, New York State Psychiatric Institute, New York, NY, USA
[2] Professor of Clinical Psychiatry, Columbia University College of Physicians and Surgeons, New York, NY
   Deputy Director, New York State Psychiatric Institute, New York, NY, USA
[3] Co-Director, HIV Prevention Training, Columbia University HIV Mental Health Training Project, New York, NY
   Research Scientist, New York State Psychiatric Institute, New York, NY, USA
[4] Assistant Clinical Professor of Psychiatry, Columbia University College of Physicians and Surgeons, New York, NY,
   USA

Introduction

More than 30 studies in the USA and Canada have documented alarmingly high rates of HIV risk behavior in adults with serious and persistent mental illness. Several studies around the world have documented rates of HIV infection among psychiatric patients that are much higher than those for the general population in the same regions (Table 8.1).

Clinicians working with patients with chronic mental illness are in a unique position to promote healthy behaviors, reduce transmission of HIV, encourage early detection and treatment, and improve care. To fulfill this role, clinicians may need to enhance their skills and comfort in delivering services to HIV-infected patients.

Case study: HIV testing of a man with a history of schizophrenia and substance abuse

Andrew is a 46-year-old African-American man with schizophrenia who spent most of his adolescence in psychiatric hospitals and substance abuse treatment clinics. When Andrew was in his mid-30s, his father died suddenly of a heart attack. After his father's death, his mother, who also suffered from schizophrenia, committed suicide. Andrew became deeply depressed and was hospitalized in a psychiatric facility. After he was

HIV and Psychiatry. A Training and Resource Manual, Second Edition, ed. Kenneth Citron, Marie-Josée Brouillette, and Alexandra Beckett. Published by Cambridge University Press. © Cambridge University Press 2005.

discharged, Andrew remained depressed and relapsed into injection drug use. His sister helped him get treatment and stay off drugs.

After having gone without psychiatric care for a few years, Andrew presents to an outpatient psychiatric clinic. As part of the initial assessment, the psychiatrist elicits Andrew's risk behaviors for HIV infection and learns of his past history of drug injection. After a few meetings during which the psychiatrist develops a trusting relationship with Andrew, the psychiatrist suggests that Andrew be tested for HIV.

How is an HIV risk assessment conducted?

The first step in the counseling and testing process is to obtain a risk history. The purpose of the risk assessment is to elicit specific information about the person's sexual behaviors and drug use. During assessment, psychiatrists should be sensitive to differences in language (including sexual vocabulary) and demonstrate cultural proficiency (see Chapter 16-A on cultural diversity). Asking "How often have you..." rather than "Have you ever..." is more likely to elicit useful risk information without implying that the clinician is judging the patient's behavior or considers it unusual, which may make the patient feel defensive. When assessing same-sex risk, it is important to ask specific questions about sexual behaviors as opposed to a single question about sexual orientation since individuals who do not label themselves "homosexual" may nevertheless have a history of sexual risk taking. The same approach should be used with substance use; risk from use of

Table 8.1. HIV seroprevalence among samples of psychiatric patients by country

Country	Seroprevalence	Number of patients	Number of studies	Sample	Source
Germany	4.8%	623	1	Inpatients	Naber *et al.*, 1994
Italy	6.5%	475	1	Inpatients	Zamperetti *et al.*, 1990
Spain	5.1%	390	1	Acute unit	Ayuso-Mateos *et al.*, 1997
Taiwan	0%	834	1	Inpatients at 2 psychiatric hospitals	Chen, 1994
Thailand	1.9%	325	1	Mentally ill offenders	Dasananjali, 1994
USA	6.9%	3917	13	Inpatients and outpatients	Cournos and McKinnon, 1997; Krakow *et al.*, 1998; Rosenberg *et al.*, 2001
Zimbabwe	23.8%	143	1	Inpatients	Acuda and Sebit, 1996

noninjected drugs (e.g., legal and illicit drugs that can be sniffed) can be easily overlooked if the assessment is focused on injected drugs. Most people, when asked in a direct and nonjudgmental way, are cooperative and forthcoming. The ease the clinician demonstrates in discussing sex and drug use will set the anxiety level for the patient. By normalizing the behaviors, the clinician can create a more relaxed tone.

Any risk history should include assessment of other sexually transmitted diseases (STDs). Some patients may have STDs without being aware of them, and may go untreated, which puts them at higher risk of acquiring HIV.

Thorough, sensitive, periodic screening for HIV risk should be a routine part of inpatient and outpatient mental health care. Included here is a sample risk screening form for use in "triage" situations (Box 8.1). More in-depth risk interviews should be conducted whenever possible. (A downloadable risk assessment is available at www.columbia.edu/~fc15/).

HIV Risk Screen

(any check in the middle or right-hand column suggests referral to testing)

1. How many sexual partners have you had in the past 10 years?

   none   ☐
   one   ☐
   more than one   ☐

2. How many men have you had anal sex (a man puts his penis into the anus of the other person) with in the past 10 years?

   none   ☐ (skip to 4)
   one   ☐
   more than one   ☐

3. How often did you use a condom when having anal sex in the past 10 years?

   never   ☐
   sometimes   ☐
   always   ☐

4. Of the following sexually transmitted diseases (gonorrhea, syphilis, chlamydia, genital warts, or genital herpes) how many have you ever had?

   none   ☐
   one   ☐
   more than one   ☐

5. In the past 10 years, how often have you given money or drugs to someone to have sex with you?

never	☐
sometimes	☐
often	☐

6. In the past 10 years, how often have you had sex with someone so that they would give you money or drugs?

never	☐
sometimes	☐
often	☐

7. How often have you injected drugs in your lifetime?

never	☐
sometimes	☐
often	☐

8. How many of your sexual partners in the past 10 years have used injected drugs?

none	☐
one	☐
more than one	☐

9. How many of your sexual partners in the past 10 years have been men who have had sex with men?

none	☐
one	☐
more than one	☐

10. How many of your sexual partners in the past 10 years ever had a sexually transmitted disease such as gonorrhea, syphilis, chlamydia, genital warts, or genital herpes?

none	☐
one	☐
more than one	☐

If the first reply is "I don't know", the patient should be prompted with, "if you had to say one way or the other, what would you say?"
(Adapted from Gerbert *et al.*, 1998)

What are the special issues involved in HIV testing of people with serious and persistent mental illness?

Voluntary testing is the norm for all patients, including those with serious mental illness. The capacity to consent to testing hinges on the patient's ability to understand the information being conveyed and to draw reasonable conclusions from it. People with serious mental illness are considered to have this capacity unless an assessment determines otherwise.

Psychiatrists can use their clinical judgment to determine when a patient is able to give informed consent and when, given his or her psychiatric condition, the person is best able to cope with any result. HIV testing often can be done when a patient is in hospital for treatment of an acute episode. In fact, testing during an inpatient stay has some advantages – if the entire process can be completed before the patient is discharged (this is more likely now that the newly approved rapid test can be used). For example, staff can ensure the patient receives post-test counseling and follow-up appointments, and address any negative impact of the test result on the patient's psychiatric condition.

Informed consent for HIV antibody testing should include explanation and discussion of:

- the test and its purpose
- the meaning of the results
- the benefits of early diagnosis and medical intervention
- the voluntary nature of the test
- the patient's right to withdraw consent at any time
- the availability of anonymous testing
- confidentiality protections
- the circumstances under which test results may be disclosed with or without the patient's agreement.

Some psychiatric conditions may interfere with the client's ability to give informed consent. In these cases, the clinician should treat the psychiatric disorder and leave HIV testing until the patient has regained the capacity to give informed consent. Substitute consent should be sought only when the clinician must establish a patient's serostatus in order to provide appropriate care or when the patient is not expected to regain the capacity to give informed consent. In these cases, consent may be given by a person who is legally authorized to do so.

People with serious mental illness usually undergo HIV counseling and antibody testing without worsening of their psychiatric symptoms (Oquendo and Tricarico, 1996).

The psychiatrist provides pre-test counseling. Andrew understands the implications of the test and decides to tell his sister that he has been tested so that she can help him cope with possible bad news. During the stressful waiting period, the psychiatrist maintains telephone contact with Andrew.

Psychiatrists can play an important role in HIV testing by being directly involved in pre- and post-test counseling. In some instances, they may choose to involve an HIV counselor in the patient's test counseling; if not, the psychiatrist has a responsibility to ensure that both pre- and post-test counseling are conducted appropriately.

How often should people with serious and persistent mental illness be tested for HIV?

Patterns of HIV risk behaviors among people with serious and persistent mental illness suggest that some patients engage in risky behaviors frequently and some do so intermittently. Psychiatrists should encourage patients who have tested negative to be retested regularly as warranted by a periodic risk assessment. HIV testing should be offered whenever a patient asks for it, and/or when a patient:

- reports current or past risk behaviors
- is pregnant
- has physical signs suggestive of HIV infection or AIDS
- has psychiatric symptoms that suggest CNS dysfunction
- is diagnosed with any other STD
- has a positive skin test for TB exposure (PPD) and resides in an area where HIV is endemic.

Andrew's HIV test comes back positive, and the psychiatrist provides post-test counseling. Despite the information Andrew receives during the counseling, he views his HIV diagnosis as a death sentence. He begins to binge on crack cocaine because he believes crack is the quickest way to die. His sister again steps in and gets him into drug treatment.

How are people with serious and persistent mental illness likely to react to a diagnosis of HIV infection?

A diagnosis of HIV infection can be made at any time in the course of the disease, from shortly after becoming infected until developing advanced AIDS. Initial reactions of shock and disbelief may be followed by depression, anxiety, and fear about having contracted a serious and still potentially deadly illness. Untreated depression and feelings of hopelessness may be associated with continuing risk behavior, even suicidal ideation (Liberman *et al.*, 1986).

Like serious mental illness, HIV and AIDS can be highly stigmatizing, and may result in the patient being rejected, abandoned, and more socially isolated than before.

If the patient's psychiatric symptoms worsen following HIV diagnosis, the clinician should offer individual counseling and supportive therapy geared to both the patient's current mental status and his or her knowledge and

understanding of HIV infection (Broder *et al.*, 1994). Pharmacological intervention also may be helpful.

Soon after his release from the detoxification program, Andrew is referred to a specialized
HIV clinic. He is attending regular appointments at a psychiatric outpatient clinic and the
HIV clinic. He reports taking all his pills "religiously". The psychiatrist and HIV physician
are in regular contact to coordinate care, simplify the medication regimen as much as
possible, and manage any drug interactions or toxicities. Andrew's regimen requires that
he take pills once in the morning, once in the afternoon, and once at night. His viral load
is undetectable.

During the course of receiving treatment, Andrew reports that he had unprotected sex
with a number of partners prior to his diagnosis. Because the HIV specialist is more
experienced with counseling contacts, he agrees to be responsible for notifying them.
Andrew collaborates well in the process and the psychiatrist provides additional support
for Andrew during this time.

Case study: An HIV-seropositive woman with schizophrenia

Jenny is a 43-year-old Latina with schizophrenia, whose mother suffered from depression
and whose father abused alcohol. Jenny has had multiple traumas in her life. She was
severely physically abused by her father, and sexually abused from age 10 through 15 by
her father and several male family friends. The abuse ended only when she ran away from
home. She has been living in single room occupancy hotels and residences but is regularly
evicted because of her disregard for drug-abstinence policies. As a result, she is often
homeless for periods of time.

By the age of 20, she had been hospitalized more than 10 times for auditory hallucinations and delusions, and currently is on psychiatric medications. However, she often stops
taking them in times of stress. Jenny has a part-time job in the patient-worker program of
the outpatient clinic she attends, but whenever she stops her medications she relapses
and trades sex for money or cigarettes.

Picked up by police for selling sex in the neighborhood because voices told her to,
Jenny is brought to the emergency room, where she is admitted to the psychiatric
inpatient unit and diagnosed with HIV infection.

What are the most common risks for HIV infection in psychiatric patients?

Psychiatric patients face the same HIV risks as other people, including unprotected
sexual activity, substance use, and social/environmental contributors. Psychiatric
symptoms and disabilities may increase HIV risk either by affecting the person's
behavior directly or by interfering with his or her ability to acquire or use HIV
information and skills to practice safer behaviors.

Sexual activity

Contrary to popular belief that the side effects of psychiatric medications reduce sexual activity, people with severe and persistent mental illness are sexually active, and often have multiple partners (Carey *et al.*, 1997). In addition, homosexual or bisexual activity, sexual victimization or coercion by others, sexual activity after substance use, sexual activity with relatively unknown partners, or trading sex for money or shelter may be more likely among psychiatric patients than in other groups (Chuang and Atkinson, 1996; Carey *et al.*, 1997; Goodman and Fallot, 1998). Most people with severe mental illness use condoms inconsistently or not at all (Carey *et al.*, 1997); only one-quarter report using condoms every time they have sex.

Substance use

A significant proportion of people with serious, persistent mental illness (up to 25% in some studies) have a history of drug injection (Carey *et al.*, 1997; Otto-Salaj *et al.*, 2001). Psychiatric patients who inject tend to do so intermittently. Because they may not be injecting at the time they are evaluated, their drug injection histories are often overlooked. Every effort should be made to capture this information during a risk assessment.

However, injecting drugs is not the only risk associated with substance use. A US review study found that psychiatric patients who have identified comorbid alcohol or other drug use disorders have a significantly higher rate of HIV infection than those who do not, even if they have never injected drugs (McKinnon and Cournos, 1998). This may be due to the impact of substance use on the person's motivation or ability to have protected sex. Any patient with an alcohol or drug-use disorder should be assessed routinely for HIV risk and offered counseling about the negative impact of substance use and about strategies to reduce risk. Even occasional drug and alcohol use can lead to unprotected sexual behavior.

Environmental and social factors

Certain environmental and social factors also may put people with serious and persistent mental illness at risk for HIV. For example, the recurrent institutionalization that is part of living with a mental illness may interrupt long-term relationships and reinforce the tendency to have unknown sexual partners. Spending extended periods of time in same-sex units in hospitals, shelters, or prisons may foster same-sex activity, which is particularly risky for men, while institutional policies that limit access to condoms may affect patients' ability to practice safer sex.

Other social/environmental factors, such as homelessness, transient living arrangements, and alienation from supportive social relationships also can increase the risk of acquiring HIV. Urban psychiatric patients often are concentrated in inner-city neighborhoods with high rates of drug abuse, alcoholism, sexually transmitted diseases, and HIV. In treatment settings in endemic areas, all sexual opportunities are high risk. High rates of unemployment also may contribute to greater risk-taking, possibly by increasing the pressure to engage in survival sex or commercial sex work (Acuda and Sebit, 1996). Any support services that help people with severe mental illness maintain stable housing, and employment may reduce their risk of acquiring or transmitting HIV.

How do psychiatric disorders contribute to HIV risk-taking?

Patients may or may not be more likely to participate in unsafe sexual and drug-use practices when their psychiatric symptoms are acute. Psychiatrists must assess this likelihood on a case-by-case basis, using information from the person's risk history. If patients are more likely to participate in risky activities when they stop their psychiatric medications, clinicians may consider several strategies to reduce HIV risk, including: early hospitalization, more vigorous treatment, or more intensive counseling for patients about how to stay safe. Patients should be taught harm reduction strategies to minimize the negative consequences of continuing alcohol or drug use. Clinicians who do not have extensive experience in counseling patients about harm reduction may consider referring patients to another staff member who has had training in this approach and who is comfortable dealing with these issues. Patients also should have unlimited access to condoms, preferably distributed in an anonymous fashion (e.g., condom baskets left around the clinic).

Jenny's physical health is monitored at the local hospital's infectious disease program. She has chosen not to take HIV medications because "she already takes too many pills". Her CD4 cell count is currently 540 cells/mm^3 and her viral load is 5000 copies/ml, so her infectious disease doctor is not pressing her to initiate antiretroviral medications at this time. Although Jenny is psychiatrically stable now, she recently tested positive for syphilis and hepatitis C.

What are the special issues involved in the follow-up of people with HIV who also have serious and persistent mental illness?

HIV infection is associated with greater sensitivity to both the therapeutic effects and side effects of psychotropic medications. Clinicians are encouraged to start with the lowest possible dose of psychotropic medications, and to increase doses slowly. Drug levels, if available, should be monitored closely, especially when patients are on complex medication regimens (see Chapter 3 on Pharmacotherapy).

Support groups, held in the community or within the psychiatric setting, are an effective way to encourage asymptomatic HIV-seropositive psychiatric patients to change their risk behavior and maintain their physical health. This kind of group intervention can prevent psychiatric symptoms from worsening, and provide a sense of community that can decrease social isolation, reinforce safer peer norms, encourage altruism, and give patients a sense of worth and accomplishment.

To help patients maintain their health, psychiatrists should ensure that biological markers, which indicate when to begin antiretrovirals and treatments for opportunistic infections, are monitored regularly.

Psychiatric patients, like medical patients, often do not adhere to medication prescriptions. This may be because they perceive medication as one of the few aspects of their lives they can control. A person's ability to adhere to psychotropic medications will be the best predictor of whether the patient can follow an HIV medication regimen. Clinicians can take several steps to improve adherence, including:

- helping the person see that following the HIV/AIDS regimen can be part of gaining control
- ensuring the psychiatrist and infectious disease specialist communicate about the person's need for and readiness to begin antiretrovirals
- timing the beginning of an antiretroviral regimen with a commitment from the person to the treatment
- selecting medications that avoid drug–drug interactions and minimize the number and doses of pills the person has to take
- coordinating the treatment plans for HIV and the psychiatric disorder.

Case study: Changing risk behaviors of people with severe, persistent mental illness

Ken is a 38-year-old man with schizoaffective disorder who tested positive for HIV 5 years ago. Since then, he has been followed jointly by a psychiatrist and an infectious disease specialist. His viral load remains undetectable. He lives alone in an apartment and has held the same job for 3 years. He has recently developed a romantic relationship with a woman who suffers from schizophrenia. Despite years of substance abuse, she is HIV-seronegative and is now sober. She and Ken would love to have a family but worry about how risky that would be for her and for the baby.

What are the determinants of HIV risk reduction among psychiatric patients?

HIV information is necessary but not sufficient to reduce risk. Information-only interventions have little impact on behavior (Kelly, 1997). The ability of US psychiatric patients to respond correctly to AIDS knowledge questions in a 1990 study (McKinnon *et al.*, 1996) was comparable with that of the general US population (Hardy, 1990). Yet many psychiatric patients had some critical gaps in information and understanding (Kelly *et al.*, 1992; Katz *et al.*, 1994; Otto-Salaj *et al.*, 1998). For example:

- 42% were unaware they could be infected by injection drug use
- 48% believed that careful cleansing after sex would provide protection from the virus
- up to 43% believed that heterosexual women cannot get AIDS
- 45% believed that a person's appearance signals whether he or she has HIV.

To ensure that all patients, regardless of their HIV status, have the information they need, clinicians should assess their understanding of HIV transmission and prevention, and clarify any misinterpretations.

Even with perfect knowledge of HIV and its transmission, however, some people may not be able to act on that information and reduce their risk. For example, a woman may know she is at risk and even be motivated to avoid infection but may not adhere to safer sex practices if these practices are not acceptable to her partner and result in rejection. Principles of cognitive–behavioral theory (Bandura, 1988) and the theory of reasoned action (Fishbein and Ajzen, 1975) have been put to the test in rigorous outcome studies of HIV risk-reduction interventions with psychiatric patients. The effective HIV prevention intervention models reported in the literature to date resemble the kinds of intervention long used in other psychosocial rehabilitation programs for people with serious and persistent mental illness (Kelly, 1997). These studies support working with patients using concepts already familiar to psychiatrists:

- Attitudes about performance of HIV-preventive acts. Encourage development of positive attitudes, perceived benefits, and positive outcome expectancies. Address perceptions of normative social support (i.e., from society, partners) for such behavior. Change perceptions of normative support and desire to comply with the opinion of others.
- Intentions to act on knowledge regarding HIV transmission and prevention. Reinforce desire to use knowledge and skills. Encourage planning for opportunities to act safely (e.g., by carrying condoms).
- Behavioral skills for performing specific HIV-preventive acts. Teach and provide opportunities to rehearse skills, including verbal and nonverbal abilities to negotiate safer sex with one's partner, to refuse to have unsafe sex, to use a condom properly (provide anatomical models), and to exit a situation if safer sex is not possible. Rehearse and reinforce skills to avoid drinking or drug use before sex or to reduce the potential harmful consequences of intoxication (e.g., by not sharing injection equipment).
- Risk behavior self-management. Reinforce and support patients' belief in their ability to use their behavioral skills. Elicit and support patients' perceptions of

their capabilities to observe safer sexual limits consistently and without relapse to unprotected behaviors.

- Risk reduction personal problem solving. Encourage field trips and trial runs to purchase condoms. Ascertain the behavioral skills that are both necessary for HIV prevention and lacking in the patient. Urge patients to model enactment of HIV-preventive skills through role-playing, subsequent feedback and reinforcement, then refining their own performance.

How can psychiatrists help patients reduce their risk of transmitting or acquiring HIV?

Intensive small-group programs can reduce high-risk sexual behaviors (including some that are substance-related) among people with severe mental illness. Psychiatrists can encourage administrative and staff facilitation of risk-reduction programs and staff training to acquire skills and comfort in conducting such interventions. Effective elements of HIV risk reduction interventions (Kelly, 1997; Otto-Salaj et al., 2001) include:

- providing HIV risk education and skills training in sexual assertiveness, negotiation, problem-solving, use of condoms, and risk self-management (including identifying and monitoring personal risk "triggers" or situations in which risk behaviors are most likely to occur)
- organizing intensive sessions, running between 6 and 15 sessions to achieve reductions in high-risk behaviors
- training participants in being AIDS educators or advocates
- offering booster or maintenance sessions, which appear to be necessary to sustain safer behaviors
- being sensitive to gender issues. Gender-specific groups can be useful for dealing with same-sex partner issues or for decreasing patients' anxiety about discussing sexual issues with the opposite sex. However, men and women should not automatically be separated for HIV prevention interventions. For heterosexual patients, mixed-gender groups may increase generalization from group exercises to real life situations, enhance men's insight into how women experience negotiations around safer sex, and allow women to practice being assertive with men about having safer sex and avoiding unwanted sex.
- including sexually abstinent patients since they may not remain abstinent forever, may share what they have learned about safer sex with friends and family members, or may validate for other patients the legitimate choice of an abstinent lifestyle.

The goal of the small group intervention is harm reduction, particularly with drug-related risk behaviors (e.g., participants can rehearse cleaning injection equipment and minimizing sexual risk while high). If a program has a large enough number of HIV-seropositive participants, clinicians can organize a separate support group to focus on the particular concerns of patients with HIV.

However, these patients can also benefit from participating in mixed groups, and need not reveal their HIV status unless they wish to do so. Whatever the group's composition, group leaders should leave time at the end of each session to discuss patients' personal issues privately and to address their needs by making appropriate referrals, including to HIV testing programs.

When clinic staff receive training in prevention interventions, they are usually highly motivated to start patient intervention groups (http://www.columbia.edu/~fc15/page2.html). However, keeping groups going can be difficult in programs that have little patient turnover. Groups work best in day programs and outpatient programs. On inpatient units, short lengths of stay may limit the number of sessions that patients can attend, but that should not discourage staff from setting up time-limited, highly focused interventions.

What is the role of individual counseling in helping patients change their risk behaviors?

The goal of individual counseling is to encourage patients to make fully informed decisions about risk and to protect others. For example, psychiatrists can encourage HIV-positive patients to disclose to sex partners and use condoms. They also can help patients overcome any specific difficulties in implementing the desired change. Problems will vary from person to person, and must be explored carefully in a nonjudgmental setting. Patients may find problem solving and role-playing useful.

During a counseling session, the psychiatrist learns that, because Ken's viral load is undetectable, he and his girlfriend thought that he was no longer contagious. When the psychiatrist explains that the risk of transmission remains, the couple decide to have protected sex and give up the idea of conceiving a child. When they discuss safer sex practices, the psychiatrist learns that, as a side effect of antipsychotic medications, Ken has developed a tremor that makes using a condom problematic. Ken also feels too shy to buy condoms. To resolve these barriers to safer sex, the psychiatrist prescribes a medication to treat the tremor and Ken's girlfriend agrees to buy the condoms. The couple regularly report that they are adhering to safer sex recommendations.

Conclusion

Psychiatrists are key actors in the lives of people with serious and persistent mental illness. They can ensure that all patients, not just those presumed to be at risk, receive thorough, periodic risk assessment. They can distribute HIV educational materials, provide risk reduction interventions, and provide pre- and posttest counseling. They also can advocate within their institutions for policies that facilitate risk reduction. For psychiatric patients with HIV, psychiatrists are the ideal liaison with the medical provider. They can help maximize adherence, minimize potential harmful medication interactions, and organize support groups.

By understanding the HIV epidemic among people with serious mental illness, psychiatrists can recognize when their patients are at risk and intervene appropriately with effective preventive, counseling, medical, and support services.

REFERENCES

Acuda, S. W. and Sebit, M. B. Serostatus surveillance testing of HIV-I infection among Zimbabwean psychiatric inpatients in Zimbabwe. *Central African Journal of Medicine*, **42** (1996): 254–7.

Ayuso-Mateos, J. L., Montanes, F., Lastra, I. *et al.* HIV infection in psychiatric patients: an unlinked anonymous study. *British Journal of Psychiatry*, **170** (1997): 181–5.

Bandura, A. Perceived self-efficacy in the exercise of control over AIDS infection. In *Primary Prevention of AIDS: Psychological Approaches*, V. M. Mays, G. W. Albee, and S. F. Schneider, eds., pp. 128–41. Newbury Park, CA: Sage.

Broder, S., Merigan, T. C. and Bolognesi, D. (Eds.) *Textbook of AIDS Medicine*. Baltimore: Williams and Wilkins, (1994).

Carey, M. P., Carey, K. B. and Kalichman, S. C. Risk for human immunodeficiency virus (HIV) infection among persons with severe mental illnesses. *Clinical Psychology Review*, **17** (1997): 271–91.

Chen, C. H. Seroprevalence of human immunodeficiency virus infection among Chinese psychiatric patients in Taiwan. *Acta Psychiatrica Scandinavica*, **89** (1994): 441–2.

Chuang, H. T. and Atkinson, M. AIDS knowledge and high-risk behaviour in the chronic mentally ill. *Canadian Journal of Psychiatry*, **41** (1996): 269–72.

Cournos, F. and McKinnon, K. HIV seroprevalence among people with severe mental illness in the United States: a critical review. *Clinical Psychology Review*, **17** (1997): 259–69.

Dasananjali, T. The prevalence of HIV infection among mentally ill offenders in Thailand. *Journal of the Medical Association of Thailand*, **77** (1994): 257–60.

Fishbein, M. and Ajzen, I. *Belief, Attitude, Intention, and Behavior: an Introduction to Theory and Research*. Reading, MA: Addison-Wesley, 1975.

Gerbert, B., Bronstone, A., McPhee, S. *et al.* Development and testing of an HIV-risk screening instrument for use in health care settings. *American Journal of Preventive Medicine*, **15** (1998): 103–13.

Goodman, L. A. and Fallot, R. D. HIV risk-behavior in poor urban women with serious mental disorders: association with childhood physical and sexual abuse. *American Journal of Orthopsychiatry*, **68** (1998): 73–83.

Hardy, A. M. National Health Interview Survey data on adult knowledge of AIDS in the United States. *Public Health Report*, **105** (1990): 629–34.

Katz R. C., Watts, C. and Santman, J. Aids knowledge and high risk behaviours in the chronic mentally ill. *Community Mental Health Journal*, **30** (1994): 395–402.

Kelly, J. A. HIV risk reduction interventions for persons with severe mental illness. *Clinical Psychology Review*, **17** (1997): 293–309.

Kelly, J. A., Murphy, D. A., Bahr, G. R. *et al.* AIDS/HIV risk behavior among the chronic mentally ill. *American Journal of Psychiatry*, **149** (1992): 886–9.

Krakow, D. S., Galanter, M., Dermatis, H. and Westreich, L. M. HIV risk factors in dually diagnosed patients. *American Journal on Addictions*, **7** (1998): 74–80.

Liberman, R. P., Mueser, K. T., Wallace, C. J. *et al.* Training skills in the psychiatrically disabled: learning coping and competence. *Schizophrenia Bulletin*, **12** (1986): 631–47.

McKinnon, K. and Cournos, F. HIV infection linked to substance use among hospitalized patients with severe mental illness. *Psychiatric Services*, **49** (1998): 1269.

McKinnon, K., Cournos, F., Sugden, R. *et al.* The relative contributions of psychiatric symptoms and AIDS knowledge to HIV risk behaviors among people with severe mental illness. *Journal of Clinical Psychiatry*, **57** (1996): 506–13.

Naber, D., Pajonk, F. G., Perro, C. and Lohmer, B. Human immunodeficiency virus antibody test and seroprevalence in psychiatric patients. *Acta Psychiatrica Scandinavica*, **89** (1994): 358–61.

Oquendo, M. and Tricarico, P. Pre- and post-HIV test counseling. In *AIDS and People with Severe Mental Illness: A Handbook for Mental Health Professionals*, F. Cournos and N. Bakalar, eds, pp. 97–112. New Haven, CT: Yale University Press, 1996.

Otto-Salaj, L. L., Heckman, T. G., Stevenson, L. Y. and Kelly, J. A. Patterns, predictors and gender differences in HIV risk among severely mentally ill men and women. *Community Mental Health Journal*, **34** (1998): 175–90.

Otto-Salaj, L. L., Kelly, J. A., Stevenson, L. Y. *et al.* Outcomes of a randomized small-group HIV prevention intervention trial for people with serious mental illness. *Community Mental Health Journal*, **37** (2001): 123–44.

Rosenberg, S. D., Goodman, L. A. and Osher, F. C. Prevalence of HIV, hepatitis B, and hepatitis C in people with severe mental illness. *American Journal of Public Health*, **91** (2001): 31–7.

Zamperetti M., Goldwurm, G. F., Abbate, E. *et al.* Attempted suicide and HIV infection: epidemiological aspects in a psychiatric ward. [Abstracts, p. 182] *VI International Conference on AIDS*. Los Angeles: American Foundation for AIDS Research, 1990.

9

Psychotherapy

Peter DeRoche, M.D.[1] and Kenneth Citron, M.D.[2]

[1] Assistant Professor of Psychiatry, University of Toronto
  Director, Clinic for HIV-Related Concerns, Department of Psychiatry, Mt. Sinai Hospital, Toronto, Canada
[2] Assistant Professor of Psychiatry, University of Toronto
  Staff Psychiatrist, Clinic for HIV-Related Concerns, Department of Psychiatry, Mt. Sinai Hospital, Toronto, Canada

Introduction

HIV infection presents a series of challenges to the psychotherapist, testing his or her ability to respond compassionately and sensitively. The psychiatrist will often benefit from a thorough working knowledge of the issues faced by people infected with HIV.

In most ways, people living with HIV do not differ significantly from other psychotherapy patients. The main differences are:
(1) the ongoing possibility of crisis
(2) uncertainty about the future
(3) The complex nature of HIV disease expression, antiretroviral treatments and associated side-effects
(4) the strong countertransference reactions these patients may evoke.

Therapists should try to adapt the psychotherapy method they are most comfortable with to the special needs of the person living with HIV. Although most forms of psychotherapy are likely to be helpful for people living with HIV, a psychiatrist's formulation of the case and knowledge of differential therapeutics should inform the method choice.

Due to its potentially fatal outcome, HIV disease has the effect of imposing time pressure on patients, which may serve as a catalyst for work in therapy and make brief models ideally suited to this group of patients. They may feel more comfortable doing one or more successive "pieces of work" in therapy as they progress through different stages of the illness and their needs change. On the other hand, with the advent of HAART, people living with HIV now have indeterminate life expectancies and may benefit from the insight and knowledge gained from open-ended psychotherapy.

This chapter will use case material to illustrate where different types of psychotherapy might be most effectively applied, both in treating those at risk for acquiring HIV, and those who are HIV positive. In reality, most therapists will use

HIV and Psychiatry. A Training and Resource Manual, Second Edition, ed. Kenneth Citron, Marie-Josée Brouillette, and Alexandra Beckett. Published by Cambridge University Press. © Cambridge University Press 2005.

an eclectic approach, tailoring therapy to a particular individual's needs at any given point in time.

What types of psychotherapy are useful in the treatment of people with HIV?

Some studies have addressed the use of particular forms of brief psychotherapy with HIV-infected individuals. In one study, Markowitz *et al.* (1995) showed that for depressed people diagnosed with HIV, interpersonal psychotherapy is superior to supportive psychotherapy and even to cognitive–behavioral therapy.

In a more recent study comparing brief interventions with cognitive–behavior therapy (CBT), psychodynamic therapy, or a psychoeducation intervention for a diagnostically diverse group of people with HIV, all three were effective, but CBT worked more quickly. Both CBT and psychodynamic therapy had more enduring effects at follow up (Lancee *et al.*, in press).

Although there is no known best method of psychotherapy for the HIV-infected patient, individual, couple, family, and group methods have all been used with significant success.

Choice of therapeutic modality will depend on:

- the therapist' training and theoretical basis of practice
- the availability of therapy options
- the goals of the therapy
- the patient's psychological resources
- the situations that arise during the course of illness.

The following discussion will describe examples of various modalities of psychotherapy applied to different situations as they arise in the course of the illness.

Case study: Gay male struggling with issues of prevention and HIV testing

Malcolm, a 29-year-old gay male who works in the advertising field, is referred by his primary care physician. He has a history of difficulties in long-term relationships with avoidance of intimacy and commitment. He often feels overwhelmed by the demands of partners for sexual fidelity and time together. He also describes feelings of inadequacy about his physical appearance. He has sought out anonymous sexual encounters in an attempt to feel "valuable and loved". Malcolm experiences anxiety about his high risk sexual activity and has declined HIV testing on several occasions.

What is the therapist's responsibility in pointing out potentially dangerous behaviors to patients?

Psychotherapists of all disciplines have a responsibility to point out potentially high-risk behaviors to their patients. With all patients, regardless of whether the therapist sees them as being at risk for HIV infection, the therapist should make gentle inquiries into their sexual practices, their drug use, or other potential risk of acquiring HIV infection. Patients should be educated about the risks for acquiring HIV infection and given appropriate information to help minimize them.

What issues impact on a person's ability to adhere to safer sex practices?

In spite of large amounts of healthcare and financial resources dedicated to educating individuals about the risks of HIV infection, people continue to practice unsafe sex. Education alone is not enough to prevent people from engaging in unsafe sex and exposing themselves or their partners to risk.

There are many reasons why people continue to put themselves at risk:

- After the advent of HAART, many individuals have come to view HIV as a chronic illness rather than a fatal disease. Feeling that a cure is around the corner, some people have eased up on practicing safer sex.
- Individuals who go to certain settings (e.g., bath houses) and engage in unsafe sex are perceived by their peers as either already infected or aware of the risks. There may be unspoken agreement that this makes negotiating safer sex unnecessary.
- Disinhibition due to the effects of a substance, a cofactor in how people behave in high-risk situations, facilitates the acting out of basic sexual desires.
- For some, anxiety about HIV is highlighted by the constant attention to safer sex, which can be associated with mounting resentment of the restrictions on their sexual expression. A kind of "burnout" can ensue leading to abandonment of safer sex. Paradoxically, this can be accompanied by a sense of relief and reduction in anxiety.
- Some people experience a sense of nihilism about maintaining safer practices over prolonged periods of time. They have the sense that infection is inevitable, which reduces their vigilance to safer sex.
- Others use massive denial to avoid anxiety about the dangers they face. Using condoms would require them to acknowledge they are taking a risk. A counter-phobic response is used to avoid the anxiety.
- Others prefer sex without condoms. Many people consider physical barriers an intrusion into their love making. Some find condoms uncomfortable. For some, the mechanics of putting on a condom precludes spontaneity and interferes with the erotic nature and passion of the encounter. Others experience the condom as a physical barrier to the intimacy of the situation and are unsatisfied emotionally by sex with a condom.
- At times, people will deliberately expose themselves to the virus to identify with someone they want to feel intimate with (i.e., a potential partner) or with a community to which they want to belong (e.g., the HIV-seropositive gay

community). Paradoxically, the individual may perceive becoming infected as a way of introducing meaning into his/her life.

- For those who struggle with chronic depressive feelings due to dysthymic disorder or major depressive illness, becoming infected with HIV may be a way out or a passive suicidal equivalent.
- A dynamic frequently encountered in psychotherapy with women, young gay men, and ethno-racial minorities is the fear of rejection if they say "no" to unsafe sex or ask about a partner's HIV status. In this scenario, issues of power in sexual politics figure prominently.
- Sex is often an opportunity to express uncomfortable unconscious conflicts or emotions. For example:
  - A victim of childhood sexual abuse might compulsively seek out receptive anal intercourse with aggressive men. Associated passivity might result in difficulties asserting his or her desire for protected sex.
  - An individual might channel the affect associated with such conflicts into aggressive behaviours. These may emerge from unconscious anger or an unconscious desire to assert control over the anxiety associated with memories of abuse. Tragically, this can manifest as disregard for the safety of sexual partners, leading the person to refuse or abandon safer sex.
  - Individuals who have low self-esteem may have little sense of control over their own lives. They may fear abandonment or rejection. They may have unmet dependency needs, and have significant difficulty asserting themselves in negotiating safer sex.
  - Unsafe sex may be associated with patterns of self-destructive, self-sabotaging behaviors resulting from early life experiences which have produced low self-esteem, anger, and chronic depression.

To help a patient become more aware of the causes of their high-risk behavior and give them a choice in future potentially high-risk situations, the clinician should explore the unconscious underlying determinants of unsafe sex.

What approach should the therapist take when the patient engages in high-risk behaviors?

The psychiatrist should use a combination of support and education in the context of the therapeutic alliance to explore the motivations for the patient's behavior, and then develop an action plan to address them. In some cases, one specific type of therapy may be useful.

Malcolm describes himself as suffering chronic low-grade depression and feelings of anxiety in social situations. He views himself as uninteresting and unattractive, which causes him to feel unappealing and unacceptable to others. Fundamentally, he feels unlovable and unworthy. To the therapist, it seems clear that these feelings originated in an early developmental history involving what Malcolm perceived as parental shaming for his less masculine behaviours and his lack of athletic prowess compared with his brothers. This was compounded by schoolyard bullying and stigmatization because he was perceived as effeminate.

What is the role of CBT in the treatment of people with HIV infection?

Cognitive–behavioral therapy is based on a premise that symptoms evolve out of and are perpetuated by dysfunctional patterns of thinking. The therapy identifies these patterns and helps the person learn to think about himself or herself and the circumstances in his or her life in ways that are more realistic and helpful. This approach is often useful with people with HIV.

Malcolm has compensated for poor self-esteem by adopting a superficial "super-masculine" persona and seeking out validating experiences through sex. In this context he has great difficulty saying "no" to men who demand unsafe sex from him. As a way to cope with his social anxiety, he frequently drinks or uses ecstasy and the occasional methamphetamine.

The therapist works with Malcolm to reformulate his presentation by elucidating the automatic thinking about himself as uninteresting and helping him understand that this originated from core beliefs that he was unlovable and unworthy of love.

In the course of CBT, Malcolm uses insights into these problems to guide him in connecting his affects to his dysfunctional automatic thinking and explores his cognitive distortions as well as more balanced and realistic ways of thinking. He is surprised to find that, in the process, his anxiety and depression diminish. Through behavioural experiments and other homework assignments, Malcolm explores alternative ways of thinking about himself and social situations. He finds he can reduce his social anxiety without using alcohol and drugs. He is also able to assert himself more in negotiating and insisting on safer sex.

At this point, Malcolm is able to revisit his resistance to HIV testing. His therapist helps him seek up-to-date information about treatment and the more optimistic prognosis associated with combination therapies. Using the techniques he learned to this point in his therapy, he is able to explore his automatic thoughts and cognitive distortions, reduce his anxiety, and decide to be tested.

What are the pre- and posttest counseling guidelines for HIV?

See Appendix I for standard pre- and posttest counseling guidelines for HIV testing. Adherence to these guidelines gives patients the greatest degree of control over what is always an anxiety-provoking situation.

Malcolm's test results reveal that he is HIV seropositive. He begins to develop severe anxiety, which progresses to panic attacks on several occasions.

What types of intervention are helpful soon after HIV is diagnosed?

In most cases, a therapy based on the principles of crisis intervention will be most helpful. The goal is to help the person return to a level of functioning that is as close to that person's premorbid level as possible. For the psychiatrist this involves:

- providing an objective but empathic environment where the person can freely express affect
- managing acute symptoms with appropriate medication
- helping the person assess or mobilize his or her resources, including family, friends, community, and religious organizations
- ensuring that the patient receives appropriate information about HIV, its natural course, and his or her treatment options.

Malcolm does well in crisis therapy. He is able to do some work around adjusting to having HIV and decides to spend some time working in another city. He terminates his relationship with the therapist. In the therapist's view, Malcolm is in the process of isolating himself from his feelings about having HIV. This is associated with what appears to be an overly optimistic view of his future. His abrupt termination of therapy and decision to move to another city are manifestations of denial.

What is the role of denial in living with HIV infection?

Healthy denial allows an infected person to live and enjoy life while not dwelling excessively on the potential negative outcomes. This implies, however, that the person tends to their medical needs and protects others through the use of safe sex practices. When infected people engage in practices that put others at risk, this can cause a therapeutic dilemma for the therapist (see Chapter 18 on Legal and Ethical Issues).

Two years later, Malcolm returns to therapy. He has moved back to town and is wondering whether he can achieve a satisfactory intimate relationship in the face of being HIV sero-positive. In view of his specific goal, his relative psychological mindedness and capacity for developing a good therapeutic alliance, the psychiatrist offers and Malcolm agrees to a course of 20 sessions of psychodynamic psychotherapy.

What potential roles does psychodynamic psychotherapy have in treating persons with HIV?

Psychodynamic psychotherapy seeks to address a patient's problems by exploring unconscious determinants of problematic behaviors and affects. Developmental history figures prominently in the generation of insight into problematic inter-personal dynamics and ways of viewing the self, others, and the world in which one lives. The clinician uses various techniques to facilitate this insight, and the therapy relies heavily on identifying and working through defenses. The therapist pays close attention to transference and countertransference. In this context, issues relating to HIV are often dealt with indirectly as the therapist and patient address fundamental problems that interfere with the patient's ability to cope with the illness.

In the course of therapy, Malcolm discusses his early life experiences growing up on a farm on the Canadian prairies. He highlights a long-term pattern of rejection by his father who could not relate to him because he was not "manly enough". His father favored his brothers who were gifted athletes and very involved in running the farm. Malcolm was always closer to his mother, feeling more affinity with her and sharing interests with her. He assumed that she knew about his homosexuality, but they never discussed it. At home and at school, he was teased for his effeminate behaviors, and throughout childhood and adolescence he felt marginalized. Ultimately, as he became aware of sexual feelings, and that they were homosexual, his sense of shame and alienation increased. Malcolm developed a pattern of avoiding intimacy and isolating himself socially in order to hide his shame. At age 19, he went to the city to university and began to experiment sexually. He was quite surprised and gratified by the attention he attracted at gay gathering places and found that he could easily attract all the sexual partners he desired. This led to promiscuity and a compulsive quality to sex, with few limits set on his sexual partners with regards to safer sex. To help deal with his anxiety about sex as well as residual social anxieties, Malcolm uses alcohol and drugs.

As the therapy progresses, Malcolm is able to identify and begin to work through his feelings about the isolation and invalidating experiences of his early years. He is able to address his anger and sadness, and is then able to begin to accept things as they are. He explores issues of stigma as they emerged over the course of his life and develops significant insight into the internalizing of homophobia and the associated self-loathing. Insight into the degree to which sex has become a way to compensate for his low self-esteem comes as a surprise to him. He and the therapist discuss the defensive nature of sex and the avoidance of intimacy. Malcolm also recognizes that HIV serves as a metaphor for feelings of unacceptability as a gay man, and he addresses his feelings that HIV felt like a punishment for his "bad" behaviour.

Finally, Malcolm is more clearly able to articulate what he wants for himself. He hopes to find someone with whom he can have a more mutually respectful relationship and with whom he can develop trust and intimacy, free of the negative expectations that he has carried into previous relationships. He wants to stop the process of projecting his self-loathing onto his partners and to stop the process of self sabotage that begins when he becomes close to someone.

What are some of the expected transference issues which might emerge in a dynamic therapy with someone with HIV?

Because people will often describe a life-long history of stigmatization and marginalization, they might expect a repetition of these experiences in therapy, particularly if they view the therapist as having a dissimilar background. For example, a gay patient who perceives his psychiatrist as heterosexual might project his negative experiences with straight society onto the therapist.

On the other hand, an isolated, frightened person who feels very alone with his or her disease might enter therapy with fantasies of rescue. The psychiatrist may be viewed as omnipotent and holding the answers for happiness. This can lead to transference rage and acting out, including prematurely terminating the sessions, if the patient feels frustrated by the psychiatrist.

People living with HIV often feel they have little control over the course of their lives and may bring these issues into the therapy in different ways. For example, they may manifest as feelings of nihilism (e.g., anticipating that the attempts at therapy are futile and that the therapist is unlikely to be effective or helpful). Alternatively, the transference may involve experiencing the therapist as controlling and distant. This could activate feelings of aloneness and ineffectualness, often originating in early life experiences, triggered by the experience of living with HIV and transferred to the therapist. Guilt may also figure prominently in some therapies, and manifest itself as concerns about taking up the therapist's valuable time, shame about not getting better, or being a burden on the psychiatrist.

What are some of the expected countertransference issues that might emerge in a dynamic therapy?

Psychiatrists working with people living with HIV may face a number of counter-transference issues including:

- Homophobia or other ethno-cultural biases. Therapists must examine the extent of their own homophobia or other stereotyped, deep-seated, racist biases in order to fully understand their potential impact on therapy.
- Attitudes towards sexuality and substance abuse. Moral judgments on the part of psychiatrists about sexual or other so-called "deviant" behaviors such as unsafe sexual practices or injection drug use may preclude empathic relationships with people living with HIV.
- Existential concerns. Psychiatrists have to examine their own issues around fear of death, meaning in life, aloneness, and control over one's destiny.
- Rescue fantasies or feelings of omnipotence. Patients sometimes come to therapy idealizing the experience as an opportunity to be saved. Likewise, they frequently present with a history of alienation and stigmatization. These experiences can easily trigger rescue fantasies in caregivers. Unless psychiatrists deal with these fantasies, they risk crossing boundaries, and attempting to do more for the patient than is therapeutically appropriate.
- Identification. Psychiatrists may identify with people living with HIV in a variety of ways. For example, they may be overwhelmed in a patient's anguish in dealing with a serious medical illness or impending death. Gay psychiatrists may struggle with feelings about their own risk of infection, or their own internalized homophobia may be triggered by others' experience of stigmatization. Female psychiatrists may identify with a female patient's rage at having been betrayed. Older psychiatrists working with younger people may develop paternalistic feelings at the thought of losing patients who remind them of their children.

- Therapeutic nihilism. At times, psychiatrists may feel hopelessness, helplessness, despair, or a sense of futility in the face of such complex issues and the possibility of early death. To be effective and helpful, psychiatrists have to come to some understanding of the meaning the therapy has for the patient, and accept treatment goals and outcomes that are often different from those more typically encountered in psychotherapy.
- Guilt. Psychiatrists may feel guilty about the limitations of therapy in relieving people's anguish. That guilt may also be associated with the psychiatrist's sense of relief at being healthy, and possibly surviving the patient and the entire HIV epidemic.
- Fears of contamination. It is very common for psychiatrists, particularly those who have had little contact with people living with HIV, to fear infection. Unless psychiatrists understand the true source of this irrational anxiety, they will feel distanced from patients and run the risk of stigmatizing the people they are trying to aid.
- Sense of inadequacy. As newer treatments for HIV have emerged, clinicians require more medical knowledge to feel comfortable treating the disease. Psychiatrists may feel inadequate in their knowledge, which may cause them to shy away from treating patients with HIV.

What are the issues associated with termination in this population?

Termination, an integral part of brief psychotherapies, can be a challenge for the psychiatrist. People living with HIV will often feel vulnerable throughout their illness and may benefit from an ongoing supportive relationship with a psychiatrist. In these cases, the psychiatrist may feel that terminating a therapy is cruel and the equivalent of abandoning the patient. Nevertheless, successfully terminating a relationship with a psychiatrist may give the patient confidence in letting go – a valuable experience because the process of dealing with a potentially fatal illness is a long series of endings and letting go.

Some months later, Malcolm again contacts the psychiatrist. Having learned that his viral load is 100 000 copies/ml and that his CD4 cell count has dropped to 250 cells/mm³, Malcolm is feeling anxious about his deteriorating HIV status. He is pursuing a promotion, but feels anxious about his bloodwork. His primary care HIV physician would like to start him on highly active antiretroviral therapy (HAART), but he is torn.

How does ambivalence relate to living with HIV infection?

Ambivalence is defined as "the co-existence of opposing feelings and thoughts". Examples include "I want to live but part of me wants to die", "I am worthy of treatments yet I feel guilty because my friends have passed away". With the advent of HAART, the therapeutic agenda for people with HIV now includes: helping them to explore ambivalence about treatments, fostering hope, and achieving a new equilibrium in which to go on living life. In assessing the pros and cons of HAART, the therapist and patient should deal with a number of sources of ambivalence, including:

- Acceptance of the illness. Taking medications for HIV requires confronting a person's denial that his or her illness has progressed to the point where they now need to take HAART. For some, medications serve as a constant reminder that they are ill.
- Complexity of the antiretroviral regime itself. The complexity of medical regimes and the multiple potential side effects contribute to ambivalence. Some medications, such as efavirenz, may have significant psychiatric side effects such as vivid dreams and risk of depression, which can be extremely disturbing to patients and may affect their ability to adhere. Before deciding to initiate HAART, a patient must reflect on how much discomfort from side effects he or she is willing to tolerate in order to benefit. This issue often has to be revisited as unforeseen side effects emerge.
- Fear of disclosure. Having to follow complex medication protocols may force patients to disclose their HIV status, which may cause them to shy away from these medications.
- Demands associated with adherence. To prevent viral resistance, the therapist should work with the patient to identify strategies to optimize adherence. This is particularly important for intravenous drug users and the seriously and persistently mentally ill, whose lives are not always routinized. Studies have shown greater than 90% adherence is required to prevent the development of drug resistance, making "life-style" issues crucial. For some patients, assessing their capacity to adhere may lead to a decision to delay HAART until their psychiatric illness or substance-abuse problem is better controlled. The therapist should also help patients work through issues of self-esteem to give them permission to assert themselves with others in order to ensure adherence.
- Body image issues. HIV-infected individuals taking antiretrovirals often deal with lipodystrophy and other cosmetic side effects of HIV (see Chapter 1, Medical overview). Some people experience these physical changes as a loss of body integrity, which constitutes a narcissistic injury. For some patients, these side effects are worse than the illness, and they will not adhere.
- Concerns about future treatability. Some patients worry that starting medications now may lead to viral resistance, which will affect their ability to find an effective combination in the future.

Malcolm works with the psychiatrist on his issues around taking HAART. When he begins to lose muscle mass, he initially balks at continuing his medications. He is switched to a regimen that minimizes this side effect. As his serum testosterone is low, he begins to take testosterone injections and follows a gym routine to improve his muscle mass. After several weeks, he feels better about himself and is more adherent, rarely missing a dose of his medication. Over several months, his CD4 cell count climbs to 350 cells/mm^{3}and his viral load becomes undetectable. Malcolm is able to stop psychotherapy, feeling more comfortable with the lifestyle decisions he has made and with hope that his medication regimen will keep his illness in check until better treatments for his HIV infection are discovered.

Case study: Long-term survivor in psychotherapy

Beth, a teacher on disability payments, presents for psychotherapy 10 years after her initial diagnosis with HIV. She had been tested because an ex-boyfriend had died with AIDS. After the initial shock of the diagnosis, she found ways of coping which largely involved avoidance.

Beth remained good friends with her ex-lover, and has strong ties to the gay community. She has also become actively involved in a community-based, peer-run program for women with HIV. Over the years, Beth has lost many friends and acquaintances to AIDS. She reports feeling burned out by all the loss she has experienced and has long ago stopped going to memorial services and funerals. She is disturbed that she largely feels numb in the face of these losses.

Beth started antiretroviral treatment in the mid-1990s when HAART emerged. She has done well medically up to this point. However, she feels guilty about her longevity, and wonders why she is the one to have survived so long.

She describes herself as chronically anxious, not knowing what lies around the corner for her medically. She wants to remain optimistic in the face of the promise of combination therapies and feels guilty that she isn't feeling more enthusiastic about her future.

She is bored with her life and can identify little that truly interests her or engages her in any meaningful way. She reports that she is quite isolated socially, and considers herself the last survivor of her cohort of friends and acquaintances affected by HIV.

What issues figure prominently in the psychotherapy of long-term survivors with HIV infection?

Paradoxically, long-term survivors are often surprised to find that they experience significant ambivalence about their health status. Many have lived through years of uncertainty, waiting for illness to emerge. They are often chronically anxious and experience varying degrees of dysphoria and anhedonia. In the early years of the illness they had to cope with the anticipation of an early death. With the advent of combination therapies, patients have had to adjust to living with a chronic life-threatening illness. Uncertainty persists, and patients often describe how difficult it is for them to get on with their lives. Given the fact that they seem to have been given a new lease on life, they experience these difficulties as incongruous.

Patients struggle with finding meaning in life. Many are on long-term disability payments and, over the years, have lost skill sets. They feel cheated for not having had the opportunity to pursue a career. Because many of their friends and associates work, they often feel isolated and marginalized.

Having experienced the loss of whole cohorts of friends and acquaintances to AIDS and not wanting to risk more loss in the future, they find it difficult to make new friends. When people experience cumulative loss, they cannot complete the work of grief, and they often describe feeling burned out and emotionally numb. Many also experience survivor guilt, wondering why they have been spared up to this point.

Many patients, particularly gay men, describe feeling marginalized within their own communities. HIV/AIDS seems to be receiving less attention in the community and in the media. Patients feel set aside and isolated. They may feel that they are being forgotten by a community which does not want to be reminded of its vulnerability.

Sero-discordant couples sometimes experience an added stress associated with the improved health of the partner with HIV. If the couple relationship had been strained, and the HIV seronegative partner continued in the relationship out of a sense of duty, they may face a crisis in the relationship when dealing with the possibility of the relationship continuing for an extended time.

What is the role of interpersonal psychotherapy in treating people with HIV infection?

Interpersonal psychotherapy (IPT) is a form of short-term psychotherapy that helps patients relate depression to events in their lives and associated changes in social roles. The therapist helps the patient view the depression as an illness and engages him or her in discussing emotionally difficult current life issues. The psychiatrist then helps frame these difficulties within one of four problem areas: grief, role disputes, role transitions, or interpersonal deficits. The therapist employs specific strategies to deal with these problem areas, focusing on the here and now. The individual explores options for achieving specific goals to help change the situation and reduce depressive symptoms.

Markowitz *et al.* (1995) have shown that IPT can be used with good success to treat people with HIV and depression.

During the assessment, it becomes obvious that Beth is depressed. She has clearly articulated difficulties with grief and role transitions. The therapist suggests that she might benefit from IPT, and she agrees to a course of 12 sessions. She is educated about the fact that her depression is a real illness, closely associated with the issues of grief and role transition. Beth's therapy focuses on elucidating these points and then supporting her through a process of exploring her options for re-engaging in a supportive social network and in activities which would help her feel more connected to meaningful activities. As she does this, she finds that her depression lifts significantly and she ends the therapy on an optimistic note.

Beth returns to therapy 8 months later. As she began to think about bringing more meaning into her life and re-engaging in society, Beth began to imagine that she might, in fact, return to work. She had left her work as a teacher 6 years earlier, when her health had seemed precarious and her time short. Up to this point Beth has been supported by a disability package from her employer which included an adequate living allowance and payment for her medications.

What issues may arise in psychotherapy with regard to return to work?

After being out of the work force for a significant time, patients with HIV face a number of important challenges. Have they lost important skills? Will they face discrimination in the work place? Could returning to work mean they lose secure income by giving up disability benefits? Will they be eligible for benefits in the new job when they are coming into it with a pre-existing illness? How will they pay for expensive medications and will there be sick time available? What if they get sick again and can no longer work? How will they support themselves then? Will the company lay them off for nonmedical reasons, leaving them without benefits?

Given the inflexibility of some insurance programs, the risk may be too great, and some patients may find themselves trapped in disability situations with no options for exploring a possible return to work.

Beth struggles with these issues for the next few months in therapy and ultimately decides not to return to work at this time because of the uncertainty. She then begins showing signs of lipodystrophy. Over time she develops sunken cheeks, an interscapular "buffalo hump", an uncomfortable increase in the size of her breasts, and an increase in her abdominal girth.

What issues does the patient face in dealing with long-term side effects of HIV treatment?

HAART is commonly associated with changes in body morphology that often raise serious ambivalence in the patient. When people with HIV notice physical changes, they often express alarm and can easily come to feel stigmatized and labelled as ill. For some, the effects of the treatment are worse than the prospect of dying.

HAART is also associated with elevated cholesterol and triglycerides as well as diabetes mellitus, which increase the risk of early death from cardiovascular events and stroke. Side effects cause many patients to feel ambivalent about their treatment.

Beth's therapy focuses on this ambivalence. She considers her options, specifically discontinuing antiretrovirals, but decides to continue after all. She grieves the changes in her body and begins to explore at a deeper level issues related to self-worth and esteem. Ultimately, she is able to come to a degree of acceptance and to tolerate uncertainty. She is better able to define her self-worth as independent of her body image.

Within a year Beth's viral load begins to rise again and her CD4 cell count declines. She tries another medication protocol but finds it difficult to tolerate the persistent nausea, abdominal cramps, and headaches. At this point, she begins to seriously consider discontinuing anti-retroviral therapy.

What issues should the therapist address in the face of a patient deciding to terminate treatment with HAART?

Many patients experience the progression of illness in the face of combination therapies as a personal failure. Sometimes this extends to a feeling of having failed loved ones or failed the memory of those who have already died. Some also feel shunned by others struggling with the illness, because they are a reminder of ongoing vulnerability. The progression of illness essentially confronts denial.

When a patient decides to terminate treatment, the therapist may be concerned about the motives behind the decision. The therapist wants to ensure that:

- the decision is based on up-to-date information
- the decision has not been significantly affected by cognitive dysfunction, psychosis, or treatable depressive syndromes
- the patient has weighed the pros and cons carefully
- the decision is not suicide-equivalent behavior.

Beth struggles with her side effects and finally decides to stop her treatments. She has some symptoms of depression but they seem to be related to demoralization resulting from the side effects. There is no evidence of cognitive impairment or psychosis. Her therapist speaks with her primary care physician who reports that, because of the extensive resistance of her viral strains, the current protocol is the last available to her. Over the next few months, Beth begins to feel better and decides to terminate psychotherapy.

She returns to therapy several months later feeling very sad about the fact that her CD4 cell count has fallen below 100 cells/mm^3, and she realizes that she is increasingly vulnerable to HIV-related illnesses. She is increasingly pre-occupied with thoughts of death and becomes extremely anxious each time she develops minor symptoms. For example, during a simple cold she finds herself driven to become even more active in order to feel safe. She has developed a concern that if she ever gives in, she will die. She feels very alone and fears she has little control over what is happening to her. Beth was raised a Roman Catholic but became disenchanted with organized religion many years ago.

What are the spiritual issues for someone faced with HIV disease?

Any patient facing death will struggle with existential concerns. In people with HIV, feelings of aloneness are aggravated by many years of having struggled with stigmatization and marginalization.

Control is also of great concern because patients often feel they have very little control over the course of their illness. Many patients feel cheated out of a happy life or as though they are being punished for their life-style choices or sexual orientation.

For many, meaning in life is a significant struggle. People with HIV are often quite young when they learn of their diagnosis. They are often unable to work or return to work, and many do not have children in whom to apply hope and to counter isolation. They often feel that, because they have been deprived of these things, they have little meaning in their lives. Many have not had life experiences with which to define personal meaning. The struggle with the finality of death is particularly difficult in this developmental stage of life, and fear of death as an existential concern presents special challenges.

Spiritual concerns, in the broadest sense, often figure prominently for people with HIV. Many have angry feelings towards religious communities. For gay men, this is usually based on religion's intolerance of homosexuality. This disenfranchisement very often extends to a disengagement from a concept of God or an afterlife. On the other hand, it is very common to encounter marked residual guilt and ambivalence, particularly when the patient comes from orthodox or dogmatic religious backgrounds. Internalized homophobia or self-blame for a "promiscuous" life style may emerge and should be recognized and dealt with in therapy

As Beth talks about her feelings of alienation from the church she begins to understand that her rejection of what she had experienced as misogynist dogma does not preclude a relationship with a creator and a supreme being. She continues to feel ambivalent, however, and occasionally has nightmares about going to hell. Over time she is able to talk spontaneously about herself as a fundamentally good person who is, in fact, deserving of care and compassion from a forgiving God.

Beth becomes interested in meditation and yoga, and is very intrigued by Buddhist concepts of being in the moment, acceptance, and compassion. Through her meditations, she is able to significantly reduce her anxiety about her illness and take more pleasure in day-to-day activities.

As Beth allows herself to accept the help offered by her friends and family, she begins to feel less alone. She takes more interest in her nieces and nephews, and realizes she can help her sister by looking after her children when she feels well enough. When helping the children with their homework, she feels she has a lot to offer given her years of experience as a teacher. She also comes to understand that there are those in her life who love her and that being in relationships with these people gives meaning to her life. She is finally able to hear them say that she brings great pleasure to others through her sense of humour and that they feel inspired by her courage.

As time passes, Beth's health continues to deteriorate. She develops *Pneumocystis carinii* pneumonia (PCP), which is treated successfully, but she never regains her strength. Her cognitive status begins to deteriorate and her therapist is shocked to see how much weight she is losing each week. During most sessions, Beth falls asleep in her chair, wrapped in a blanket that the therapist keeps on her sofa.

The therapist worries that Beth is putting too much pressure on herself to come to sessions, but her sister reports that Beth values these sessions immensely.

What concerns arise for the psychiatrist in the face of impending death?

As the therapist faces a patient's impending death, countertransference feelings can become particularly prominent. Helplessness, hopelessness, and therapeutic nihilism can surface. The problems facing the patient and therapist may be no more difficult, but the options for addressing them may seem less obvious. Without effective techniques in this situation, the therapist may feel ineffectual and incompetent, which may lead to guilt, which may manifest itself in a reawakening fear of contagion or in finding the patient physically repulsive. To continue to be available to the patient in helpful ways, the therapist must address these experiences and associated feelings. It may be necessary for the therapist to grieve the loss of the person as he or she had been up to this point.

Through peer support, the therapist recognizes her feelings and becomes more comfortable with Beth's impending death. She confronts her own feelings of omnipotence and guilt about surviving Beth. This letting go in the therapist allows her to be more present for Beth.

Beth develops hepatic failure and finally becomes homebound. Her therapist decides to visit her at home weekly. She listens as Beth talks about her fears of dying, encourages her in a process of life review, and helps her continue to explore ongoing interpersonal issues. The therapist is also able to provide support to Beth's sister and good friends who visit her regularly.

What are the implications for psychotherapy when it moves to the person's home?

The nature of the therapy changes when it moves to a person's home. Although the supportive component of the therapy may become more prominent, the therapist should not abandon the opportunity for further psychodynamic exploration. The therapist should be aware of what it means to the person to have the therapist in his or her home and be conscious of boundaries, while still allowing considerable flexibility.

When treatment moves to the person's home, therapists should ask their patients whether it is appropriate to involve caregivers in the therapy. Caregivers often face significant anxiety and can benefit from the therapist's support and insights.

Therapists who do not feel comfortable going into patients' homes should accept these feelings and make suitable referrals to community outreach groups.

After Beth's death, her sister meets with the therapist and confirms that Beth's therapy helped greatly. Her anxiety and depression had improved, and she seemed more open in her relationships with others. Beth's sister feels that, as a result, Beth's friends were genuinely more available and loving toward her. The changes in Beth affected the lives of those around her.

Conclusion

Psychotherapists who work with people living with HIV infection consistently report that their patients make satisfactory gains. Clinical practice demonstrates that any psychotherapy appropriately prescribed and competently applied can help an individual through crisis, critical decision making, the pursuit of insight, and the working through of problematic affects, behavior, and interpersonal patterns. People with HIV have a lot at stake and are often motivated to do the work of therapy. For many, HIV serves as a catalyst for this work. Living and dying with HIV provides the opportunity to work through long-standing intrapsychic and interpersonal difficulties. Although the work can be challenging for therapists, it has the potential to be extremely gratifying.

REFERENCES

Markowitz, J., Klerman, G. and Perry, S. Interpersonal psychotherapy of depressed HIV-positive outpatients. *Hospital and Community Psychiatry*, **42** (1992): 885–90.

Weiss, J. J. Psychotherapy with HIV-positive gay men: a psychodynamic perspective. *American Journal of Psychotherapy*, **51**(1997): 31–44.

SUGGESTED READING

Blechner, M. *Hope and Mortality: Psychodynamic Approaches to AIDS and HIV*. Hillsdale, NJ: The Analytic Press, 1997.

Cartwright, D. and Cassidy, M. Working with HIV/AIDS sufferers: "When good enough is not enough". *American Journal of Psychotherapy*, **56** (2002): 149–66.

DeRoche, P. Pyschodynamic psychotherapy with the HIV-infected patient. In *Dynamic Therapies for Psychiatric Disorders (Axis I)*, J. P. Barber and P. Crits-Christoph, eds., pp. 420–43. New York: Basic Books, 1995.

Harrison, G. *In the Lap of the Buddha*. Boston, MA: Shambhala, 1994.

Markowitz, J., Klerman, G., Clougherty, K. *et al.* Individual psychotherapies for depressed HIV-positive patients. *American Journal of Psychiatry*, **152** (1995): 1504–09.

Schaffner, B. Modifying psychoanalytic methods when treating the HIV-positive patient. *Journal of the American Academy of Psychoanalysis*, **25** (1997): 123–41.

10

HIV and substance use disorders

Fabrizio Starace, M.D.[1], Annunziata Ciafrone, M.D.[2] and
Giuseppe Nardini, M.D.[3]

[1] Director, Consultation Psychiatry and Behavioral Epidemiology Service, Cotugno Hospital, Naples, Italy
[2] Assistant, Consultation Psychiatry Unit, Cotugno Hospital, Naples, Italy
[3] Assistant Director, Consultation Psychiatry Unit, Cotugno Hospital, Naples, Italy

Introduction

Drug use is a significant risk factor for HIV infection. In fact, substance users and their partners account for the majority of new HIV infections in western industrialized countries (Table 10.1).

Substance users may acquire or transmit HIV infection as a direct result of their substance use (i.e., by sharing needles or paraphernalia used to inject drugs) or indirectly (i.e., through unprotected sexual intercourse while under the influence of drugs or alcohol) (Table 10.2).

According to UNAIDS (2000), "most of these infections could have been averted". Prevention programs that promote safer sex and provide thoughtful drug treatment, including methadone maintenance and needle exchange services, have proven effective in reducing the risk of HIV infection.

Substance use is also a risk factor in disease progression. Substance users often find it difficult to adhere to complex antiretroviral treatment regimens, and some of the substances they use may affect their response to treatment.

Patients who use substances should be carefully assessed for their drug use patterns and related physical, psychological, and social problems. Psychiatrists can play a key role in coordinating multidisciplinary assessments and planning appropriate addiction interventions.

Case study: HIV-seropositive woman with heroin addiction

Simona, a 25-year-old woman who has been HIV-seropositive for 8 years, has difficulties adhering to her prescribed antiretroviral therapy. Her physician refers her to a consulting psychiatrist. In the interview, the psychiatrist learns that, since her childhood, Simona has shown rebellious behavior, and inability to accept rules at home or at school. When she

HIV and Psychiatry. A Training and Resource Manual, Second Edition, ed. Kenneth Citron, Marie-Josée Brouillette, and Alexandra Beckett. Published by Cambridge University Press. © Cambridge University Press 2005.

was 15, her father, to whom she was deeply attached, was diagnosed with cancer. At about the same time, she met a man, much older than she was, who introduced her to substance use. After her father's death, Simona increased her substance use, which led to both needle sharing and prostitution. As a result of these behaviors, she acquired HIV infection.

When she received the diagnosis, she started attending the drug unit for methadone treatment, but has been unable to change her lifestyle. Despite a gradual increase of her daily methadone dose to 60 mg, she has not been able to stop using substances. She continues to take drugs – usually heroin, but also cocaine and benzodiazepines. When using these substances, she often does not adhere to her HIV treatment regimen. She is aware of the risks she is taking by not looking after her health, but appears to be unable to stop using substances. She even asked her mother to shut her up at home, but she could not last more than 2 days. Simona is worried about changes in her physical appearance as a result of HIV disease progression, which prevent her from having a social life.

Based on the clinical evaluation, the psychiatrist determines that Simona has a personality disorder. She also suffers symptoms of withdrawal, especially on days when she takes the antiretroviral therapy as prescribed. The withdrawal symptoms, which she associates with antiretroviral therapy, cause her to take substances and substance use causes her not to take the antiretroviral therapy.

Table 10.1. HIV/AIDS statistics and main modes of transmission (UNAIDS, 2000)

Region	Adults and children living with HIV/AIDS	Main mode(s) of transmission for those living with HIV/AIDS
Sub-Saharan Africa	24.5 million	Hetero
North Africa and Middle East	220 000	Hetero, IDU
South and South-East Asia	5.6 million	Hetero, IDU
East Asia and Pacific	530 000	IDU, Hetero, MSM
Latin America	1.3 million	MSM, IDU, Hetero
Caribbean	360 000	Hetero, MSM
Eastern Europe and Central Asia	420 000	IDU
Western Europe	520 000	MSM, IDU
North America	900 000	MSM, IDU, Hetero
Australia and New Zealand	15 000	MSM
Total	34.3 million	

Hetero: heterosexual transmission; IDU: transmission through injecting drug use; MSM: sexual transmission among men who have sex with men.

Table 10.2. Most frequently abused substances and their relationship with HIV infection

Substance	Desired effects	Undesired effects	Relationship with HIV
Alcohol	Euphoria, lightness	Anxiety, depression, irritability, insomnia, appetite loss	Unsafe sex, sexual violence
Opiates	Analgesia, sense of tranquillity, decreased sense of apprehension	Nausea, vomiting, depression of respiration, changes in the neuroendocrine system	Needle sharing
Cocaine and crack	Euphoria, enhanced vigor, hyperactivity, interpersonal sensitivity, aphrodisiac effect	Coronary vasoconstriction, impairment of myocardial function, panic attacks, bouts of anxiety and suspiciousness, anorexia	Unsafe sex, sexual violence, needle sharing
Marijuana	Euphoria, increased talkativeness, feeling of elation, rapid flow of ideas	Anxiety (rare)	No proven relationship
MDMA and other stimulants	Heightened states of introspection and intimacy	Trismus, bruxism, restlessness, anxiety, decreased appetite, tachycardia, palpitations, dry mouth, insomnia	Unsafe sex

What is a harm reduction strategy?

The treatment of drug abuse and drug dependence is a long-term process. Often drug users either do not want or are not able to stop using drugs. In those cases, the main goal of treatment is to reduce the risk of HIV infection and the negative social impact of the drug abuse (i.e., harm reduction). The harmful biological consequences of drug abuse are rarely due to the effect of the drug itself. They are usually due to the modes of administering the drugs and to the presence of adulterants. Examples of harm-reduction strategies include:

- providing sterile injection equipment (needle exchange services)
- providing methadone maintenance therapy, which will reduce the use of illegal substances and, therefore, the risk of adulteration, and help shift the person to an oral substance, thereby reducing the risk associated with injecting drugs
- administering heroin under strict medical control, which reduces the risks associated with both administration and adulteration. A national program in Switzerland showed the effectiveness of this approach in nonresponders to traditional methadone maintenance programs. Similar programs are being developed in the Netherlands, Germany, and Spain.

How important is adequate dosage of methadone?

Substance abuse is associated with an irregular lifestyle which, in turn, does not allow the substance user to develop the behavioral skills needed to manage complex regimens like highly active antiretroviral treatment (HAART). Patients who receive an adequate dose of methadone are more likely to remain in treatment, use fewer illicit drugs, and enjoy a more stable lifestyle. Less than 40 mg per day of methadone is generally considered a low dose. The vast majority of people abusing heroin require a daily dose ranging between 50 and 100 mg (Dole, 1989; Kleber, 1989; Ball and Ross, 1991). However, several factors, including chronic diseases (especially liver disease), pregnancy and other pharmacological treatments (see below) may affect methadone metabolism and therefore, efficacy.

The psychiatrist recommends gradually increasing Simona's dosage of methadone from 60 mg a day up to 80 mg a day, and arranges another appointment. When Simona returns 15 days later, she is well groomed and has a new haircut. She reports feeling better. She is taking her antiretroviral therapy correctly and taking care of her physical health. However, she has not completely given up using substances. She no longer takes cocaine and has reduced her use of heroin, but she is still taking benzodiazepines to help her deal with the withdrawal symptoms she continues to experience, usually in the afternoon.

How does antiretroviral therapy affect methadone metabolism?

Several antiretroviral drugs can affect methadone metabolism. Methadone is mainly metabolized by cytochrome P450 CYP3A4 and glucuronidation. Sub-enzymes

CYP 2D6, 2C9, and 2C19 also exert minor metabolic influences. Researchers have documented drug interactions, especially with non-nucleoside analogues (NNRTIs) nevirapine and efavirenz, and the protease inhibitors (PIs) ritonavir, nelfinavir, amprenavir, and lopinavir/ritonavir. These agents may decrease plasma levels of methadone. In patients on methadone maintenance, the initiation of one of these agents may result in withdrawal symptoms that can only be managed by substantially increasing methadone dosage.

The psychiatrist recommends gradually increasing Simona's daily methadone dose to 100 mg. Over the next 7 days, Simona's toxicological urine tests are negative. However, she is not able to remain abstinent over the long-term. Two weeks later, she reports that she is again using heroin and has stopped taking methadone and the antiretroviral drugs.

Does antiretroviral therapy affect the metabolism of recreationally used drugs?

Interactions between recreationally used drugs and the antiretroviral agents (particularly the NNRTIs and the PIs) have been reported or can be predicted based on known metabolic pathways of these substances. Some of these interactions are potentially life threatening. For this reason, it is crucial that patients:

- be informed about the importance of adequately reporting to their physicians the recreational substances they are using
- refrain from experimenting with new drugs before verifying their safety with the HIV specialist.

For more information about the potential interactions between antiretrovirals and recreationally used/abused substances, see Chapter 3, Table 3.4.

Can the presence of psychiatric comorbidity affect the patient's ability to adhere to treatment?

Treatment of HIV-seropositive patients is particularly difficult when the patient has a comorbid substance abuse disorder and personality disorder. These conditions are associated with poor adherence to treatment and outcome. Patients with triple diagnosis (HIV infection, drug abuse, personality disorder) show diminished:

- self-concept (the dynamic system of learned beliefs, attitudes, and opinions that each person holds to be true about his or her personal existence)
- self-efficacy (the ability/competence to deal with challenges)
- coping skills (the skills to deal with difficult situations and be more positive about the future).

The psychiatrist recommends increasing Simona's daily methadone dosage to 120 mg, and offers Simona behavior therapy and her family a psycho-educational intervention.

At the 6-month follow up, Simona demonstrates a greater ability to take care of herself. Her physical appearance has improved, she is reading again. She and her mother get along better.

She has decided to attend a course to learn computer skills and is looking for a job. With regard to her substance use, she reports occasional craving episodes which she is able to control.

What are the different models of care for people with a dual or triple diagnosis?

Patients who have dual or triple diagnosis may find professional help from different health agencies confusing, and treatment may have to be adapted to meet their needs. Three different models of care have been applied: serial treatment, parallel treatment, and integrated treatment.

- In a serial model, one treatment (either psychiatric or for addiction) is followed by the other. The drug unit and the mental health centre plan different programs based on their own guidelines and resources. Serial treatment works with patients who are able to achieve normal or nearly normal mental status for significant periods under appropriate psychiatric treatment, and for mild to moderate drug and/or alcohol abuse. Serial treatment does not work well for patients who have major psychotic disorders with significant psychosocial and functional consequences or for patients with both severe substance use disorder and antisocial personality.
- In a parallel model, the patient receives concurrent but separate treatment for both psychiatric and addiction disorders. This approach requires close cooperation between the two separate units: psychiatry and drug dependency. Parallel treatment works with patients whose psychiatric (e.g., schizophrenia, bipolar disorder, major depression) and addiction disorders have been stabilized.
- In an integrated model, the patient receives concurrent, integrated treatment for physical, drug-related, and psychiatric disorders. The model applies the core concepts and methods from both psychiatric and addiction treatment. This intervention model, based on the interaction between different professional skills, offers the patient coordinated *pharmacological* protocols (e.g., detoxification, methadone maintenance, support and/or treatment of psychiatric comorbidity, as well as treatment of HIV infection and other concomitant pathologies), *psychotherapeutic* interventions (e.g., counseling, individual or group psychotherapy), and *psycho-educational* interventions (i.e., for patients and their families). The integrated model is the most appropriate approach for patients with HIV who also have dual diagnoses.

In a patient not already involved with the healthcare system (i.e., methadone maintenance), how would the intervention have been different?

People with a substance use problem may mistrust established authority figures, including healthcare professionals. Their previous encounters with the healthcare system may have been negative, leading them to avoid seeking healthcare. When they do go to a clinic, it may take several months for them to establish a trusting relationship with the care provider, a first necessary step in dealing with a substance use problem. Consider the following example:

Lina was using heroin on a regular basis. She often missed appointments with the physician, only to appear a few days later at the clinic in need of food, money, medication, or shelter. As much as possible, the clinic helped her meet these basic needs. Over time, she developed a strong positive relationship with her physician and the clinic's nurse and social worker. Although she had previously refused to even discuss her use of heroin and its impact on her health, she is now willing to do so.

What is the Stages of Change model?

When working with people with substance abuse problems, care providers should recognize that they will be at different stages in dealing with their addiction, and meet them where they are. According to the Stages of Change model (Prochaska et al., 1991), individuals go through five stages to change behavior, and movement through these stages is not linear but cyclical (Table 10.3).

The healthcare provider's role varies, depending on the person's stage. For example, with people who are either unaware of the need to change or not yet ready to commit (pre-contemplation and contemplation), the clinician's role is one of motivator. With patients who have decided to change (preparation and

Table 10.3. The Stages of Change Model

Stage	Definition	Intervention
Pre-contemplation	The patient denies the problem and doesn't want to change	Inform the patient, take time, maintain an alliance
Contemplation	The patient is aware that the problem exists but is still not committed to take action	Maintain motivation. Inform. Balance the positive and negative effects of the desired change
Preparation	The patient decides to act and begins to plan his/her program	Support decision to change. Help find a good strategy
Action	The patient modifies his/her lifestyle to overcome the problem	Make a list of "at risk" situations. Discuss the difficulties. Prepare a plan in case of relapse
Maintenance	The patient works to prevent relapse and to reinforce the acquired skills and behavioral models	Be tolerant. De-dramatize relapse. Reinforce support network

action), the physician's role is to provide personalized assistance that will enable patients to successfully replace the addictive behavior with healthier habits. With patients who are trying to maintain new behaviors (maintenance), the physician's main role is to focus on relapse prevention.

> ## Case study: HIV-seropositive man with alcohol addiction
>
> Marco, age 37, is referred to the psychiatric unit by the infectious diseases centre where he was diagnosed with HIV infection a year ago. He has recently quarrelled with his physician about the issue of alcohol abuse. He has become angry, verbally aggressive, and very critical of his antiretroviral treatment. He cannot understand why it is so important to follow the medical prescription. He feels well, and finds remembering to take the medication bothersome. He also claims that the HIV drugs aren't helping. When the consulting psychiatrist raises the issue of alcohol abuse, Marco becomes nervous. He claims that drinking is a way to ease his anxiety. Drinking makes him feel better than all the antiretroviral medications he takes.

To what extent does alcohol abuse influence adherence to treatment?

Alcohol abuse can produce profound alterations in behavior and cognition. It is also a significant factor in nonadherence to medical prescription. Patients who abuse alcohol are more likely to develop nonadherent behavior than heroin users (Starace et al., 2000).

While people with HIV report that drinking helps them manage the emotional turmoil, anxiety, and depression associated with being HIV-seropositive, alcohol intoxication is associated with mood lability, depression, agitation, disinhibition, and impaired judgment. Alcohol abuse affects people's ability to take their HIV medications correctly. Alcoholic patients often show low levels of self-efficacy and tend to believe that treatment with antiretroviral drugs is too complex to be included in their daily routine. Because of the unpleasant withdrawal symptoms, many are not able to give up alcohol in order to take care of their HIV disease.

When treating patients who abuse alcohol, it is important to manage withdrawal symptoms adequately. Treatment of alcohol abuse should not begin until the patient is stable and no longer experiencing withdrawal symptoms.

In the absence of serious medical complications, an alcohol withdrawal syndrome is usually transient and self-limited. Treatment for withdrawal is symptomatic and prophylactic. At the current time, long-acting benzodiazepines are the drugs of choice for treating withdrawal. In patients with liver disease, oxazepam is recommended. Treatment for withdrawal symptoms must include large doses of vitamins, particularly thiamine, to prevent peripheral neuropathy and Wernicke–Korsakoff syndrome.

Treatment of alcoholism has two goals:
- achieving sobriety
- improving psychiatric conditions associated with alcoholism.

Many patients find the deterrent effect of disulfiram helpful in maintaining abstinence. Some patients may profit from the Twelve Step program or other psychotherapeutic approach.

The psychiatrist prescribes Marco chlordiazepoxide and recommends a Twelve Step program, but Marco refuses. Two weeks later, Marco comes back to the psychiatric unit. He is sorry for what happened during the previous interview. He reveals that, since his last visit, he has had sexual intercourse with women he barely knows, using no precautions. This risky behavior always occurs after drinking at parties.

Can alcohol abuse affect sexual behaviour?

Several studies have documented the effect of alcohol abuse on sexual behavior associated with HIV transmission (Petry, 1999). Individuals who abuse alcohol have more negative attitudes towards condom use and are more likely to have sexual intercourse with a large number of partners than people who do not abuse alcohol. This is likely due to alcohol's disinhibiting effect on sexual behaviour.

When the psychiatrist explores Marco's knowledge about HIV and its modes of transmission, he learns that Marco is confused and has only a fragmentary understanding of these issues. In addition, the role of antiretroviral therapy is unclear to him. Marco's motivation to change his lifestyle and adhere to HIV medications is poor, and he does not appear to have the skills required to change his behavior. The psychiatrist uses a structural interview based on the Information–Motivation–Behaviour (IMB) Skills Model (Fisher and Fisher, 1992) to assess gaps in Marco's information and motivation, and to identify the behavioral skills he needs.

What is the Information–Motivation–Behavioral (IBM) skills model?

The IMB model is a valid and reliable theoretical construct for understanding and modifying HIV risk behavior across different populations. This model gives caregivers a theoretical framework to assess the crucial relationship between information, motivation, and behavior in the patient's efforts to prevent the spread of HIV or adhere to treatment, and to develop appropriate interventions.

Information

Preventive behavior is associated with the level of information about HIV infection. The more HIV-seropositive patients know about the disease, the more likely they are able to prevent transmission and to adhere to treatment.

Motivation

While knowledge helps, information alone is not sufficient to prevent the spread of HIV. Well-informed individuals may not necessarily be motivated and/or have the behavioral skills to prevent HIV transmission or adhere to treatment. Personal and social sources of motivation are the main factors influencing risk behavior and/or nonadherence. Motivation is affected by personal attitudes, social rules for or against prevention, the patient's perception of the seriousness of the consequences of not adhering to the "rules", and the patient's perception of his/her vulnerability.

Behavioral skills

In addition to information and motivation, patients need specific behavioral skills to prevent HIV infection (e.g., being assertive with a potential sexual partner) or to maintain optimal adherence (e.g., the ability to tell the doctor their difficulties in taking medications on schedule). Patients who do not have these skills (e.g., the ability to cope with stressful situations without taking alcohol) will likely show dysfunctional behaviors.

Having identified Marco's needs for information, motivation, and improved behavioral skills, the psychiatrist is able to work with Marco to address all three areas. He confronts Marco's understanding of the frequency and intensity of side effects of antiretroviral agents, the "beneficial" effects of alcohol on anxiety and depression, the tractability of symptoms associated with alcohol withdrawal, and the negative consequence of nonadherence. In his efforts to improve Marco's motivation, the psychiatrist chooses a rational, nonmoralistic approach to avoid giving rise to Marco's aggressive-avoidant behavior. Using role playing, the psychiatrist helps Marco develop the skills to effectively communicate with the doctor about his emotional problems and to avoid alcohol abuse before and after sexual practices.

Conclusion

Both alcohol and drug abuse are risk factors for HIV infection and can substantially influence the course of diseases associated with HIV. Harm reduction strategies, based on a less restrictive legal approach, combined with community-based treatment and education programs may significantly improve the clinical management of patients with HIV and substance use disorder.

HIV care and drug/alcohol management should ideally be provided by an integrated service that carefully assesses and addresses medical, psychological, and social factors contributing to the substance use disorder. Multidisciplinary, theoretically grounded interventions have proven to be effective in helping alcohol and drug users change behavior.

Mental health professionals may play a key role in coordinating the multidisciplinary efforts to manage the personality, psychological, and cognitive difficulties so frequently experienced by HIV-seropositive substance users.

REFERENCES

Ball, J. C. and Ross, A. *The Effectiveness of Methadone Maintenance Treatment.* New York: Springer-Verlag, 1991.

Dole, V. P. Methadone treatment and the acquired immunodeficiency syndrome epidemic. *Journal of the American Medical Association,* **262**(12) (1989): 1681–2.

Fisher, J. D. and Fisher, W. A. Changing AIDS-risk behavior. *Psychological Bulletin,* **3**(3) (1992): 455–74.

Kleber, H. D. From theory to practice: the planned treatment of drug users. Interview by Stanley Einstein. *International Journal of Addiction,* **24**(2) (1989): 123–66.

Petry, N. Alcohol use in HIV patients: what we don't know may hurt us. *International Journal of STD,* **10**(9) (1999): 561–70.

Prochaska, J. O., diClemente, C. C. and Norcross, J. C. In search of how people change: applications to addictive behaviours. *American Psychologist,* **47** (1991): 1102–14.

Starace, F., De Gaetano, A., Chirianni, A. *et al.* (2000). *Non-adherence in HIV-seropositive persons: Psychosocial factors and implications for treatment.* XII International AIDS Conference, Durban, South Africa, July 9–14, 2000.

UNAIDS. HIV-AIDS statistics. Geneva: UNAIDS, June 27, 2000.

SUGGESTED READING

Dingle, G. A. and Oei, T. P. (1997). Is alcohol a cofactor of HIV and AIDS? Evidence from immunological and behavioral studies. *Psychological Bulletin,* **122**(1)(1997): 56–71.

Fitterling, J. M., Matens, P. B., Scotti, J. R. and Allen, J. S. Jr. (1993). AIDS risk behaviors and knowledge among heterosexual alcoholics and non-injecting drug users. *Addiction,* **88**(9) (1993): 1257–65.

Gordon, C. M., Carey, M. P. and Carey, K. B. Effects of a drinking event on behavioral skills and condom attitudes in men: implications for HIV risk from a controlled experiment. *Health Psychology,* **16**(5) (1997): 490–495.

Lowinson, J. H., Ruiz, P., Millmann, R. B. and Langrod, J. G. *Substance Abuse. A Comprehensive Textbook.* Baltimore: Williams and Wilkins, (1997).

Prochaska, J. O. and diClemente, C. C. *The Transtheoretical Approach, Crossing Traditional Boundaries of Therapy.* Homewood, ILL Dorsey Professional Books, (1984).

Ries, K. R. (1995). Assessment and treatment of patients with coexisting mental illness and alcohol and other drug abuse. *Treatment Improvement Protocol Series 9.* Department of Health and Human Services Publication No. 95-3061. Rockville, MD: Department of Health and Human Services, 1995.

11

Psychiatric issues in pediatric HIV/AIDS

Kevin J. Lourie, Ph.D., L.M.H.C.[1], Maryland Pao, M.D.[2]*,
Larry K. Brown, M.D.[3] and Heather Hunter, B.A.[4]

[1] Director of Youth and Family Services, East Greenwich, RI, USA
[2] Deputy Clinical Director, Intramural Research Program, National Institute of Mental Health, National Institutes of Health, Bethesda, MD, USA
[3] Professor, Bradley/Hasbro Research Center, Department of Psychiatry, RI Hospital and Brown University, Providence, RI
[4] Department of Psychology, University of Kansas, Lawrence, KS, USA

Introduction

Human immunodeficiency virus (HIV) transmission now occurs at a higher rate among women and youth than other groups. Worldwide, about 2.7 million children under age 15 and more than 10 million aged 15–24 are afflicted, and half of all new infections occur among young people (UNAIDS, 2001). In the USA, for example, there are at least three HIV-seropositive youths for every known case of adolescent AIDS, and the number of reported pediatric HIV cases more than doubled from 2000 to 2001 (Centers for Disease Control and Prevention, 2001).

More than 90% of pediatric infections occur through vertical (mother-to-child) transmission. Most adolescents (ages 13–24) who become infected acquire HIV through sexual transmission, followed by injection drug use (Centers for Disease Control and Prevention, 2001).

Despite improvements in antiretroviral therapies, child mortality due to AIDS remains significant. As of 2000, more than 4.3 million children under 15 had died of AIDS, and more than 13 million had lost their mothers or both parents to AIDS (UNAIDS, 2000). Fortunately, recent developments in antiretroviral therapy have helped decrease the incidence of vertical transmission, and reduce the treatment burden on those infected, more than doubling their life expectancy. More children

---

* Dr. Pao's views are her own and do not necessarily reflect the opinions of the US Government.

HIV and Psychiatry. A Training and Resource Manual, Second Edition, ed. Kenneth Citron, Marie-Josée Brouillette, and Alexandra Beckett. Published by Cambridge University Press. © Cambridge University Press 2005.

with HIV are living past 10–15 years of age. Even without medical treatment, many HIV-infected children may remain asymptomatic for as long as a decade.

Although more than 95% of all new infections in 2000 occurred in developing countries where antiretroviral therapies are less accessible, pediatric AIDS continues to gradually shift from being an acute terminal childhood disease to a chronic long-term disease. Pediatric AIDS will continue to be of great significance to pediatricians, child psychiatrists, psychologists, and allied professionals (Brown *et al.*, 2000).

> ## Case study: Entering school with neurocognitive problems
>
> Crystal, a 5-year-old girl infected with HIV through vertical transmission, has lived with her foster mother, two half-siblings and two foster brothers since the age of one. She was placed in foster care because her biological mother, who abused cocaine, had died of AIDS. Crystal has been healthy, but her foster mother brings her to the pediatrician with concerns about her behavior. The school staff complaining that Crystal does not participate well in class because she is "withdrawn at times, but overall, too active and can never sit still to pay attention". In addition, her foster mother is most disturbed that Crystal is enuretic 3–4 nights a week. Although Crystal is hyperactive and has a short attention span, her foster mother does not want her to receive psychotropic medications. Crystal is referred for psychological testing and found to be functioning in the mildly retarded to borderline cognitive range.

What neurocognitive disorders are seen in young children with HIV?

Less than one-quarter of HIV-infected children will develop HIV-associated cognitive motor complex (HACM). HACM is characterized by a triad of cognitive, motor, and behavioral changes. In children, it manifests itself as impaired brain growth, progressive motor dysfunction, and loss or plateauing of developmental milestones. Although many children with HIV are asymptomatic, a significant proportion will experience at least some cognitive and language delays associated with HIV by the age of 5 or 6 (Papola *et al.*, 1994). Children with HIV have academic achievement scores that are significantly below average, as well as associated impairments in psychological functioning. Their visual–motor skills are also frequently impaired. Children who are infected perinatally have more difficulties than those infected later via transfusion or sexual intercourse.

Fortunately, the use of antiretroviral therapies appears to delay the onset of HACM. When diagnosing HACM, it is important to distinguish HIV-associated disorders from impairment and mental retardation secondary to other causes, such as prenatal exposure to drugs and alcohol, inadequate prenatal care, and neglect.

How do neurocognitive deficits present in younger children?

The clinical presentation of neurocognitive deficits in toddlers and school-aged children is highly variable. A child may be unable to speak or barely able to walk without assistance and fail to progress developmentally despite multiple interventions, or the neurocognitive problems may present later in the form of difficulties at school. In fact, it is not uncommon for the children's behavioral symptoms to be identified first in the school setting. For example, school staff may observe that the child is not progressing in schoolwork or is unable to remember lessons that she had previously learned.

Because the development of HACM is highly variable, it is critical that clinicians evaluate the neurocognitive abilities of HIV-infected children regularly. Progressive impairments in cognition may indicate a worsening of HIV disease itself rather than a concurrent infection or other process.

What is the standard evaluation of a child suspected of having neurocognitive impairment secondary to HIV?

The standard evaluation consists of the following:

(1) Comprehensive medical and psychiatric history
   At what point in brain development did HIV infection occur, if known?
   What are the neurocognitive symptoms?
   Has there been a loss of previously attained developmental milestones?
   Were there prenatal injuries such as in utero exposure to drugs (e.g., cocaine, alcohol) or viral infection?
   Is there any genetic predisposition for neurocognitive disorders (e.g., Down syndrome)?
   Is there a history of learning disability?

(2) Social history
   Are there any environmental circumstances contributing to the current difficulties?
   Is there a lack of cognitive stimulation due to a chaotic living environment?

(3) Detailed mental status examination

(4) Standard medical/neurological evaluation with additional HIV-related tests
   CD4 lymphocyte count
   Viral load
   HIV genotyping to determine patterns of drug resistance

(5) Neuropsychological testing
   What are the cognitive strengths and weaknesses?
   If present, are the impairments consistent with those typically seen in HIV disease?

(6) Neuroimaging

Are there intracranial abnormalities (e.g., atrophy, mass lesions, white matter abnormalities) suggestive of infection, malignancy, or other neuropathologic process?

Crystal's investigation reveals no reversible cause for her cognitive difficulties. Her viral load is undetectable and HIV treatment is felt to be optimal. Crystal is placed in a special education program more appropriate for her cognitive abilities, and receives behavioral treatment. However, she continues to have a flat affect, and to manifest problem behaviors, such as provoking siblings at home, calling out impulsively at school, and poor attention, which make it difficult for her to complete her work. The enuresis does not resolve with the behavioral treatment. After a child psychiatrist prescribes nortriptyline, the enuresis resolves, Crystal's attention and mood improve, and she becomes more socially engaged. Over time, the clinician develops a trusting relationship with Crystal's foster mother, who agrees to a trial of psychostimulants.

What are the treatment options for neurocognitive disorders in HIV-infected children?

Highly active antiretroviral therapy (HAART) is the mainstay of treatment for HIV-associated cognitive motor complex (Brouwers *et al.*, 1996). Antiretroviral drugs reduce HIV-related neurotoxicity, the underlying cause of HACM. These drugs can arrest neurocognitive deterioration and often improve function. In a seminal study by Brady *et al.* (1996), the cognitive status and adaptive functioning of children with AIDS improved over 36 months of antiretroviral treatment. The improvement was most pronounced for patients 6 years and older. Whenever possible, it is essential to start children with HACM on HAART, and make every effort to ensure adherence to the medication regimen (see discussion of adherence below).

Regular neurological and psychometric testing may help clinicians track illness progression and response to therapy. Such testing may also be useful in determining whether problematic behaviors stem from organic brain disease, and in facilitating long-term planning (e.g., for education, foster care).

What other treatments are effective for managing HACM?

Once HAART has been optimized, clinicians should treat psychological and behavioral dysfunction related to HACM symptomatically. Psychostimulants, antidepressants, antipsychotics, anticonvulsants, and other mood stabilizers may all have a role in the care of children with HACM. The clinician should keep in mind potential drug interactions between medications used to treat HIV and its complications, and psychotropic medications (see Chapter 3 for more information).

With the addition of methylphenidate, Crystal shows functional improvement in concentration, impulsivity, and hyperactivity. She continues to have social difficulties at school but seems generally more settled.

> ## Case study: Adolescent with depression
>
> Tamika, a 16-year-old girl with vertically transmitted HIV, presents to the primary care clinic complaining of hopelessness. She expresses suicidal ideation with a plan to overdose.
>
> Prior to this, Tamika has been generally healthy. Despite a tumultuous social history, she continues to attend high school and hold a part time job at the mall. Tamika, who lived with her mother until she died, has no contact with her father and now lives with her aunt. Having witnessed her mother's rapid death from AIDS, Tamika has become depressed. She was also recently hospitalized for the first time with medication-related pancreatitis. While in hospital, she agrees to start an antidepressant but refuses to resume antiretroviral medications which made her feel sicker. After being discharged, Tamika is unable to return to school. She cries frequently and sleeps most of the day. She complains of poor concentration and memory lapses, and fears she is developing "AIDS dementia".

How common is depression among HIV-infected children and adolescents?

Over the last decade, overt stigmatization of HIV/AIDS has diminished, and medical advances have significantly improved survival and quality of life for people with HIV disease. Nonetheless, pediatric HIV patients continue to experience significantly more subjective distress than their uninfected peers (Hansell et al., 1998). In addition to the emotional distress related to the physical signs of illness (e.g., wasting, dermatologic conditions), they must also cope with the emotional distress of social stigmatization, isolation and hopelessness, forced disclosure, loss and bereavement, and anxiety about their medical prognosis.

In both adults and children living with HIV, psychological stress, repression of anger, external locus of control, and low social support are associated with poorer coping overall (Grassi et al., 1998). The inability to cope may lead to greater social withdrawal and the worsening of psychological symptoms. Children are especially vulnerable to believing that their illness is a consequence of being bad.

A recent study of adolescents attending an HIV clinic found that 44% had major depression, and 85% had at least one DSM-IV Axis I diagnosis as determined by a structured clinical interview (Pao et al., 2000).

How do depressed HIV-seropositive children and adolescents typically present?

Depressed teenagers with HIV are likely to present to the medical team "in crisis". They may also present with somatic complaints and conduct problems (e.g., risky sexual behaviors, substance abuse, and/or poor compliance with medical care). Younger children may present with irritable mood, poor concentration, disruptive behaviors, and school failure (Bose et al., 1994).

What should be included in the evaluation of an HIV-seropositive child or adolescent with depression?

Depression is diagnosed using the standard DSM-IV criteria. When evaluating a child or adolescent with HIV for depression, clinicians should also consider the following:

- Count fatigue or anorexia toward the diagnosis of depression, even though they may be consequences of HIV-related medical illness.
- Evaluate for potentially treatable organic causes of depression, which are especially relevant in the immunocompromised child:
  infection
  metabolic or electrolyte abnormality
  psychoneurotoxicity due to medications or illicit substance use
  intracranial infection, malignancy
  HACM.
- Find out important HIV-related medical information:
  CD4 cell count
  viral load
  history of HIV-related symptoms and illnesses
  history of hospitalizations
  quality of relationship with medical providers
  antiretroviral regime – including adverse effects (especially neurological/psychiatric side effects), tolerability of medication regime, and adherence to medication regime
  other medications, including herbal, and over the counter remedies
  alternative therapies for HIV
  substance abuse.
- Inquire about suicidal ideation and suicidal behaviors.
- Evaluate for pain. Pain is a common and often under-recognized concomitant of HIV/AIDS, and chronic pain predisposes people to depression. Pain negatively affects quality of life and sleep patterns. Children and adolescents with HIV who are withdrawn because of physical pain may be incorrectly diagnosed as depressed. In these cases, good medical management combined with adequate analgesia will often clear depression.

When taking a social history, clinicians should bear in mind the special circumstances many children and adolescents with HIV face. For example, some may have a parent or other family member who is seriously ill, and be uncertain about their future living arrangements and guardianship. Some may have substitute caregivers, be in foster care, or be involved with child protection agencies.

Clinicians should also explore any history of sexual, emotional, or physical abuse. They should discuss the child's disclosure history (i.e., who has been told about the patient's HIV infection, who has done the disclosing). They should also determine whether the child has any concerns about sexuality that may affect his or her mental health.

What is the differential diagnosis of depression in children and adolescents with HIV/AIDS?

- Medical illness as described above.
- Depression spectrum DSM–IV disorders: adjustment disorder with depressed mood, dysthymic disorder, bipolar depression, substance-induced mood disorder.
- Bereavement.

Because of concerns about her suicidality, Tamika is hospitalized on a medical floor with a one-to-one sitter. Abnormal lab values include a markedly elevated amylase, CD4 of 10 cells/mm^3, and viral load of 350 000 copies/ml. Based on the degree to which Tamika's immune system is compromised and her cognitive complaints, the psychiatrist recommends an MRI of the brain which is unremarkable. Given the absence of fever or any localizing signs, the clinician decides that no further neurological work up is needed.

After several days of treatment with analgesia and complete bowel rest, Tamika's pancreatitis resolves. The psychiatrist initiates treatment with citalopram and, after a week, Tamika's mood and affect begin to improve. She agrees to start a new antiretroviral regimen.

Tamika also works with her therapist to address her belief that her illness and pain are punishment for being a bad person, and her fear that she will die in pain like her mother.

What psychological themes underlie the presentation of pain in younger individuals?

As in other chronic illnesses, clinicians should assess pain within a developmental context and identify preventive and therapeutic intervention strategies to reduce distress. Children and adolescents understand the meaning of pain in vastly different ways. Beyond managing the pain pharmacologically, caregivers should try to understand any psychological meaning the pain may have for the child. For example, for a child who fears being abandoned by her caregivers, pain may be a form of communication aimed at keeping caregivers close by. Developing family or individual psychotherapeutic interventions that strive to understand what is being communicated and address the pain's meaning can improve the child's emotional well-being and minimize the need for pain medication.

What principles should be followed when prescribing psychotropic medications for depressed HIV-infected children and adolescents?

When prescribing psychotropic medications, clinicians should bear in mind that youth with HIV are thought to be more sensitive to side effects and to require lower doses than their uninfected peers. In addition, safety considerations often dictate the choice of agent for patients on multiple medications. The clinician should be aware of the potential for clinically significant drug–drug interactions between antiretroviral agents and psychotropic agents (see Chapter 3).

The choice of antidepressant medication also depends upon symptomatology. If the child's prominent symptoms are low energy and/or hypersomnia, a more activating agent is appropriate. If the adolescent has sleep problems, a medication with sedating properties can be given at bedtime. Psychostimulants, such as methylphenidate or dextroamphetamine may be useful adjuncts for children with symptoms of refractory depression, apathy, malaise, mental slowing, or attention deficits.

Judicious use of psychotropic medications in children and adolescents may improve the functioning and quality of life of many youth with HIV. British, Canadian, and US regulatory agencies have announced new warnings and precautions to strengthen safeguards for children and adolescents treated with antidepressant medications. When introducing these medications to the HIV treatment regimen, clinicians should present information about the indications for which the drugs are approved or if use is "off-label" but appears to be clinically indicated. As always, a balanced discussion of the risk–benefit ratio for a particular child's situation should be reviewed. Clinical improvement or worsening, suicidality, and other unusual changes in behavior should be closely monitored, particularly in the early stages of treatment.

What types of psychotherapy and systemic interventions are useful for depressed children and adolescents with HIV?

Cognitive–behavioral techniques are used to teach "active" strategies, such as problem-solving and help-seeking, rather than "passive" strategies, such as self-blame, resignation, and acting-out. This approach is useful in improving coping skills.

Insight-oriented psychotherapy allows children and teens to describe their experience with HIV, explore difficulties in relationships, and mourn losses (e.g., parents and other loved ones with HIV, hope for future romance, childbearing).

Interpersonal psychotherapy has demonstrated efficacy in depressed adolescents (Mufson et al., 1994) and has been used successfully in HIV-seropositive depressed adults (Markowitz et al., 1991).

Social support of family and peers is another important factor in adolescents' emotional well-being and their ability to cope. Early assessment and intervention with the family can help shore up the adolescent's support system. Common themes that arise include: biological mothers who are also ill, feeling guilty and self-critical; grandparents and surrogate parents who feel overwhelmed or unwilling to raise a second family; siblings who either fear contagion or resent the special attention the ill child receives.

Tamika's maternal aunt, her main caregiver, meets with the team social worker alone and with Tamika. In the hope that her biological father will be supportive, Tamika decides to re-initiate contact with him.

Tamika recovers sufficiently to return to work and, for a brief time, goes on national tour as a spokesperson for adolescents living with HIV. Over the next 2 years, she has recurrent depressions during which she discontinues all her HIV medications. Her already fragile health deteriorates rapidly, and she is diagnosed with an aggressive lymphoma. During her last hospital stay, Tamika refuses all treatments as well as hospice care. Her aunt and father request full resuscitation and have difficulty visiting Tamika in the hospital. The psychiatric consultation team works with both the family and medical staff to help them come to terms with the irreversibility of Tamika's condition. Three months later, Tamika dies of pneumonia.

How does age affect a child's reaction to issues of death and dying?

Children's understanding of death and dying, regardless of its cause, varies with age (Lewis, 1996). Very young children associate physical symptoms, such as pain, with punishment, and exhibit magical thinking about the idea of death, to the extent that they can understand it. All pediatric patients must be reassured that their symptoms are not their fault. With the youngest, chronic patients, every attempt must be made to reinforce attachment to family members, in order to prevent acute separation anxiety and withdrawal as a response to the disease.

Children between 5 and 10 years of age express more confusion about mortality and the causes of acute symptoms, and experience greater conflict about their bodies and early sexual development as a result of chronic illness. While their response is often denial and a regressive tendency, parents and clinical staff can help by attempting to alleviate perceived guilt and to contradict a negative self-concept. Positive cognitive coping strategies will help reduce their level of despair.

Older children, between 11 and 15 years of age, often understand the finality of terminal illness and death, although they have great difficulty regulating their daily tasks and thought processes as part of living. They are more prone to express anger and exhibit acting out behaviors, and to resort to dysfunctional thinking and risky behaviors as a way to cope with ingrained hopelessness.

How can mental health professionals help an HIV-seropositive child cope with the death of a parent?

Children with HIV who have recently lost a family member may develop a number of symptoms, including depression, suicidal ideation, somatization, conduct disturbance, poor academic performance, and low self-esteem (Rotheram-Borus et al., 2001). They often lack the support of their own ill parents and may be deprived of other social support. They may also experience stigmatization.

Pediatric AIDS patients need to be able to express their fears and fantasies, deal with their reaction to a parent's illness, and adequately grieve after the parent dies. If children do not have the opportunity to communicate their fear and grief, they may develop pathological grief reactions. Any unresolved anger they may feel toward their infected parent can undermine the emotional support available to the child. When children cannot express their grief, then the symptoms associated with mourning (e.g., depression, conduct disturbance) may worsen, leading the child to believe that the parent's death was shameful.

To help a child express grief and cope with death, the clinician should elicit the support of friends, siblings, and members of the child's extended family. If a child has lost a parent, his subsequent caretaker should be someone with whom the child can effectively bond and who will reciprocate the attachment. In addition to working with the child, the treatment team must also help the infected child's family members cope with their sense of loss and fears about the child's mortality.

Workshops or family sessions on coping skills and bereavement can encourage communication. For example, they can support parents and help them develop the skills to disclose their serostatus to their children. They can also help family members and friends adapt to the illness, and provide the support infected children need to express their feelings about losing a parent or caregiver as well as their fears about their own illness and mortality.

Case study: Issues in adherence

John, a 14-year-old with vertically transmitted HIV, has been living with his elderly grandmother since his mother died of AIDS several years ago. Because of her age, his grandmother has become more forgetful. She has also stopped monitoring his medication, because he is "grown".

As a child, John adhered to his medications with little supervision. However, as an adolescent, he wants to be "normal" (i.e., like the other kids) and sometimes "forgets" to carry his medications with him. Although John takes most of his medications each day, it is not always convenient for him to take all his doses and he does miss some. No one has ever discussed with him what to do when he misses or sleeps through a dose.

John's willingness to adhere to his treatment regimen is also affected by the fatigue, diarrhea, and abdominal bloating he experiences when on medication, and by the fact that medication did not save his mother's life (although HAART was not available at that time). He often wonders whether the medication makes any difference for him.

What adherence issues are seen among HIV-positive children and adolescents?

Complex antiretroviral regimens suppress virus replication, decrease patients' viral load, and improve their immune status. To maintain a certain level of drug in their system, people on antiretroviral therapy must adhere rigorously to their drug regimen. Any drop in drug levels due to a missed dose may allow drug resistance to develop.

Some antiretroviral regimens are very cumbersome to follow, even for the most conscientious patient. When working with children and adolescents with HIV, mental health providers should evaluate both the caregiver's understanding and commitment to adherence, and the child's ability and willingness to take medications. They should also assess the setting in which the child is cared for, and the extent to which people are aware of the child's HIV status. If the family is trying to keep the child's HIV infection secret, they may be relabeling or hiding medication bottles, allowing the child to miss doses when not at home, or avoiding filling prescriptions at the local pharmacy. In fact, social stigma and fear of disclosure may have as much influence on adherence as other factors, such as socioeconomic status and high-risk lifestyles.

Children tend to be fairly adherent when they have a good relationship with their primary care provider. Clinicians may seek behavioral consultation to help with pill-swallowing techniques.

At first John resists his caregivers' attempts to get him to take his medications more regularly. However, over time, he develops a trusting relationship with workers at the HIV clinic, who repeatedly explain to him the importance of taking his medication. John feels more cared for, and his acting-out behavior decreases.

Which techniques facilitate adherence in children and adolescents?

Adolescents with chronic medical illnesses tend to experiment with their medications, so clinicians should expect some non-adherence with HAART. However, an adolescent's level of risk behavior does not predict nonadherence (Belzer et al., 1998).

Threatening young people or trying to "scare" them into being adherent is not usually effective. It is more effective to work with adolescents to develop common goals, and provide repeated nonjudgmental explanations about the benefits of adherence.

To facilitate adherence, many treatment and drug trials occur in family-centered, multidisciplinary settings (Remafedi, 1998), which are associated with better clinic attendance and less use of emergency services. Given that, it may be helpful to create the same type of treatment setting for children with HIV. Facilitated peer support groups are also an effective strategy. Not only do they provide a way for infected youth to learn stress management techniques for coping with HIV, they also give them the opportunity to develop and share specific strategies for taking their medications.

Clinicians should remember that adherence is not a fixed state. Young people often regress in times of stress. It is important to continually reassess pediatric patients for adherence, and to develop targeted inventions to limit stresses that may affect their willingness or ability to take their medications as prescribed. To provide effective care for HIV-infected youth and their families, the treatment team must be willing to persevere and be flexible.

> ## Case study: Child working on disclosure
>
> Darrell is a 7-year-old boy, infected through vertical transmission. His mother, who has told very few people about her own serostatus – not even her current boyfriend – will not agree to disclose Darrell's infection to him or to others. Because she brings her boyfriend to Darrell's appointments, clinicians have to be careful about the information they discuss.

When is it appropriate or necessary to disclose HIV serostatus?

Parents or guardians often withhold information about HIV serostatus from children out of fear that the information may cause depression, anxiety, and a decline in health. Because disclosure often involves discussing sexual activities or drug use, many families try to keep it secret. The stigma and shame of keeping HIV a secret may cause families to feel more isolated, and impair a child's emotional well-being.

There is no single, easy guide to deciding when and/or who to tell about HIV infection, although clinicians generally agree that a child's cognitive and emotional maturity are more important than age in determining when to disclose. By disclosing developmentally appropriate facts about the illness, clinicians and families can help children adapt psychologically and reduce feelings of distrust, isolation, confusion, and depression (American Academy of Pediatrics, 1999). Less secrecy about HIV helps children feel less shame and leads to greater intimacy in family relationships. In certain instances, disclosure may not be in a child's best interests. For example, when a child is critically ill, or too impulsive or disinhibited due to HACM or pre-existent cognitive difficulties, clinicians and families may choose not to disclose to the child. There is a concern that indiscriminate disclosure by the child would increase stigma and discrimination. However, the child's HIV status must be disclosed and discussed before he or she becomes sexually active.

How do you prepare a child for disclosure?

Disclosure work is done over multiple individual and family sessions. It is geared to providing developmentally appropriate information, and should include: what a virus is, who can get it, how it is transmitted, and the difference between "virus" and "disease". After each session, the clinician should tell other caregivers what has been discussed and how to handle questions as they come up. Ultimately, the child learns that he is infected and what can be done to help.

To ensure the child understands what he is being told, the clinician should provide information in small increments, and ask the child to repeat it back. Depending on the age and cognitive abilities of the child, the information can be communicated using visual aids, stories (such as "Jimmy and the Eggs' Virus"), coloring worksheets or videos (National Pediatric and Family HIV Resource Center, 1999). For more information about disclosure strategies for different developmental stages, please consult www.pedhivaids.org/education.

What do you do when a family refuses to disclose to the child?

Some parents or guardians cannot be convinced that disclosure is helpful. In these cases, the team should continue to support the family and try to understand the fears that make them unwilling to disclose. Over time, by working with the family and joining with them in common goals, the clinician may be able to help them address their fears and change their view.

Clinicians begin to work on disclosure when they feel Darrell is developmentally able to understand the information without indiscriminately revealing it to everyone. Eventually they are able to convince his mother he needs this information to decrease his anxiety. The therapist also addresses Darrell's mother's need to disclose her own status to her current boyfriend.

How do you prepare a child and family to transfer from a pediatric setting to an adult setting?

All children with chronic medical illnesses and their families find moving from a pediatric setting to an adult setting difficult. The transition goes most smoothly when clinicians from each clinic setting can demonstrate to the patients and their families that:
- they communicate well with each other
- valuable medical information will not be lost.

For any patient who has attended the pediatric clinic for any length of time, work on the transition should begin as early as a year in advance. Clinicians from the two clinics should be familiar with each other's services and how they differ in order to prepare patients for any changes.

During the transition from the pediatric to adult setting, some children may "act out" by being non-adherent. Clinicians should address this potential risk openly and discuss the risks with the child. To help ensure the child does not feel cast aside or forgotten, clinicians should explore a number of different strategies, such as arranging for the child to make a "check-back" visit to the pediatric clinic or establishing a photo board of "graduates" from the pediatric clinic.

Conclusion

For many children and adolescents who have access to antiretroviral therapies, HIV has become more a chronic disorder and less a lethal illness. However, antiretroviral treatment regimens can be cumbersome, and adherence is a serious problem for some young people. Mental health clinicians can play a key role in increasing adherence to drug regimens, managing pain, and providing psychiatric treatment for the family.

As children with HIV live longer, their ability to meet normal developmental milestones and their educational needs take on new significance. Mental health clinicians can assist in addressing developmental issues by, for example, helping families plan appropriate education programs for children with mild cognitive impairment, helping adolescents and their families manage emerging sexuality issues, and providing education to reduce behaviors that may put others at risk.

Effective treatment of children and adolescents living with HIV requires cooperation among pediatricians, social workers, psychologists, psychiatrists, case managers, and occupational, physical, and language therapists. Whenever possible, a child's treatment strategies and case management should be coordinated with community-based agencies.

REFERENCES

American Academy of Pediatrics. Disclosure of illness status to children and adolescents with HIV infection. *Pediatrics*, **103**(1) (1999): 164–6.

Belzer, M., Fuchs, D., Tucker, D. and Slonimsky, G. High risk behaviors are not predictive of antiretroviral non-adherence in HIV+ youth. *12th World AIDS Conference*, Geneva, June 28–July 3, 1998.

Bose, S., Moss, H. A., Brouwers, P. *et al.* Psychologic adjustment of HIV-infected school-age children. *Developmental and Behavioral Pediatrics*, **15** (1994): S26–33.

Brady, M. T., McGrath, N., Brouwers, P. *et al.* Randomized study of the tolerance and efficacy of high- versus low-dose zidovudine in human immunodeficiency virus – infected children with mild to moderate symptoms (AIDS clinical trials group 128). *Journal of Infectious Diseases*, **173**(5) (1996): 1097–106.

Brouwers, P., Charles, D., Heyes, M. P. *et al.* Neurobehavioral manifestations of symptomatic HIV-1 disease in children: can nutritional factors play a role? *Journal of Nutrition*, **126** (1996): 2651S–62S.

Brown, L. K., Lourie, K. J. and Pao, M.. Children and adolescents living with HIV and AIDS: a review. *Journal of Child Psychology and Psychiatry*, **41**(1) (2000): 81–96.

Centers for Disease Control and Prevention, *HIV AIDS Surveillance Report*. Mid-year edition, **13** (2001).

Grassi, L., Righi, R., Sighinolfi, L. *et al.* Coping styles and psychosocial-related variables in HIV-infected patients. *Psychosomatics*, **39** (1998): 350–9.

Hansell, P. S., Hughes, C. B., Caliandro, G. *et al.* The effect of a social support boosting intervention on stress, coping and social support in caregivers of children with HIV/AIDS. *Nursing Research*, **47** (1998): 79–86.

Lewis, M. (ed.) *Child and Adolescent Psychiatry: A Comprehensive Textbook*, 2nd edn. Baltimore: Williams and Wilkins, 1996.

Markowitz, J. C., Klerman, G. L. and Perry, S. Interpersonal psychotherapy of depressed HIV-seropositive outpatients. *Hospital and Community Psychiatry*, **43** (1991): 885–90.

Mufson, L., Moreau, D., Weissman, M. *et al.* Modifications of interpersonal psychotherapy with depressed adolescents (IPT-A): Phase I and II studies. *Journal of the American Academy of Child and Adolescent Psychiatry*, **33**(5) (1994): 695–705.

National Pediatric and Family HIV Resource Center (NPHRC). (1999). Complex issue of HIV disclosure to children and adolescents in the forefront. www.thebody.com/nphrc/disclosure.html

Pao, M., Lyon, M., D'Angelo, L. D. *et al.* Psychiatric diagnoses in HIV seropositive adolescents. *Archives of Pediatrics and Adolescent Medicine*, **154**(3) (2000): 240–4.

Papola, P., Alvarez, M. and Cohen, H. Developmental and service needs of school-age children with human immunodeficiency virus infection: a descriptive study. *Pediatrics*, **94**(6) (1994): 914–18.

Remafedi, G. The University of Minnesota Youth and AIDS Projects' Adolescent Early Intervention Program. *Journal of Adolescent Health*, **23** (1998): 115–21.

Rotheram-Borus, M. J., Lee, M. B., Gwadz, M., and Draimin, B. An intervention for parents with AIDS and their adolescent children. *American Journal of Public Health*, **91**(8) (2001): 1294–302.

UNAIDS. Global summary of the HIV/AIDS epidemic, December 2000. World AIDS Campaign, 2000. (Available as a living document at www.unaids.org/wac/2000).

AIDS Epidemic Update. Children and young people in a world of AIDS. Joint United Nations Program on HIV/AIDS, (2001). (Available as a living document at www.unaids.org/epidemic_update)

WEB SITES

Disclosure strategies for different developmental stages (Available as a living document at www.pedhivaids.org/education.)

12

Uninfected children of parents with HIV

Cynthia J. Telingator, M. D.

Instructor in Psychiatry, Harvard Medical School, Cambridge, MA Training Director, Division of Child and Adolescent Psychiatry, Cambridge Hospital/Cambridge Health Alliance, Cambridge, MA, USA

Introduction

According to a report presented in a special session on HIV/AIDS at the United Nations in June 2001, "The total number of children orphaned by the epidemic since it began −13.2 million − is forecast to more than double by 2010" (UNAIDS/WHO, 2001). The largest number of orphans live in sub-Saharan Africa, but the Caribbean and Asia are expected to experience large increases in the number of children orphaned by AIDS. Children whose parents have HIV must cope, often in silence, with the emotional, economic, social, and physical sequelae of this disease. These children lose their parents, their communities, and other important sources of support. They experience multiple losses and feelings of shame, responsibility, and isolation. In most parts of the world, the societal infrastructure for dealing with HIV is compromised and overwhelmed.

Working with these children and their families can be difficult, but also rewarding. Many of their issues are similar to those faced by children dealing with grief due to other causes, but many are unique.

Case study: An uninfected preschool child

A woman with HIV, who was receiving treatment at a multidisciplinary HIV clinic, was concerned about her 3-year-old daughter's speech and language delays, and asked that the child, Angela, be evaluated. Although her parents were first generation immigrants from Haiti, Angela was born in the USA. Her parents spoke primarily Creole, but were also able to converse in English. Staff at the clinic learned that the father was also infected with HIV although he wanted his diagnosis to remain a secret from his wife.

A child psychiatrist in the clinic began an evaluation. Concerned that the child presented with echolalia as well as echopraxia, the psychiatrist arranged for Angela to be seen by a neurologist and a speech therapist. Based on the evaluation, the psychiatrist was able to understand the child's behaviors as a manifestation of anxiety.

HIV and Psychiatry. A Training and Resource Manual, Second Edition, ed. Kenneth Citron, Marie-Josée Brouillette, and Alexandra Beckett. Published by Cambridge University Press. © Cambridge University Press 2005.

Angela had been exposed to domestic violence, but she was also watching her parents change due to the impact of HIV on their physical and emotional health.

Soon after the referral, Angela's mother's health rapidly deteriorated. She developed cognitive difficulties and became psychotic. The mother's psychosis and dementia confused Angela who helplessly watched her mother's physical and emotional deterioration. Angela was placed in a preschool setting with other children whose parents had HIV. A psychiatrist involved with the clinic saw her twice a week for group therapy in that setting. Over time Angela was taught how to name and identify feelings and, as she developed the tools to describe her experience, she began to emerge from her shell. The psychiatrist and teacher worked with her and the other children, validating the changes they saw in their parents and naming these changes as a consequence of their illness. As Angela's anxiety and posttraumatic stress disorder (PTSD) were addressed in therapy, most of her presenting symptoms subsided. Over time, the clinician built trust with Angela, her parents, and the extended family.

When Angela's mother was placed in a long-term medical facility, the child remained with her father in their apartment. However, within a month of her mother's departure, her father was diagnosed with Kaposi's sarcoma and his health declined rapidly. The father's deterioration compromised his ability to care for his daughter. No guardianship plans had been made for Angela because her mother had believed that the father was healthy. His secrecy precluded the involvement of other family members in either the child's or the parent's care. With the father's consent, clinic staff made emergency plans to place Angela in a pre-adoptive home. As he neared death, he made the decision to disclose the nature of his and his wife's illness to the family. Angela was then moved from the pre-adoptive home, where she had lived for 2 months, to a relative's home. Several weeks later her father died, and on the eve of her father's wake, her mother died. She was orphaned at the age of four because of AIDS.

How should a clinician approach a young child who is HIV affected?

An evaluation of any child or adolescent affected by HIV must be within the context of the family. According to many studies of the psychological impact of the death of a parent in two-parent families, the surviving parent's ability to cope and support the child through the grieving process is one of the single most important factors in the child's psychological well-being (Raveis et al, 1999). Children like Angela who are orphaned, unlike children of war who lose a parent, often do not have a community to support them. The shame and stigma which surround HIV can isolate families, and the isolation often persists after the parent's death.

In this situation, long-term intermittent contact with a therapist can be of great benefit to the family. Although the family may initially reject the mental health clinicians' invitation to speak about their experience, they will often accept help negotiating an overwhelming system to access benefits and services. With gentle persistence, the clinician can gain the family's trust, and the family will often reach out, particularly when parents become concerned about their children's well-being. At this point, the clinician should discuss with parents their wishes about addressing the child's questions about the parents' and/or siblings' illness. This is an opportunity for the therapist to discuss ways to validate what the child is witnessing, even if the illness is not named, and to invite parents and children to express their feelings, fears, and hopes for their future and the future of other family members.

How should Angela be assessed?

Angela's clinically complicated presentation is likely a result of internal and external factors. In assessing her, the clinician would:

- consider the many factors before the onset of HIV-related illness that might have affected her early development, including domestic violence, maternal depression, and poverty
- determine how witnessing her parents' physical and psychological demise would compound the psychological insults she had already endured
- rule out a medical cause of her presentation
- understand the cultural and language issues which may have contributed to Angela's behavior and language delays.

Angela's guardians gave permission for the relationship with the clinician to continue after her parents' death. Despite the tragedy she endured, Angela, unlike many AIDS orphans, had a stable home environment after the death of her parents. She also had an ongoing therapeutic relationship with her psychiatrist. This helped to provide some continuity in her life and a foundation, which enabled her to move ahead developmentally.

What cultural issues should the clinician consider when treating children of HIV-positive parents?

Clinicians must educate themselves and be sensitive to the cultural and religious beliefs of the families they are treating. Cultural awareness and sensitivity will further the alliance with the families, and enhance the clinicians' ability to work with families of different cultural backgrounds (see Chapter 16A on cultural diversity).

To accept psychiatric care for their children, many parents must overcome the stigma and shame of their illness, as well as their own sense of inadequacy and guilt as a parent for having contracted HIV disease. This can be a major obstacle in doing preventive work with these families. Parents often need extensive individual counseling before they will allow their children to be treated.

Angela's parents had to overcome many obstacles in order to accept psychiatric treatment. Angela's mother was concerned that others might think Angela was "crazy". This arose from a belief by many in her community that anyone needing psychiatric care was "crazy". Angela's mother was unusual in her ability to overcome this stigma, and seek what she felt would be the best intervention for her daughter in the long term.

What role will a child's capacity to form attachments play in her ability to utilize treatment?

A child's early attachment history, and her capacity to form attachments will likely affect her ability to successfully grieve the loss of her parents and proceed developmentally. Formulating an intervention strategy for children affected by HIV should include an awareness of the child's capacity to form attachments, and utilize treatment modalities that address this issue.

Is disclosure necessary for therapy to be successful?

Treatment for HIV-affected children should be tailored to the individual child's needs within the context of the family. The clinician must be aware of and respect the parent's wishes around disclosure. Whether or not the name of the parent's illness is disclosed, it is important for the clinician to find a means to speak about what is occurring in the lives of all family members. By validating the social, economic, and physical changes the child has witnessed as a consequence of the illness, the clinician can lessen the child's sense of personal responsibility and confusion. This dialogue can also help the parent make guardianship plans, and foster attachment to new caregivers.

How might Angela's life have been different if she had an HIV-seropositive sibling? Is there a difference between the experience of siblings of those infected with HIV versus those who have siblings with other chronic illnesses?

An uninfected child in a family with an infected child has to deal with the fear of another loss as well as survivor guilt. This experience is not so different from that of children who have siblings with other chronic illnesses. In those countries where HIV treatment is available, the course of HIV disease has changed, from an acute terminal illness to a more chronic disease. As in families with other illnesses, siblings learn to tolerate the chronicity of the illness and the intermittent medical interventions, and family dynamics shift. In families with HIV, the difference is that one or both of the parents have the same disease.

The guilt parents feel about transmitting the disease is often played out in their relationship with an ill child. Uninfected siblings can feel both guilty and relieved for being HIV negative, and jealous of the time and attention the ill child receives. Uninfected siblings also are often asked to maintain the "secrecy" of the illness. They are likely to feel responsible for protecting the "ill" child in situations where the parents are not present. Because of their need to maintain the family's privacy, uninfected children can become isolated from peers and other adults who may otherwise be able to give them emotional and developmental support.

Case study: Working with an uninfected adolescent

Wendy is a 15-year-old Caucasian girl whose mother has a history of drug abuse. Wendy and her siblings were removed from their mother's home when they were preschoolers because of neglect. Wendy was sexually abused while in foster placement. She was returned to her mother after her mother stopped using drugs. Currently, the family consists of Wendy, her brother Joe, who is 8, her 13-year-old sister, Jan, who is in a long-term psychiatric facility, and her mother.

When her mother was diagnosed with HIV, she told Wendy and asked her not to tell her siblings, thus isolating Wendy in her grief. Recently Jan was informed by staff at the psychiatric facility of her mother's diagnosis without her mother's permission and has subsequently refused all contact with her. Wendy and her mother believe that Joe "doesn't know", although he has been in situations where his mother's diagnosis was openly discussed.

Since learning of her mother's diagnosis, Wendy has made two suicide attempts, both times using medications prescribed for her mother's HIV and related illnesses. In these suicide attempts she expressed both her despair and rage at her mother, and her identification with her as sick and dying. Following her second suicide attempt, Wendy was referred for psychiatric evaluation.

When Wendy meets with a psychiatrist, she talks about the painful process of watching her mother deteriorate, and her struggle to maintain a connection to her in face of her rage, guilt, and sorrow. The changes she has witnessed in her mother have been frightening and confusing. Wendy describes her mother to the psychiatrist with fear in her eyes; "she has chicken legs and a big belly. Why doesn't she do something so she could look more normal? She can fit into my clothes now."

The weekend after this session, Wendy's mother took her to buy school clothes. Wendy wanted to buy pants a size too small for her as a way of differentiating herself from her mother who was physically and emotionally regressing to a point that was too terrifying for Wendy to bear. A fight ensued between the two of them, and Wendy ran away from home for 2 days. In a family meeting after her return, Wendy was able to express some of her fears and ask that her mother begin to consider the question of where the children would live after she dies. Wendy has been more able to express her concern about her own future, her dreams, and her fears. Because she has aspirations to do more than her mother has done, she struggles with feelings of betrayal and loyalty. She worries about who will raise her younger brother. She knows her mother's fantasy is for her to assume the role of parent after her mother dies.

As with many female teenagers in her position, Wendy is at high risk for pregnancy, substance abuse, and HIV. In a recent session she stated, "I wanted to leave my house when I was 16, but if I'm going to have to take care of my brother, I might as well have my own kid." She has begun to drink and has become sexually active. Although she knows about safe sex practices and has been adhering to them so far, she recently commented, "Well I may get pregnant, but I won't get HIV." This statement reflects her struggles with her ambivalent feelings towards her mother, and her identification with her in face of an impending loss.

What role will Wendy's capacity to attach play in her ability to utilize treatment?

Unlike Angela, Wendy was insecurely attached to her mother before her mother's illness. Her attachment behaviors were recreated in the context of the therapy. Wendy was only able to use her therapist intermittently, as she could tolerate, to work through her feelings towards her mother.

What developmental issues are significant for an adolescent affected by HIV?

Because feelings of aggression and sexuality are heightened during adolescence, HIV infection itself is a concrete threat. It is a means of identifying with a dying parent, a way of joining them to avoid abandonment, a way of striking out against a parent, and a way of striking out against oneself due to survivor guilt. Teenagers normally struggle with developmental issues of separation and individuation. For teenagers with an HIV-infected parent, the struggle is intensified and complicated by the knowledge that the separation may represent a permanent loss.

Adolescents in HIV-affected families may have contact with the law as they unconsciously seek a more powerful person or persons to contain feelings of aggression, rage, and fear. Acting out in adolescents may also manifest with increased sexuality, which is a way to punish oneself for the parent's illness and expected death, as well as serve the unconscious wish to replace the lost object with a baby. The adolescent may hold the fantasy that a grandchild will give the parent a reason to live, an unconscious offering to the ill parent to fill a void the adolescent is incapable of fulfilling. Each adolescent's coping style will vary, but most are vulnerable for high-risk behaviors.

Wendy eventually got pregnant while involved with a young man who physically abused and rejected her. After her child was born, her mother invited her back home, and Wendy returned with the gift of a granddaughter. Her mother was stabilized medically by the introduction of protease inhibitors. Because her mother told her that the therapist would attempt to have her daughter removed by the department of social services, Wendy stopped seeing him. She sacrificed the therapist in order to preserve her newly constructed family and the hope of keeping her mother alive.

Wendy returned to the therapist several years later to seek help with anxiety. She had stopped using drugs, and created a life of her own. She went back to school to attain a college degree, and held a full time job. Soon after she returned to therapy, she got pregnant for the second time.

As is true with many families with HIV, Wendy's story includes multigenerational losses which have not been acknowledged or grieved as each generation repeats the previous generation's story without the hoped-for brighter outcome.

What are the countertransference issues the therapist may have been dealing with?

The countertransference issues are complex and the feelings often overwhelming. The mental health clinician must confront her own feelings of helplessness in the face of a disease that can devastate and destroy families. The therapist, like the child, may regress and experience the HIV-infected adult and/or child's deterioration as a result of her own action or inaction. To defend against this fear as well as the expression of her own dependent longings, the therapist is likely to unconsciously deny the impact of these losses.

To help facilitate the grief process, the therapist must be able to bear the effect of grieving a multitude of losses. The therapist must acknowledge both the usefulness, as well as the destructiveness of her denial in her own effort and ultimately the family's effort to mourn. Working with HIV-affected families, the therapist is apt to struggle with complicated feelings arising from her identification with the parents and the children, who are attempting to cope with complex medical and psychosocial issues. She will also have to contend with her guilt of surviving.

The therapist must be attentive to the vicarious traumatization she may experience as it may cause her to become either overinvolved or detached and unavailable. Support and supervision are necessary to help the therapist cope with:

- the child's wish, the parent's wish, and her own wish to fulfill the role of parent
- the guilt associated with having the wish, and for not being able to fulfill it.

This work is long term, and the ramifications of this illness will be felt within the family system for a long time.

How has the course of treatment changed in parts of the world where HIV medications are available?

Treatment for uninfected children is likely to continue over a long period of time. Early contact can benefit the family, by allowing the clinician to participate in preventive mental health care. Brief interventions may assist with emotional struggles, which can become entwined with developmental issues. Different members of the family may reconnect with the therapist again and again at different points of their lives.

The treatment begins with the diagnosis, but does not end with the death of a family member. Every effort must be made to maintain a therapeutic connection with the uninfected children after the death of a parent or sibling. In too many clinic settings, the case is closed when a family member dies. To provide continuity for the family, arrangements must be made, within or outside the clinic, for the same clinician to provide mental healthcare during the infected patient's illness and after the death. The family may be hesitant to reach out for mental healthcare after the death of the parent due to feelings of shame, stigma, and the lack of awareness of how grief manifests in children. But, when a clinician is already involved with the family, the new guardians will know that the clinician has become a trusted member of the care team, and will allow the clinician to continue working with the uninfected children after a parent's death.

Conclusion

The impact of HIV on families is devastating. It is a war without armor, and the orphans are left to grieve for a person whom the community has often shunned. Therapists provide a setting where uninfected children can stay connected to their parents in love and in rage. This can make an important difference in allowing children to meet developmental challenges while contending with their grief. HIV is an epidemic that continues to have a profound impact on the lives of many families across the globe, but each small intervention can help to give a child, an adolescent, and an adult hope for the future.

REFERENCES

Raveis, V. H., Siegel, K. and Karus, D. Children's psychological distress following the death of a parent. *Journal of Youth and Adolescence*, **28**(2) (1999): 165–180.

UNAIDS/WHO. Fact Sheet: Orphans and Children in a World of AIDS. *United Nations Special Session on HIV/AIDS*, New York: June 25–27, 2001. Available at www.unaids.org

SUGGESTED READING

Boyd-Franklin, N., Danovsky, M. and Lowrie, K. (eds.) *Children, Families, and HIV/AIDS.* New York: Guilford Press, 1995.

Committee on Pediatric AIDS. Disclosure of illness status to children and adolescents with HIV infection. *Pediatrics,* **103** (1999): 509–10.

Foster, G. Supporting community efforts to assist orphans in Africa. *New England Journal of Medicine*, **36**(24) (2002): 1907–10.

Gabelle, S., Greendel, J. and Andieman, W. (eds.) *Forgotten Children of the AIDS Epidemic.* New Haven: Yale University Press, 1995.

Michaels, D. and Levine, C. Estimates of the number of motherless youth orphaned by AIDS in the United States. *Journal of the American Medical Association,* **268** (1992): 3456–61.

Schuster, M. A., Kanouse, D. E., Morton, S. C. *et al.* HIV-infected parents and their children in the United States. *American Journal of Public Health,* **90**(7) (2000): 1074–81.

Telingator, C. Children, adolescents, and families infected and affected by HIV and AIDS. *Child and Adolescent Clinics of North America,* **9**(2) (2000): 295–312.

13

Psychological issues faced by gay men

Peter E. Kassel, Psy.D.[1] and Stephen Knowlton, Ph.D.[2]

[1] Assistant Professor of Psychiatry, Harvard Medical School, Cambridge, MA
Staff Psychologist, Massachusetts Institute of Technology Medical Department,
Private Practice in Brookline, MA, USA
[2] Licensed Psychologist, Private Practice in Somerville and Boston, MA, USA

Introduction

In Western culture, many of those with HIV infection are gay men. To help psychiatrists better understand the psychological context of their gay patients, this chapter:

- reviews historical and contemporary theories of gay male development, discusses psychoanalytic theory of male homosexuality, presents a critique of certain aspects of more traditional psychodynamic theory, and discusses newer theories
- describes the difference between sexual orientation and gender identity
- discusses the impact of growing up gay on psychological development, paying particular attention to: poor self-esteem and internalized homophobia, and their relationship to shame and widespread inhibition; the impairment of normal relational development and the splitting off of sexuality from relationships; the particular importance of adolescence in gay male development; and the palliative effects of new opportunities that arise for many gay men during adult development.

Review of psychoanalytic theory

Throughout his career, Freud thought and wrote about male homosexuality (e.g., Freud, 1905, 1922, 1935), exploring the topic from a number of different perspectives. He saw homosexuality as reflecting arrested psychosexual development in the context of the constitutional bisexuality of all humans, and thus as somewhat pathological. Freud also conflated the concepts of sexual orientation and gender identity (discussed at greater length below). However, his attitude remained humane and measured.

HIV and Psychiatry. A Training and Resource Manual, Second Edition, ed. Kenneth Citron, Marie-Josée Brouillette, and Alexandra Beckett. Published by Cambridge University Press. © Cambridge University Press 2005.

Subsequent psychoanalytic thinkers, culminating with many active in the USA after the Second World War, such as Irving Bieber (1962) and Charles Socarides (1968, 1978), assumed increasingly homophobic stances. Bieber (1962) postulated that male homosexuality resulted from a "triangular family constellation" consisting of a close-binding, intimate relationship with the mother and a detached, hostile father. Socarides (1968), on the other hand, saw homosexuality as preoedipal in origin, resulting from a boy's failure to separate and individuate from his mother. For Socarides and others, the failure to reach a healthy "oedipal resolution" resulted in the boy choosing to love men just as his mother did, instead of identifying with his father in loving women. The main problems with both theories include:

- their failure to account for the substantial number of heterosexual men with similar developmental histories
- their generalization from a small clinical sample
- the confusion of correlation with causality (e.g., gay sons may disproportionately elicit closeness from mothers and detachment from fathers).

Nonpsychoanalytic approaches to understanding homosexuality have generally been less pathologizing, beginning from the earliest theories of Havelock Ellis (1900) and Magnus Hirschfeld (1914). Important contributions include:

- Kinsey *et al.*'s (1948) well-known assertion that the high frequency of homosexual behavior precludes its consideration as pathological.
- Hooker's (1957) study in which psychological testing of heterosexual and homosexual men failed to demonstrate measureable differences in levels of pathology.
- Saghir and Robins's (1971) finding that gay and straight subjects did not differ significantly in terms of psychopathology.
- Bell *et al.*'s (1981) exhaustive social psychological study of gay and straight men which found that family differences similar to those described by Bieber do exist, but fail to account for differential outcome in sexual orientation.

It is worth noting that certain psychoanalytic researchers during this period also approached homosexuality with fewer negative preconceptions (e.g., Stoller, 1973).

More contemporary theories regarding the psychological development of gay men reflect several changes. First, theorists no longer equate homosexuality with psychological maladjustment. The vast majority of contemporary psychological theorists and authors understand homosexuality to be one of several forms of sexual orientation which, in and of itself, has nothing to do with psychological health. In this regard, sexual orientation and psychopathology have been rightly understood by such mainstream organizations and publications as the *Journal of the American Psychoanalytic Association* as independent dimensions of psychological functioning

(Friedman and Downey, 1998). Furthermore, the expression of homosexuality is seen as one point of a spectrum of healthy human sexuality that is not only broad, but also somewhat flexible across the life span. This perspective reflects the integration of scientific findings beginning with Kinsey *et al.* (1948) which describe a varied rather than fixed range of expression of sexual behaviors and orientations throughout life.

Interestingly, these changes follow a shift from more traditional (drive) theory to more contemporary relational and interpersonal psychoanalytic thinking. They reflect a growing awareness of the association between psychological health and an interest in intimate relationships in general, irrespective of the gender of the object. Theorists such as Mitchell (1981), Chodorow (1989), Isay (1989), LeVay (1993), LeVay and Hamer (1994), Butler (1995), Dimen (1995), Frommer (1995), Corbett (1996, 1998), and Layton (1998) have also shed light on the importance of the complex interplay of biology, family, and culture on sexual orientation and gender identity.

More contemporary theorizing has focused on understanding the *impact* of growing up gay in a predominantly heterosexual culture in which difference and, in particular, gender nonconformity in boys, is often vilified. The consequences of growing up gay are always profound and usually complicate psychological development for gay men (Isay, 1989; Corbett, 1996, 1998; Kassel and Franko, 2000; Phillips, 2001). It is very difficult for gay individuals to mature without significant scars to their self-esteem. Their childhood experiences with peers and family members, especially fathers, are frequently characterized by isolation, rejection, shame, and an absence of a sense of belonging, and can foster the poor self-esteem, and sense of inadequacy and defectiveness many gay men experience.

The issue of gender identity

The issue of gender nonconformity has often been conflated with homosexuality (Freud, 1930; Socarides, 1968), but it is important to distinguish between these two concepts. Homophobia is driven primarily by "hatred and fear of what is perceived and labeled as feminine in men" (Isay, 1989) rather than relating essentially to sexuality. To simplify a complex set of ideas, many earlier psychoanalytic authors presented several concepts as unidimensional that are, in reality, multidimensional and multivariant. For example, they held that to love men was the exclusive domain of women. From this point of view, loving men is in itself feminizing. Separating out the two dimensions (i.e., gender identity and sexual orientation) permits one to see the possibility of being a man, having a masculine gender identity, and loving men. Gender theorists (Layton, 1998; Chodorow, 1999) have illustrated how devaluing gay men because of a perceived feminine gender identity reflects a general devaluation of what is feminine.

Case study: Gender nonconformity, stigma, and shame

Paul is a 35-year-old gay white man who works as an investment adviser. He has been HIV-seropositive for 6 years and has been taking HAART since seroconverting. He remains asymptomatic with a low but detectable viral load.

Paul is the youngest of four children from a middle-class family. He describes his family as combining a fierce sense of loyalty with a great deal of emotional inarticulateness, unacknowledged vulnerability, hurt, and rage. Paul has always felt loved by his parents but he has also felt deeply injured by their inability to express their love in a supportive manner. For instance, when he was in kindergarten, he tearfully told his mother that other children had taunted him as "femmy" to which his mother replied, "Well, honey, you are femmy" and referred to some of his "girlish mannerisms" and his tendency to play with the girls in the neighborhood. He still feels a considerable amount of humiliation and anger about this. When he discussed the incident with his mother as an adult, she explained that she was "just trying to be honest".

The family has a significant history of alcohol abuse and dependence. Paul himself became alcoholic in high school. He reports being aware that drinking helped boost his self-confidence and numb feelings of anxiety and self-consciousness about his attraction to other boys. He succeeded academically in high school and college. During college he came out to himself, and then to friends and family, who reacted supportively. After graduation from college, Paul began working and did well professionally. In spite of his achievements and support from friends and family, Paul continued to struggle with feelings of being inadequate and unlovable, and his drinking worsened. He became involved with a lover who was HIV-positive and "partied" extensively (i.e., used various recreational drugs, often in sexually charged situations like circuit parties and bath-houses). Paul and his lover consistently practiced safer sex with each other, but Paul often had unprotected sex with other men while intoxicated. It seems likely that he became infected from one of these encounters.

When he found out he was HIV-seropositive, Paul stopped drinking and started attending Alcoholics Anonymous. As his boyfriend continued to use drugs, Paul found it increasingly untenable to maintain both his sobriety and his relationship. He broke up with his partner, and feelings of depression and anger re-emerged. Without alcohol to ameliorate these feelings, he sought psychotherapy.

How do shame and stigma concerning early childhood gender-nonconformity affect psychological development?

During their psychological maturation, repeated experiences of difference and rejection play a central role in the development of shame and inhibition in gay men. Numerous studies (Bell *et al.*, 1981; Zuger, 1984; Bailey *et al.*, 1995; Whitman, 1977) have demonstrated that "pre-homosexual" boys (i.e., boys who grow up to be gay) experience themselves as significantly different from their peers in a general way, and ascribe these differences to such dimensions as not liking sports, feeling "feminine," enjoying solitary activities associated only indirectly with gender (e.g., reading, drawing, music), and being far less likely to enjoy traditional boys' activities such as football and baseball. This sense of difference is frequently translated into "defectiveness" and can be carried into adulthood.

These "nonerotic behaviors" suggest the differing developmental pathways of heterosexual and homosexual boys (Friedman, 2001). Behaviors which are more gender-atypical or reflect "gender nonconformity" are more frequent among boys who grow up to have a gay sexual orientation (Zucker and Bradley, 1995). Owing to traits coded as "different", gay boys and young men often experience bullying and abusive treatment by male peers, siblings, and fathers, and suffer from the prolonged effects of these traumas well into adulthood (Friedman *et al.*, 1991; Corbett, 1996; Phillips, 2001). While most contemporary analytic theorists believe that homosexuality no longer falls within the category of "disease", the stigma and traumatization many gay men experience because of their boyhood gender role atypicality can and do lead to anxiety and depression which may, in turn, result in psychological difficulties or even psychiatric syndromes. Current thinking about homosexuality and pathology holds that sexual orientation itself is no longer understood to reflect pathology. If difficulties or even illnesses arise, they are understood to be consequent to the repetitive traumas associated with growing up gay in a society which is heterosexist and anti-homosexual. The experience many gay men have of their fathers as "distant" can compound their perception of childhood difference and may reflect a father's (conscious or not) awareness of and reaction to his son's pre-homosexuality. In a hopeful vein, however, the ways in which "growing up gay" may incline certain boys and men to socially advantageous behaviors such as altruism and less-encumbered creativity are less well understood. These areas seem very worthy of investigation.

Weekly individual therapy focused initially on supporting Paul's sobriety and helping improve his affect tolerance. Gradually, Paul became more able to address longstanding feelings of shame due to internalized homophobia rooted in narcissistic vulnerability about appearing and acting inadequately masculine. Paul came to understand that he sought out frequent casual sexual contact as a way to experience acceptance by other men, and to validate his attractiveness. The delicate task for the therapist was to empathize with his longing for the validation he sought and often felt from these encounters, while helping him reflect on the consciously unintended side effects (e.g., acquiring other sexually transmitted diseases) which not only affected his physical health but paradoxically undermined the project of improving his self-esteem.

Case study: Relational development – inhibition and the splitting-off of sexuality

Al is in his mid 40s. The third of four children who were first generation Americans, he grew up in a close-knit, religious family of Arab-American émigrés. He recalls knowing he was "different" from his earliest memories, by which he means "different" from other boys because of his attraction to them rather than to girls. He felt "different" from the other men in the family, for his interests and temperament were more in line with those of his sisters and mother.

He recalls being extremely modest about his body as a young boy and very anxious about appearing unclothed around other people. In this regard Al was different from his older brother, who seemed to share his father's comfort and sensibility regarding his own body and its exposure. His father, apparently out of a desire both to tease and to help remedy the situation, threatened to "walk in on" him when Al was naked after bathing. While Al knew his family's actions were meant to be affectionate, he found them humiliating and scary.

The family had deep religious beliefs and practices. Al recalls that sex was never talked about other than as "dirty" and something that only "impure sorts" would do. He recalled his mother admonishing him to "scrub his penis very well in the bath" one night, because "it is important to clean all the 'dirty' off it". His dawning awareness of his homosexuality posed a threat in at least two regards: he had strong sexual feelings and thoughts, themselves somewhat taboo in his family, and these outlaw desires concerned boys instead of girls. He spent years promising himself, and praying, that he would "stop being that way".

Al's modesty about being seen without clothing was compounded by his own hunger to "see" other boys. As he matured and became more aware of his sexual feelings, he became riveted by looking at other partially dressed or unclothed boys and men. On a few occasions, other boys at school would notice him looking at them longingly, and he was teased and humiliated. He became much more careful about letting others notice his looking. In his mid-adolescence he had several close friendships with girls and even a "girlfriend" whom he liked greatly and felt very close to, although he felt no romantic interest in her. At the same time, he remembers continuing to date her in hopes that he could be "won over or converted" to heterosexuality.

When Al reached college, his self-image was extremely poor, and he was very surprised that other men showed an interest in him. His first sexual experiences were accompanied by a tremendous amount of excitement and guilt. After each of the three times he had sex, he showered with very hot water, soaped himself repeatedly, and afterwards vowed to "never do that again".

Upon graduating from college, he moved to a larger city and felt a freedom to explore gay life and make friends with others like him. It was at this time that the AIDS epidemic began. He became tremendously fearful that he had been or would be exposed to HIV, and began a 12-year "monastic existence" without sexual contact with another person. In his late 30s, he dated once in a while, and on rare occasions became sexual with other men.

> In his 40s, Al was successful professionally yet had turned down several interesting promotions, instead nominating subordinates. At that point in his life, he began his most serious romantic relationship. He and his boyfriend shared many common interests, and enjoyed each other's company and lives immensely. Although strongly attracted to his new boyfriend, Al felt unable to be sexual with him. At first, these difficulties manifested themselves in a lack of desire. Despite feeling very drawn to his boyfriend, Al found himself thinking and believing "I'm not really turned on by him," and even wondered if he suffered from a testosterone deficiency accounting for his diminished sexual desire (he did not). His strictly sexual involvements with other men demonstrated to him that he did indeed experience sexual desire, but was afraid to be sexual with his boyfriend. He decided to seek psychotherapy.

How does growing up gay lead to inhibition and the splitting off of sexuality from relationships?

Another frequent psychological effect of growing up gay is an inhibition of healthy narcissistic aims, such as personal and professional initiative. Frequently, a man's awareness of his homosexuality can have a negative effect on aspects of healthy exhibitionism, such as drawing attention to oneself, ambition, creativity, agency, and willingness to pursue romantic relations. Because gay boys and men sense there is something fundamentally different about themselves, they grow up experiencing relatively little affirmation of their desires and interests. This sense of "badness of desire", combined with what children hear and learn about homosexuality as they mature, can lead them by inference to the conviction that there is something terribly wrong with them. They may despise and hide aspects of the self that may draw the focus of others and betray these differences. As they grow older, gay boys' and young men's resultant shame, disavowal, caution, and sneakiness often lead to conflicts in the expression of healthy exhibitionism.

Another manifestation of this conflict involves learning to "split off" or keep sexuality separate from relationships. Gay boys and men experimenting with their sexuality usually begin to do so within a context of tremendous furtiveness, anxiety, shame, and self-loathing. The young gay man's early sexual experiences frequently take place away from the scrutiny of his usual peer group. In this way, painful disapproval and humiliation are avoided, but so too are the potentially validating effects of peer encouragement and approval. Over time, this can lead to a more pronounced separation of sexuality from other forms of social and romantic relating.

Because gay men often keep sexuality and relationships separate in their early sexual lives, normal relational development may be derailed. Due to the occult nature of gay boys' sexual experimentation, they do not usually experience courting and dating in a more "normalized", safe, and reinforcing environment until the post-college years – considerably later than for their non-gay peers. This is a primary reason why many relationships between men in their 20s or early 30s can appear intense or immature. Socially and romantically, gay men at these ages are experimenting with and accomplishing what their non-gay cohort did normatively in their teens and 20s.

In psychotherapy, Al realized that he was deeply afraid that he had become infected with HIV in the past, and he could not bear to put his boyfriend at risk. He later came to understand that his fears of being HIV infected, and the early coupling of sexuality and "dirtiness" led to his conflicts about being sexual with a boyfriend he loved. Al internalized the belief that "sex was something you did not do to or with 'nice' people". As a result, he had grown up keeping sex and relationships separate.

Al used his psychotherapy to understand the connections between his childhood experiences of "difference" and a broader inhibition which protected him from "standing out". He became aware of how conflicted he had been until that point about pursuing his own professional advancement.

What is the specific importance of adolescence in gay male development?

For the young gay man, adolescence is the developmental stage when much of the turmoil associated with same-sex feelings becomes conscious. This period is frequently marked by painful longing, secrecy, and a cycle of excitement followed by shame and dread. "Desire" can be a problematic affect: if unrestrained, the consequences may be complicated and uncomfortable. During adolescence, the "back and forth" between desire, the need to hide that desire, and consequent shame, guilt, and frustration can be painful. Sporting matches and locker rooms occupy a very evocative place in the memory of many gay men, as the physical and/ or visual contact with peers gives rise to excruciating yearning. Young gay men, manifesting a hidden longing and lack of experience feeling appreciated and desired (in the same way most of their peers do), often begin their erotic and sexual lives feeling deficient. They experience *other men* (and not themselves) as those who are longed for, and their own desires as shameful.

This set of dynamics has a particular relevance for gay men with body image disturbance (Kassel and Franko, 2000). For many gay men, these painful developmental experiences are normative and lead them to experience themselves and their bodies as damaged or something about which to be self-conscious or ashamed. The focus among some gay men on becoming lean and muscled, without excess fat or body hair, reflects a nearly perfectly re-worked ending: as an adult, the muscled gay man has the power to become the object of affection and idolatry of other men, turning the tables on his own adolescence and early adulthood.

How do homophobia and low self-esteem influence the practice of safer sex?

The psychological sequelae of societal homophobia have profoundly affected how gay men address safer sex and HIV. While men vary in terms of the psychological determinants of their approaches to safer sex and the meanings of HIV, three themes deserve mention:

- Many men practice safer sex quite consistently, repeatedly test negative for HIV, and yet have a hard time psychologically internalizing or "believing" their seronegativity (Rofes, 1998). This seems to reflect an experience of "taint" related to their sexuality, which can lead to a feeling of inevitability about becoming infected (see Chapter 9 on psychotherapy).
- Low self-esteem can lead gay men to place themselves in harm's way by intentionally having unprotected anal sex, aware of the possibility of, and at times even desiring, HIV infection.
- Gay men may have sex that includes some risk of HIV infection in a way which is essentially healthy and life-affirming (Rofes, 1998). In important ways, "unprotected" sex is also the same as "regular" sex, especially for the generations of people who were sexual long before condom use became part of "recommended regular sex practice". Very few sexual behaviors carry absolutely no risk of HIV infection, so every gay man must calculate the trade-off that is healthiest for him. It may be important and psychologically healthy (and even unavoidable) to accept some risk of HIV infection when pursuing a behavior or relationship that holds significant meaning or gratification.

What specific developmental issues exist for gay men as they move from adolescence to adulthood?

Just as adolescence is often considered a second period of individuation (Blos, 1962) where "childlike notions about the nature of sexuality are revised" (Levy-Warren, 1996), the postadolescent and early to mid-adult periods often represent a "delayed adolescence", where a more authentic and positive sense of the self is consolidated. During this period, gay men may at first appear more immature than their peers as they practice with social grouping and dating, but this is often the first time that many gay men are able to experience being genuinely themselves.

In adulthood, gay men have opportunities to develop their more authentic social, relational, and sexual selves, and the importance of the peer group cannot be overestimated. For young adult gay men, the peer group is a place for practicing or "trying on" different ways of being, and receiving social approval for them (rather than the opprobrium they experienced as children and adolescents). In early adulthood, many gay men develop their first deeply intimate and nonsexual social friendships, as well as their first romantic relationships. These relationships can provide a context for healing and growth-enhancing object relationships, and may even form the basis for a more supportive "selected family" in the event that a gay man's family of origin is not able to affirm his sexual orientation. Within these relationships, many men choose to cohabitate, to purchase property together, and (increasingly) to raise children.

Case study: Deciding to raise a child

Tony was 45 and Bill 41 when they met, and they have been together for 8 years. When Tony met Bill, it had been 3 years since his previous lover had died of AIDS, and Tony questioned whether he wanted or could find someone to love as fully again. In Tony's previous relationship, he and his partner were newly diagnosed with HIV when they met. Although they had both been healthy and sick at different times in their relationship, Tony's overall health had remained good while his partner became sicker and died.

When Bill met Tony, he was leaving a relationship of 11 years. Bill had known he was seropositive for 6 years, and his previous partner was HIV-seronegative.

Tony and Bill took great pleasure in their mutual interests: arts and culture, world politics, and the outdoors. From their early childhoods, each had hoped to raise children. As adults, they assumed that their homosexuality and their HIV status posed two insurmountable obstacles to adoption. In light of all they shared in common, both expressed a sense of surprise and also bittersweetness at having met the other, for they had lost many friends and loved ones to AIDS, and each had suffered serious declines in his own health within the last year.

A few years into their relationship, Bill's physician recommended that he begin HAART. Not long after, Tony's physician did the same. Since that time, both of them have enjoyed robust health, renewed energy, and hopefulness. Bill began lengthy studies in pursuit of a career he had always longed for, and they took long and physically demanding trips to locations that challenged their endurance.

Bill and Tony both have siblings with children, and they also have several gay and lesbian friends (individuals and couples) who have chosen to raise children. With improved and stable health, they questioned whether their HIV status would necessarily limit their physical and emotional capacity to be fathers.

What issues should a gay man with HIV consider when deciding to raise a child?

When trying to decide whether to raise a child, a gay HIV-infected man should consider:

- the state of his health and likelihood that he will continue in good health
- any legal issues that might arise in the event of his death (if single), or for gay couples, if one partner survives the other
- resources available to support their decision (e.g., same-sex parenting networks, social service agencies).

Bill and Tony began careful research on the topic of same-sex adoption, talking with many people, agencies, and resources. They also spoke at length with their physicians. For both of them, being healthy, and physically and emotionally "up to the task", was essential before pursuing adoption. They also consulted legal experts about adoption to clarify any legal issues. They made the decision to adopt and are currently on a waiting list and expect to be new fathers within the next year.

Conclusion

The developmental pathways outlined here may be "generational" in that they describe gay men presently in their 20s, 30s, and beyond rather than adolescents and postadolescents. Younger gay men may experience less strife, stigma, and consequent self-hatred – and if so, this is a welcome, hopeful and much-needed change given the hostile environment, both socially and intrapsychically, in which gay men mature. In many urban areas, there are gay youth organizations, many of which are located in or affiliated with schools or universities. The spectre of growing up gay is no longer accompanied only by shame, secrecy, self-hatred, and expectations of a life lived in misery as was commonly the case even 15 years ago. In increasing numbers, gay men and women live their lives "in the open" without fear of social difficulty or legal barriers (witness the number of gay politicians and celebrities who are increasingly comfortable with being public about their lives). Political parties court gay men and lesbians for their votes and social clout. In many municipalities, discrimination on the basis of sexual orientation is now illegal, and legal systems have increasingly confirmed the rights of gay people to form unions, share property, and possess legal and financial rights regarding their domestic partnerships, property, medical decision-making and, often, children.

Young gay men growing up today have a greater chance to feel better, if not even good about themselves, sooner. Now that homosexuality is no longer seen as "pathological" or "deviant" and with the support of changes in the social sciences (especially psychology and psychiatry), culture, and the law, adulthood can provide gay men can with a healthy and affirming context in which to overcome years of internal and sociocultural difficulties.

REFERENCES

Bailey, J. M., Nothnagel, B. A. and Wolfe, B. A. Retrospectively measured individual differences in childhood sex-typed behavior among gay men: correspondence between self- and maternal reports. *Archives of Sexual Behavior*, **24**(6) (1995): 613–22.

Bell, A., Weinberg, M. and Hammersmith, S. *Sexual Preference: Its Development in Men and Women.* Bloomington: Indiana University Press, 1981.

Bieber, I. *Homosexuality.* New York: Basic Books, 1962.

Blos, P. *On Adolescence: A Psychoanalytic Interpretation.* New York: Free Press, 1962.

Butler, J. Melancholy gender-refused identification. *Psychoanalytic Dialogues* 5(2) (1995): 165–80.

Chodorow, N. *Feminism and Psychoanalytic Theory.* New Haven, CT: Yale University Press, 1989.
   The Reproduction of Mothering: Psychoanalysis and the Sociology of Gender, Berkeley: University of California Press, 1999.

Corbett, K. Homosexual boyhood: notes on Girlieboys. *Gender and Psychoanalysis,* 1(4) (1996): 429–61.
   Cross-gendered identifications and homosexual boyhood: toward a more complex theory of gender. *American Journal of Orthopsychiatry,* 6(8) (1998): 352–60.

Dimen, M. On "our nature": Prolegomenon to a relational theory of sexuality. In *Disorienting Sexuality,* T. Domenici and R. Lesser, eds. New York: Routledge, 1995.

Ellis, H. *Studies in the Psychology of Sex: Sexual Inversion.* London: University Press, 1900.

Freud, S. *Three essays on sexuality;* 7 (1905): 135–243, Standard edn. London: Hogarth Press, 1953.
   Some neurotic mechanisms in jealousy, paranoia and homosexuality 18 (1922): 221–232, Standard edn. London: Hogarth Press, 1953.
   Civilization and its Discontents; 21 (1930): 59–145, Standard edn. London: Hogarth Press, 1953.
   Letter to an American mother (1935). In *Homosexuality and American Psychiatry* Bayer, R. ed. Princeton: Princeton University Press, 1987.

Friedman, R. C. and Downey, J. I. Male homosexuality: a contemporary psychoanalytic perspective. *Archives of Sexual Behavior,* 20(2) (1991): 219–20.
   Psychoanalysis and the model of homosexuality as psychopathology: a historical overview. *American Journal of Psychoanalysis,* 58(3) (1998): 249–70.

Frommer, M. Countertransference obscurity in the treatment of homosexual patients. In *Disorienting Sexuality,* ed. T. Domenici and R. Lesser, eds. New York: Routledge, 1995.

Hirschfeld, M. *Die Homosexualitaet des Mannes und des Weibes. Handbuch der gesamten Sexualwissenschaft in Einzeldarstellung,* 3. Berlin: Lorius Marcus, 1914.

Hooker, E. The adjustment of the male overt homosexual. *Journal of Projective Techniques,* 21 (1957): 18–31.

Isay, R. *Being Homosexual: Gay Men and their Development.* New York: Avon Books, 1989.

Kassel, P. E. and Franko, D. F. Body image disturbance and psychodynamic psychotherapy with gay men. *Harvard Review of Psychiatry,* 8(6) (2000): 307–17.

Kinsey, A. Pomeroy, W. and Martin, C. *Sexual Behavior in the Human Male.* Philadelphia: Saunders, 1948.

Layton, L. *Who's that Girl? Who's that Boy? Clinical Practice Meets Post-Modern Theory.* New York: Aronson, 1998.

LeVay, S. *The Sexual Brain.* Cambridge, MA: MIT Press, 1993.

LeVay, S. and Hamer, D. Evidence for a biological influence in male homosexuality. *Scientific American,* 270(5) (1994): 44–9.

Levy-Warren, M. *The Adolescent Journey.* Northvale, NJ: Aronson, 1996.

Mitchell, S. The psychoanalytic treatment of homosexuality: Some technical considerations. *International Review of Psychoanalysis*, **8** (1981): 63–80.

Phillips, S. The overstimulation of every day life: new aspects of male homosexuality. *Journal of the American Psychoanalytic Association*, **49**(4) (2001): 1235–67.

Rofes, E. *Dry Bones Breathe: Gay Men Creating Post-AIDS Identities and Cultures*. New York: Harrington Park Press, 1998.

Saghir, M. and Robins, E. Male and female homosexuality: natural history. *Comprehensive Psychiatry*, **12** (1971): 503–10.

Socarides, C. *The Overt Homosexual*. New York: Grune and Stratton, 1968.
   Homosexuality. New York: Jason Aronson, 1978.

Stoller, R. The impact of new advances in sex research on psychoanalytic theory. *American Journal of Psychiatry*, **130** (1973): 241–51 and 1207–16.

Whitman, F. L. Childhood indicators of male homosexuality. *Archives of Sexual Behavior*, **6** (1977): 89–96.

Zucker, K. and Bradley, S. *Gender Identity Disorder and Psychosexual Problems in Children and Adolescents*. New York: Guilford Press, 1995.

Zuger, B. Early effeminate behavior in boys: outcome and significance for homosexuality. *Journal of Nervous and Mental Disorders*, **172** (1984): 90–7.

14

Women and HIV

Lorraine Sherr, Ph.D.

Professor of Clinical and Health Psychology, Head of Health Psychology Unit, Department of Primary Care and Population Sciences, Royal Free and University College School of Medicine, London, UK

Introduction

At the end of 2001, UNAIDS estimated that there were 37.1 million adults living with HIV/AIDS. Of those, 18.5 million or about 50% were women. In sub-Saharan Africa, more women than men are infected. Epidemiological studies indicate that women can and do become infected with HIV through sexual transmission more easily and at higher rates than men. For biological, psychological, and/or social reasons, the course of HIV disease may differ in women (Kilian *et al.*, 1999), and the mental health impact of infection has its own place in the study of women.

While women represent a significant and growing part of the pandemic, knowledge and services specific to women continue to lag behind those specific to other HIV-infected populations (Gorna, 1995). For many years, papers on HIV and women were the exception rather than the norm (Sherr, 1996), and women were rarely included in clinical trials. In the late 1990s, research tended to focus on the role of women in vertical (i.e., mother to child) transmission (Mofenson, 1999; Shafer *et al.*, 1999; Wiktor *et al.*, 1999; McIntyre and Gray, 2002) and on child outcomes, rather than addressing women's issues (Pinch, 1994) or tracking maternal outcomes.

This chapter discusses the mental health implications for women living with HIV, which are often inextricably bound with their physical health concerns. It discusses a number of factors to consider in caring for women with HIV, including relationships, sexual behavior, parenting, pregnancy, treatment and adherence, and emotional impact (such as anxiety, depression, grief, bereavement, and coping).

What are the risk factors for HIV transmission in women?

Women are at risk of HIV transmission through sexual contact and through injection drug use. There is also growing evidence that a significant number of

HIV and Psychiatry. A Training and Resource Manual, Second Edition, ed. Kenneth Citron, Marie-Josée Brouillette, and Alexandra Beckett. Published by Cambridge University Press. © Cambridge University Press 2005.

women in Africa may have been infected through the practice of reusing needles for immunizations.

In terms of sexual transmission, women appear to be at greater risk of HIV infection than men. Viral load is higher in semen than in vaginal secretions, semen remains at body temperature longer in the vagina than vaginal secretions do on the penis (which means that women have longer exposure to HIV), and HIV can easily penetrate vaginal mucous membranes. Other factors that affect women's risk of sexual transmission are:

- the number of sexual partners women have
- the stage of HIV disease in the sexual partner (more advanced stage associated with increased transmission)
- the practice of anal intercourse
- the presence of genital ulcers or other sexually transmitted diseases.

Plummer et al. (1991) pointed out the risks associated with the presence of cervical ectopy, while De Vincenzi (1994) recorded some sexual practices such as avoidance of ejaculation in the vagina as protective.

The effects of contraception on HIV transmission are unclear. Some researchers have seen associations with oral contraception (Plummer et al., 1991), while others have failed to establish links (Kapiga et al., 1994). With regard to specific forms of contraception, studies to date have shown no association between intrauterine devices and HIV transmission (Kapiga et al., 1994, 1998; Sinei et al., 1998). A meta-analysis of available studies (Stephenson, 1998) reveals the level of conflicting findings. The definitive answer to the role of oral or other contraceptives in HIV transmission is yet to be determined. However, contraception may be a surrogate marker for women who are more sexually active and that behavior, rather than the contraceptive, may be a key factor in transmission risk.

Violence against women may also be a risk factor for HIV transmission. Quigley et al. (2000) noted a risk for HIV transmission from males to females associated with sex against the woman's will. Women who are forced to have sex are usually not in a position to take precautions to protect themselves from exposure to HIV or other sexually transmitted diseases. The risks of HIV transmission during rape would be affected by the level of physical trauma experienced, the rate of HIV in the population, and the number of assailants. Although the association between rape and HIV transmission has not been well documented, the emotional trauma of rape is enhanced by the fear of transmission, the unpleasantness of postexposure prophylaxis (PEP), and the fact that exposure to antiretroviral therapy during PEP may affect the efficacy of the drugs should the woman become infected and need treatment in the future. Studies of cohorts of HIV-seropositive women have shown that many of them experienced violence prior to diagnosis, and also experience both physical and sexual violence after the diagnosis (Sowell et al., 2002b).

Only a single case of female to female sexual transmission of HIV has been documented in the literature. However, other confounding and potential risk-exposure factors, such as injecting drugs and needle sharing, should not be dismissed (Kilian *et al.*, 1999).

Women are vulnerable to HIV from sharing needles. This appears to be one of the main modes of transmission in Russia, and in women in some developed countries.

Case study: The effect of testing HIV seropositive on relationships

Jeannette and Ben have been in a relationship for 4 years. They have no children. Jeannette, who is quiet, softly spoken, and fairly needy, has not had many previous relationships. Her last partner had multiple sexual partners, was a former drug user, and treated Jeannette poorly. The more difficult he was to engage, the more Jeannette became dependent on him. When he left her, she was depressed and lonely. Jeanette met Ben at a folk-dancing class, which her neighbor had encouraged her to join. They developed an easy relationship, which grew from strength to strength. Ben is very involved in his hobbies and has a job that takes him out of town for periods of time. Although Jeannette feels very lonely when he is gone, she distracts herself with her job as a library assistant.

When she hears that her old partner has become ill, she becomes concerned about HIV and hepatitis. Ben and Jeannette test together, and this is the first time he really understands about her previous partner and his drug-use history. She tests HIV seropositive, and he tests negative. Although he says he will stand by her, he withdraws, does not want to talk about HIV, and throws himself into his work. Jeannette is physically quite well, but emotionally shaken. She is depressed at times and finds it difficult to return to work. Their sexual relationship has not resumed since the HIV test result.

What is the impact of HIV on women, sex, and relationships?

HIV can have dramatic, far-reaching effects on women's relationships, and its impact can be compounded by issues of dependence and blame. Because discordancy (i.e., the woman is HIV seropositive, her partner is seronegative) is not uncommon, the fear of rejection is often an issue. Many women fear that they will be abandoned by existing partners if they disclose their status, and the literature shows that some of their fears are founded. HIV can also create a barrier in negotiating new relationships. Women are often uncertain when and whether to tell new partners. If they disclose early, they risk rejection. If they do not disclose early, they find it difficult to do so later on.

The issues of sex and relationships are inextricably linked. Several studies have documented that a significant proportion of women diagnosed with HIV refrain from sex, or lose enjoyment or desire. Even when women do continue or resume sexual activity, most report sexual adjustment problems (Hankins, 1995). Research has shown that HIV-seropositive women are exposed to multiple stressors, some of which are unique to women while others are common between the sexes (Semple, 1993, 1998).

In this case, Jeannette has specific needs in her relationship, and sex plays a key role in sustaining her behavior. Her counseling needs to address a number of factors. Brief support would focus on helping her:

- come to terms with her HIV status
- value her current health and develop coping strategies to sustain her health
- explore her dependency roles, and ways of becoming more self-sufficient
- understand how to gather mutual support from a relationship
- rehearse worst possible scenarios in case the relationship does crumble
- see that there is life beyond the relationship
- look at sex in the presence of discordance, safe sex, and future reproduction issues.

Case study: A woman struggles with disclosure and self-image

Mariana is HIV seropositive and is currently on a triple combination therapeutic regimen. Her CD4 cell count is good, and her viral load is low. However, her treatment regimen has a high pill burden and food requirements which she finds difficult – particularly during the week at work. She has a job in a fashion store and spends much of the day on her feet at the shop front. Although she is supposed to have regular lunch breaks, her manager often asks her to change her lunch times when the store is busy. Because Mariana has not disclosed her status to her manager or co-workers, she stores her medications at home in case anyone finds them. This means she has to travel home to have her lunch and her pills. Mariana also suffers from lipodystrophy associated with her medication, which has affected the shape of her breasts and thighs. She has responded by wearing loose clothing and spends so much time hiding the effects that she keeps reminding herself of her condition. She hates to look in the mirror, and she feels that no-one will ever love her again.

Do women respond differently than men to HIV treatments?

There is no evidence that females show a lower virological, immunological, or clinical benefit from HAART compared with males. However, Rezza *et al.* (2000) noted that women have lower viral load measures than men, although it is unclear how meaningful this is in terms of treatment planning. Many treatment and care guidelines do not take women and their needs into account, and women's access to therapy and outcomes may be affected by a complex array of factors, including recognition of HIV status, knowledge of available treatments, real or perceived risk of discrimination, and sociocultural conditions.

Toxicity profiles related to antiretroviral therapy seem to have a gender effect (d'Arminio Monforte *et al.*, 2000). Females are at greater risk of developing forms of lipodystrophy. When this conditions leads to marked changes in the body and appearance, it has specific implications for women's quality of life, adherence to medications, and self-image/esteem.

In this case, Mariana is managing her HIV well on combination therapies, but needs to look at the effects of lipodystrophy on her self-esteem and body image, and how that affects areas of her life. Adherence counseling may also be useful. Low self-esteem, poor social support, and side effects are all factors associated with diminished adherence to treatment regimens. Support and counseling may be crucial to help Mariana maintain her life-sustaining medications.

What health issues do women with HIV infection face?

HIV is associated with an increased incidence of cervical dysplasia, which can progress to extensive cervical cancer. Women with HIV also have an increased risk of cervical abnormality, invasive cervical cancers, other infections and STDs, and fertility problems. Cervical carcinoma *in situ* is an AIDS defining diagnosis. Although abnormal bleeding has been reported in women being treated for HIV, no studies have yet reported on the association between HAART and menstrual function. Any of these conditions will have an impact on women, and therapists should explore their emotional effects.

How does stigma affect women?

The experience of illness is affected by society's reaction or perceived reaction to the condition. HIV is associated with "pervasive and extensive discrimination" (Van de Ven *et al.*, 1996), and this stigma can have a far-reaching influence in women's lives (Haour Knipe and Rector, 1996; Price and Hsu, 1992; Sherr, 1996b). Stigma and reactions to stigma may be an important point of discussion and support for HIV-positive women.

Sankar *et al.* (2002) noted that fear of stigma could "constitute a moral justification for selective adherence" as a means of protecting from stigma. On the other hand, stigma may be a marker for a lack of identification with the disease. Reminders of illness triggered by taking medication may create an uncomfortable dilemma for women struggling to come to terms with infection.

What factors can influence adherence in women?

Adherence is key to successful HAART treatment, but studies rarely examine the role of gender in adherence. Most current studies are cross-sectional in nature and few give systematic clarity on the efficacy of interventions in improving adherence (Sherr, 2001). However, adherence is associated with reduced viral load and certain factors – including side effect, lowered mood, reduced social support, and isolation – may affect adherence. Sankar *et al.* (2002) noted that women who were categorized as "always adherent" were surrounded by sources of influence which were generally supportive. They point to the importance of identifying influences that both support or undermine adherence in the daily lives of women with HIV. Addressing these is crucial in maintaining good physical health. Issues to remember when considering adherence include:

- good preparation for commencing treatment
- timely decision making, taking into account physical and psychological need
- understanding lifestyle and the extent to which various regimens fit into the routines
- understanding motivation, beliefs, and commitment to treatment
- exploring barriers to adherence and creating strategies to overcome and manage these
- providing adherence support
- addressing any concerns regarding side effects.

Case study: Issues of parenting, relationships, and sexuality

Patience is an HIV-seropositive woman who was diagnosed with HIV 7 years ago. She originally resided in Zambia, but has lived abroad for 8 years. While her extended family is far away, her immediate family is around her. She is currently well and on a triple combination regimen. Her husband, Joseph, has three children from a previous marriage. His first wife died. Patience has an 11-year-old daughter from an earlier relationship.

Joseph has not tested for HIV. Patience believes that he is unfaithful to her. She is afraid to have sex with him for fear of becoming ill, but she is economically reliant on him. Patience used to work as a clerk in a large company but, since her diagnosis, she has been unemployed. Money is tight. Joseph often leaves her on her own, and Patience often feels lonely and scared. In spite of this difficult situation, she would like to have another child.

What parenting issues do HIV-positive women face?

Parenting in the presence of HIV is a challenge. It is critical to understand the role of women as mothers. Women with HIV face the same parenting issues faced by all women, and may have additional burdens directly or indirectly associated with HIV, including:

- disclosure (i.e., keeping secrets is a burden for young children, matched only by the strain of not being told the truth in the first place)
- testing the children (and management of multiple family infections if a child has HIV),
- the burden of hospital and clinic visits
- the needs and demands on everyday life from adherence to treatment regimens
- the emotional energy and distraction caused by coping with HIV.

Parenting in the presence of anxiety, depression, panic, or other mental health disorder adds to the burden. Facing mortality (Graham and Newell, 1999) and preparing a future life for children may be overwhelming. It is also not uncommon for people with HIV to reconstitute families, which adds additional challenges for parenting, stability, and emotional growth.

According to the literature, women with HIV report very positive experiences of mothering, and often re-engage in living on the arrival of children. However, the literature also shows that women often prioritise caring for others over their own care, and the very individual who is at the core of the family and its emotional health is not sustained either emotionally or in terms of her physical health needs.

Cowdery and Pesa (2002) note that quality of life issues for HIV-seropositive women have been understudied, especially given that women take on social and work roles which are different and distinct from men. They found that age was a significant factor as was social support and employment status.

Counseling support and the availability of self-help organizations can help women with HIV manage parenting issues. This is especially true if the organization provides an environment where all family members can share their situation, realize that they have similar issues to other families, and receive both practical and emotional support.

In this case, Patience would benefit from brief counseling to help her adjust to life with HIV. The therapist would help her look at power, self-reliance, and personal meaning. By exploring what the family can do to improve their life and plan for the future, counseling can help Patience shift from a focus on "death from HIV" to "living with HIV".

What are the reproductive/sexual health concerns of HIV-positive women?

All HIV-seropositive women should have an opportunity to discuss and explore sexuality and reproduction. Some may be reluctant to talk about their views for fear of discrimination and preset attitudes condemning or discouraging childbirth. However, many women with HIV desire a child, many have unprotected intercourse and, for many women, conception is not only possible but desirable.

Counselors providing support for women with HIV should have an understanding of the multiple factors associated with pregnancy decision making.

In discordant couples (i.e., one partner is positive and the other negative) conception and pregnancy poses a risk of exposure to HIV. Many women also fear that they will experience discrimination in the face of HIV infection, and that having a baby will compound the stigma (Sherr et al., 1999, 2000).

The advent of improved diagnosis, treatment, management, and prognosis may affect women's decisions about becoming pregnant (Ergin et al., 2002). Sowell et al. (2002a) noted that traditional gender role orientation and motivation for childbearing were significant factors in predicting pregnancy intention among women with HIV. Pregnancy decision making is also affected by a number of contextual factors (Nyamathi and Stein, 1997), such as social expectation (Pinch, 1994; Semple, 1998), partner influences, psychosocial factors, traditional gender roles (Sowell et al., 2002a), and a wish to create something of value which will survive beyond the woman's death (Kurth and Hutchinson, 1990; Kline et al., 1995; Ahluwalia et al., 1998). Motherhood has special meaning for women (Kurth, 1993) both in terms of its fulfilment as well as its vision as a career in itself (Merrick, 1995).

Women with HIV may experience fertility problems. A routine gynecological and psychosexual interview should be offered to all women on a regular basis.

Case study: A HIV-seropositive pregnant woman

Miral, a 27-year-old woman, tests HIV seropositive during routine pregnancy care. She is married with a 4-year-old child and is currently 17 weeks pregnant. Because her HIV test was part of a battery of pregnancy tests, she received minimal HIV counseling. She has no obvious risk factors for HIV, and is currently well.

What is involved in the diagnosis and care of pregnant women with HIV?

Offering HIV testing to all pregnant women is a standard of prenatal obstetrical care. (Lawsuits have occurred in cases where testing was not been offered and women were subsequently found to be HIV positive.)

Testing during pregnancy is important because interventions are available to reduce vertical transmission (Dabis et al., 1999; Ergin et al., 2002). Treatment currently revolves around three elements (Van de Perre, 1995):

- the use of antiretroviral treatment in pregnancy, labor, and to the infant to reduce transmission
- the use of cesarean section to avoid exposure to vaginal secretions (however this is being examined in the light of reduced risks if women have undetectable viral loads)
- the avoidance of breastfeeding.

Pregnancy in antiretroviral naive women who do not require therapy may be managed differently than in those who do require therapy, or those who are on therapy when they conceive.

In some developing countries, using one drug (monotherapy) to prevent vertical transmission may compromise the mother's viral resistance status. If a woman's medications are either inadequate to suppress the virus or not continued after childbirth, she may experience viral rebound with a new resistant strain of HIV (Phillips *et al.*, 2001).

The issue is different for women who conceive while on HAART. There are currently no data on the teratogenicity of HAART. In the absence of such information, clinicians usually follow local protocols for continuation, cessation, dosage, and regimen. As new data emerge, these guidelines should be updated. Given the concerns about the longer-term effects of any substances administered during pregnancy, the optimum regimens, and the long-term management needs of the woman, it is important for clinicians to keep up-to-date with new developments and recommendations.

The decision to have a cesarean section or avoid breastfeeding should be explored with the mother, both from a psychological and physical perspective.

Data seem to show no relationship between pregnancy and disease progression (Coley *et al.*, 2001). However, longer-term studies do show that there are other negative effects. As women with HIV succumb to their disease, orphanhood is a particular problem, exacerbated by the lack of medications in developing countries.

Case study: A pregnant woman struggles with termination of pregnancy issues

Joanne, a 28-year-old woman, tested negative during her first pregnancy but tested HIV seropositive during her second pregnancy. She is currently 14 weeks pregnant and is suddenly overwhelmed by a number of issues she needs to address. Should she continue with the pregnancy or terminate? If she proceeds, what are her views on treatment, interventions, and delivery? She cannot really focus on these questions at the moment because she keeps thinking about herself. Will she live to see the baby born? How can she think of a life with HIV infection? She is frightened by the diagnosis and overwhelmed by all the information. She cannot understand the complexities of the disease and finds it difficult to grapple with the needs of the pregnancy and her own turmoil.

What are the effects of HIV diagnosis during pregnancy?

Both Miral and Joanne must deal with their HIV diagnosis without preparation and without the benefits of full HIV pretest counseling. Most prenatal (antenatal) testing regimes either do not deal with the important elements of in-depth pretest counseling or cover these in a cursory manner. The result is a woman with scant emotional preparation, risk assessment, adjustment, and potential coping.

What is the role of pre- and post-test counseling?

There is no substitute for good pre- and posttest counseling. Given the potential to address risk, prevention and adaptation, test counseling is an investment for women who test negative as well as positive. Effective HIV test counseling for pregnant women should follow the guidelines outlined in Appendix I, with the following additions:

Pretest counseling

- Ensure tests are only carried out if there is an HIV management infrastructure in place prior to the test.
- Discuss partner testing.
- Explain array of interventions available.
- Assure the woman that, regardless of her decision, her pregnancy care will not be jeopardized.
- Explore risk exposure, risk management, and risk reduction.
- Explore preparation, emotional support, planning, and decision making.

Post-test counseling

HIV negative

- Discuss safe sex during pregnancy.
- Discuss emotional responses and ongoing concerns or worries.
- Explain the need for repeat testing and risk exposure issues.

HIV positive

- Give the result without delay.
- Refer women for HIV care immediately.
- Be prepared for an extreme emotional response.
- Pace decision making needs according to the time of the test.
- Discuss involving partners, weighing the balance between support and rejection.
- Discuss issues of trust, disclosure, and discrimination.
- Introduce clearly planned management, with named individual caregivers and access to peer and professional support.
- Ensure woman has access to crisis management and brief therapy. (Remember that most women do not consider termination of pregnancy. However if they wish to discuss this, it should be open for them.)
- Discuss testing of partner and other children.

Is decision making more difficult at a time of heightened anxiety?

When a woman is diagnosed with HIV during pregnancy, she faces many decisions regarding management, treatment, sexual behavior, disclosure, and adjustment, which often absorb enormous time, support, and emotional energy, and require pacing. However, because of the pregnancy, some decisions have to be made relatively quickly. To make these decisions, women need information about the virus, transmission, and infection control that is comprehensible. Information is a basic building block for decision making. However, at times of anxiety, a person's ability to process, recall, and comprehend information may be adversely affected.

When making decisions about their pregnancy, women should be encouraged to consider the risk–benefit analysis of multiple interventions. The way information is provided can affect the decision-making process. For example, if survival information is framed positively (e.g., the baby has a 95% chance of being born virus free) women may respond differently than when the same information is framed negatively (e.g., the baby has a 5% chance of being born with HIV). Decision making can be aided by clarity, pacing, and facing up to (and thinking through) fearful or anxiety-provoking potential situations. Good use of peer support, community support, and counseling approaches are useful. It is important for women to have time to reflect, rehearse, and change decisions – not only to help them make good decisions but to help them adjust emotionally when they revisit their decisions.

Counselors should help women address instrumental and support concerns. Women may need multiple opportunities with a sensitive care provider (i.e., a safe environment) to weigh options around treatment for both themselves and their children.

What are women's concerns about wider family infection?

When a woman is diagnosed with HIV during pregnancy, this may raise questions about the HIV status of her partner and any older children. While pregnant women are routinely tested, their male partners are rarely tested. This is a limited approach because fathers may well be infected and may infect mothers during pregnancy. Relationship problems often stem from blame in the (mistaken) belief that the person who first tested positive brought HIV into the relationship (Postma *et al.*, 2000).

Multiple HIV infection in a family is not uncommon, yet the emotional impact of such sudden knowledge can be significant. Pacing is a key element at this point. Some women would be reassured by addressing any uncertainties, while others may want to deal with the current situation initially and then slowly plan for other members of the family.

What is the nature and extent of emotional trauma at the time of HIV diagnosis?

Mental health considerations are crucial at this time. Women report heightened anxiety, depression, and problems with psychosexual function at the time of diagnosis. It is crucial for therapists to help women explore and deal with any suicidal thoughts or depression. Depression affects a pregnant woman negatively, and can also have developmental consequences for her infant. When coping with emotional trauma around diagnosis, women may need emotional support from a variety of sources.

How can care be prioritized?

The literature suggests that the needs of the unborn baby are seen as paramount, and the mother's needs may be overlooked. A family approach provides a more holistic view and, in the long term, serves the baby better as well as the mother, father, other siblings, and perhaps even the wider family. Ideally, care for infected infants and mothers will be provided concurrently, and will include access to appropriate childcare to allow mothers to receive their care.

How can women maximize their coping skills?

There is good evidence that social and emotional support aids coping, that women cope in a variety of ways, and that some use different coping methods and styles for different challenges. Women benefit from continuity of care, good support, and nonjudgmental input linked with trust.

What is involved in planning care for women with HIV?

Care for women is based on available evidence, and current practices and premises. It is important to take stock of these, to apply findings on a general level to individual women, and to reassess approaches. Given the emerging literature, clinicians should challenge concepts, question assumptions, and ensure that information gleaned from other infected groups (e.g., gay men) is not simply transferred to women. Often a set of facts or presumptions may result in action and implications – especially for women – that may jeopardize their health. Table 14.1 sets out a number of presumptions that may have specific implications for caring for women.

What are the guiding principles for planning care?

- Focus on the individual needs.
- Ensure women-centered care is available.
- Understand women and their family or life role and provide treatment in context.

Table 14.1. Implications of presumptions for women's care.

Presumptions	Action	Implications for women
HIV is a male disease	Concentration of research on men and treatment models in relation to men's needs	Understudied (increase from 3% to 5% of HIV studies mentioning women in MEDLINE search over 15 years) Models not user-friendly therefore not used
Women with HIV do not want babies	Termination of pregnancy offered.	Termination of pregnancy is not the option of first choice and those who did terminate conceived again within 1 year (Sunderland *et al.*, 1990).
	Presumption of avoidance of pregnancy	Pregnancy was not avoided but was sought. Women were willing to conceive even if the act of conception exposed them to infection.
Women with HIV-seropositive baby would avoid further pregnancy	Reproductive advice not high on the HIV clinic agenda	On the contrary, Temmerman *et al.* (1990) found that women with an HIV-seropositive baby were more likely to conceive a subsequent child than the other way round
Women lacked power	Programmes to empower women	Not necessarily a lack of power. It is important to appreciate women's roles and how they may bring different strengths to situations besides power. Programmes dealt with the wrong problem and programmes did not listen to women and what they were saying
Women were primarily responsible for infecting infants	Programmes targeted women for HIV antenatal testing for treatment to prevent vertical transmission and not for their treatment	First identified seen as first infected so antenatal female testing only disadvantaged women in their relationships. Women exposed to monotherapy (virus-free baby seen as more desirable than orphanhood – both could and should be avoided)

Table 14.1. (cont.)

Presumptions	Action	Implications for women
Treatment for women could be inferred by data from male research	Women were not included in many early trials	Female-specific ramifications, such as cervical pathology, were recognized late. Women-specific cohort studies were set up (e.g., Wits, Hers). Treatment variations and implications still unclear
Disclosure of HIV status did not pose a risk for women	Issues of disclosure not sufficiently planned for or counseled	Studies have shown that women's concerns were based on fact, and that they were often abandoned, abused, or held responsible. Couple testing has not taken off, despite its clearly protective effect on women

- Avoid generalizing directly from the male literature as there may be gender-specific responses and reactions which would benefit from different approaches.
- Recognize that women's needs are complex and include physical, emotional, psychosexual, reproduction, family, and individual needs.

What are the issues surrounding the concept of women and power?

It is a commonly held presumption, well articulated in both the literature and the design of interventions, that "women lack power". The notion is so widespread that it may be accepted as an inescapable truth. Indeed the very action of couching female action in terms of "lack of power" may have the effect of perpetuating the very imbalance it aims to describe or prevent (Sherr, 1995). The cluster of findings in relation to women and HIV infection may be reinterpreted to provide a better, or at least different, understanding of the ways women react to HIV-related events (Sherr, 1996a,b). A list of research findings, core concepts, and alternative explanations are set out in Table 14.2. Although not an exhaustive examination of women and power issues, it does provide an array of examples where reframing is possible. Such an approach may allow clinicians to reframe the reactions women have, rather than interpret these within a power (i.e., lack of power) paradigm. This may help women to receive the understanding and insight needed at the time and appreciate their life circumstances and their strengths as well as their weaknesses.

Table 14.2. Alternative explanations for research findings on women and power issues.

Study	Finding	Reinterpretation
Worth (1990)	Women are less likely to leave their partner if he becomes HIV positive than the other way round	Not a lack of power, rather can be seen as commitment
Kamenga et al. (1991)	Women are more likely to be exposed to unprotected sex from an HIV-positive male partner than the other way round	Not a lack of power, rather it represents male disregard
Sherr (1995)	Women are more likely to be tested for HIV during pregnancy than the fathers of the baby	This is not a lack of power, but shortsighted policy, despite the fact that male testing is cost effective (Postma et al, 1999, 2000; Sansom et al., 2003) and desired by women (Sherr et al., 2003).
Hankins (1992)	Women are more likely to attend for treatment later in their disease course	This is not a lack of power, but self-sacrifice. Often women prioritize child medical care. The provision of family clinics can address their needs (Melvin and Sherr, 1993).
Sherr et al. (1993)	Women are more likely to bring their children to HIV clinic appointments than themselves	This too is a form of self-sacrifice and commitment to their children
Kamenga et al. (1991)	HIV-seronegative husbands are more likely to abstain from sex than when the woman was seronegative. Husbands who were abstinent from sex within their marriage reported extramarital sex which was invariably unprotected	No women with HIV in this study reported extramarital sex
White et al. (1997)	In an audit of HIV seropositive children, 46% of fathers' HIV status was unknown as they were untested or unavailable	Women are prepared to establish their HIV status and be available for caring for their HIV-seropositive children. This is not a lack of power, but relates to the serious role and responsibilities of mothering

Table 14.2. (cont.)

Study	Finding	Reinterpretation
Greig and Koopman (2003)	HIV prevention behaviors (notably condom use) were not associated with empowerment education but with economic factors and negotiation	Empowerment programs may need to be tailored to cultural realities. Provision of economic resources may be more effective
Wilson et al., (2003)	573 couples studied showed that background risk from sexual contacts other than primary partner was higher for males (7.4 vs 1.4).	This is not a lack of power, but one of many studies that shows female vulnerability as a result of male sexual behavior
Sweat et al., 2000	Cost-effectiveness of voluntary testing and counseling (VCT) was enhanced for couple testing	Often it is not the lack of power that results in a predominance of women-only testing programmes, but a gender bias in researchers, despite the well-established efficacy of couple testing

The problem can be seen as power, but if seen as something else such as women's approaches, their way of conducting relationships or economic/social pressures, then understanding and intervention may be more clearly focused.

Conclusion

There is a strong link between the medical and emotional care of women with HIV. Mental health elements overlap at every juncture, and quality care for women should be based on a model of preventive provision in terms of mental health support. In the era of new treatments, improved prognosis, and reduced vertical transmission, more and more women will survive with a good quality of life to play a key role in their family and community. While the base of knowledge needs to expand to provide true evidence-based healthcare for women with HIV, women's needs are no longer being overlooked and women are playing a central role in HIV prevention, treatment, and care.

REFERENCES

Ahluwalia, I., DeVellis, R. and Thomas, J. Reproductive decisions of women at risk of acquiring HIV infection. *AIDS Education and Prevention*, **10**(1) (1998): 90–7.

d'Arminio Monforte, A., Cozzi Lepri, A., Rezza, G. *et al.* Insights into the reasons for discontinuation of the first highly active antiretroviral therapy (HAART) regimen in a cohort of antiretroviral naive patients. *AIDS*, **14** (2000): 499–507.

Coley, J. L., Msamanga, G. I., Fawzi, M. C. *et al.* The association between maternal HIV-1 infection and pregnancy, outcomes in Dar es Salaam, Tanzania. *BJOG: an International Journal of Obstetric and Gynaecology*, **108**(11) (2001): 1125–33.

Cowdery, J. and Pesa, J. Assessing quality of life in women living with HIV infection. *AIDS Care*, **14**(2) (2002): 235–45.

Dabis, F., Msellati, P., Meda, N. *et al.* Six month efficacy tolerance and acceptability of a short regimen of oral zidovudine to reduce vertical transmission of HIV in breastfed children in Cote d'Ivoire and Burkina Faso: a double blind placebo controlled multicentre trial. *Lancet*, **353** (1999): 786–92.

De Vincenzi, I. A longitudinal study of human immunodeficiency virus transmission by heterosexual partners. *New England Journal of Medicine*, **331**(6) (1994): 341–6.

Ergin, A., Magnus, M., Ergin, N. and He, J. Short course antiretroviral treatment in the prevention of perinatal HIV-1 transmission. A meta-analysis of randomized controlled trials. *Annals of Epidemiology*, **12**(7) (2002): 521.

Gorna, R. *Vamps, Victims and Virgins.* London: Cassell, 1995.

Graham, W. and Newell, M. L. Seizing the opportunity: collaborative initiatives to reduce HIV and maternal mortality. *Lancet*, **353** (1999): 836–9.

Greig, F. E. and Koopman, C. (2003). Multilevel analysis of women's empowerment and HIV prevention quantitative survey. Results from a preliminary study in Botswana. *AIDS Behaviour*, **7**(2) (2003): 195–208.

Hankins, C. Public policy and maternal fetal HIV transmission. *Psychology and Health*, **6**(4) (1992); 287–96.

Haour Knipe, M. and Rector, R. *Crossing Borders, Migration Ethnicity and AIDS.* London: Taylor and Francis, 1996.

Kamenga, M., Ryder, R., Jingu, M. *et al.* Evidence of marked sexual behaviour change associated with low HIV l seroconversion in 149 married couples with discordant HIV 1 serostatus – experience at an HIV counselling center in Zaire. *AIDS*, **5** (1991): 61–7.

Kapiga, S., Shao, J., Lwihula, G. and Hunter, D. Risk factors for HIV infection among women in Dar es Salaam, Tanzania. *Journal of Acquired Immune Deficiency Syndrome*, **3** (1994): 301–9.

Kapiga, S. H., Lyamuya, E. F., Lwihula, G. K. and Hunter, D. J. The incidence of HIV infection among women using family planning methods in Dar es Salaam, Tanzania. *AIDS*, **12**(1) (1998): 75–84.

Kilian, A., Gregson, S., Ndyanabangi, B. *et al.* Reductions in risk behaviour provide the most consistent explanation for declining HIV-1 prevalence in Uganda. *AIDS*, **13**(3) (1999): 391–8.

Kline, A., Strickler, J. and Kempf, J. Factors associated with pregnancy and pregnancy resolution in HIV seropositive women. *Social Science and Medicine*, **40**(1) (1995): 1539–47.

Kurth, A. Reproduction issues, pregnancy and childbearing in HIV infected women. In *Women, Children, and HIV/AIDS*. F. L. Cohen and J. D. Durham, eds., pp. 104–33. New York: Springer, 1993.

Kurth, A. and Hutchinson, M. Reproductive health policy and HIV – where do women fit in? *Pediatric AIDS/HIV Infection*, **1** (1990): 121–6.

McIntyre, J. and Gray, G. What can we do to reduce mother to child transmission of HIV? *British Medical Journal*, **324** (2002): 218–21.

Melvin, D. and Sherr, L. The child in the family – responding to AIDS and HIV. *AIDS Care*, **5**(1) (1993): 35–42.

Merrick, E. Adolescent childbearing as career choice perspectives from an ecological context. *Journal of Counseling and Development* **3** (1995): 288–95.

Mofenson, L. M. Short course zidovudine for prevention of perinatal infection. *Lancet*, **353** (1999): 766–7.

Nyamathi, A. and Stein, J. Assessing the impact of HIV risk reduction counseling in impoverished African American women – a structured equation approach. *AIDS Education and Prevention*, **9**(3) (1997): 253–73.

Phillips, A. N., Staszewski, S., Lampe, F. *et al.* Human Immunodeficiency Virus Rebound after suppression to < 400 copies/ml during initial highly active antiretroviral therapy regimens, according to prior nucleoside experience and duration of suppression. *Journal of Infectious Diseases*, **186**(8) (2002): 1086–91.

Pinch, W. Vertical transmission in HIV infection/AIDS – a feminist perspective. *Journal of Advanced Nursing*, **19** (1994): 36–44.

Plummer, F. A., Simonsen, J. N., Cameron, D. W. *et al.* Cofactors in male-female sexual transmission of HIV type 1. *Journal of Infectious Diseases*, **163**(2) (1991): 233–9.

Postma, M., Beck, E., Hankins, C. *et al.* Cost effectiveness of expanded antenatal HIV testing in London. *AIDS*, **14** (2000): 2383–6.

Postma, M., Beck, E., Mandalia, S. *et al.* Universal HIV screening of pregnant women in England – cost effectiveness analysis. *British Medical Journal*, **318** (1999): 1656–60.

Price, V. and Hsu, M. Public opinion about AIDS policies – the role of misinformation and attitudes towards homosexuals. *Public Opinion Quarterly*, **56** (1992): 29–52.

Quigley, M., Morgan, D., Malaba, S. *et al.* Case control study of risk factors for incident HIV infection in rural Uganda. *Journal of Acquired Immune Deficiency Syndrome*, **23** (2000): 418–25.

Sankar, A., Luborsky, M., Schuman, P. and Roberts, G. Adherence discourse among African American women taking HAART. *AIDS Care*, **14**(2) (2002): 203–18.

Sansom, S., Jamieson, D. J., Farnham, P., Bulterys, M., and Fowler, M. HIV retesting during pregnancy costs and effectiveness in preventing perinatal transmission. *Obstetrics and Gynecology*, **102**(4) (2002): 782–90.

Semple, S. Women. In *HIV Nursing and Symptom Management*, M. E. Ropka and A. B. Williams, eds. pp. 615–31, Boston: Jones and Bartlett, 1998.

Semple, S. J., Patterson, T. L., Temoshok, L. R. *et al.* Identification of psychobiological stressors among HIV-positive women. Neurobehavioral research center (HNRC) group. *Women Health*, **20**(4) (1993): 15–36.

Shafer, N., Chuachoowong, R., Mock, P. *et al.* Short course zidovudine for perinatal HIV-1 transmission in Bangkok Thailand – a randomised controlled trial. *Lancet*, **353** (1999): 773–80.

Sherr, L., Petrack, J., Melvin, D. *et al.* Psychological trauma in female HIV infection. *Counselling Psychology Quarterly*, **6**(2) (1993): 99–108.

Sherr, L. *The Psychology of Pregnancy and Childbirth*. Oxford: Blackwell Publications, 1995.

The person behind the virus. Migration, human factors and some moral and ethical questions. In *Grossing Borders, Migration Ethnicity and AIDS*, M. Haour. Knipe and R. Rector, eds., pp. 70–85. London: Taylor and Francis, 1996a.

Tomorrow's era – gender psychology and HIV infection. In *AIDS as a Gender Issue*, L. Sherr, C. Hankins and L. Bennett, eds., pp. 16–45. London: Taylor and Francis, 1996b.

Sherr, L., Bergenstrom, A., Bell, E., *et al.* Adherence to policy guidelines – a review of antenatal screening policies in the UK and eire. Psychological Health and Medicine, **6**(4) (2001): 463–72.

Sherr, L., Hackman, N., Mfenyana, K., Chandia, J. and Yogeswaran, P. Ante-natal HIV testing from the perspective of pregnant women and health clinic staff in South Africa – implications for pre and post test counselling. *Counselling Psychology Quarterly*, **16**(4) (2003): 337–47

Sherr, L., Bergenstrom, A., Bell, E. *et al.* Ante-natal HIV screening and ethnic minority women. *Health Trends*, **30**(4) (1999): 115–20.

Sherr, L., Bergenstrom, A. and Hudson, C. N. Consent and antenatal HIV – testing the limits of choice and issues of consent in HIV and AIDS. *AIDS Care*, **12**(3) (2000): 307–12.

Sinei, S. K., Morrison, C. S., Sekadde-Kigondu, C. *et al.* Complications of use of intrauterine devices among HIV-1 infected women. *Lancet*, **351** (1998): 1238–41.

Sowell, R., Murdaugh, C., Addy, L. *et al.* Factors influencing intent to get pregnant in HIV infected women living in the southern USA. *AIDS Care*, **14**(2) (2002a): 181–92.

Sowell, R., Phillips, K., Seals, B., Murdaugh, C. and Rush, C. Incidence and correlates of physical violence among HIV infected women at risk for pregnancy in the southeastern US. *Journal of the Association of Nurses in AIDS Care*, **13**(2) (2002b): 46–58.

Stephenson, J. M. Systematic review of hormonal contraception and risk of HIV transmission. *AIDS*, **12**(6) (1998): 545–53.

Sunderland, A. Influence of Human Immunodeficiency Virus infection on reproductive decisions. *Obstetrics and Gynecology Clinics of North America*, **17**(3) (1990): 585–94.

Sweat, M., Gregorich, S., Sangiwa, G. *et al.* Cost effectiveness of voluntary HIV-1 counselling and testing in reducing sexual transmission of HIV-1 in Kenya and Tanzania. *Lancet*, **356** (2000): 113–21.

Temmerman, M., Moses, S., Kiragu, D. *et al.* Impact of single session post partum counselling of HIV infected women on their subsequent reproductive behaviour. *AIDS Care*, **2**(3) (1990): 247–52.

Van de Perre, P. Postnatal transmission of HIV type 1 – the breast feeding dilemma. *American Journal of Obstetrics and Gynecology* **173** (1995): 483–7.

Van de Ven, P., Turtle, A., Kippax, S. *et al.* Trends in heterosexual tertiary students knowledge of HIV and intentions to avoid people who might have HIV. *AIDS Care* **8**(1) (1996): 43–53.

White, J., Melvin, D., Moore, C. and Crowley, S. Parental HIV discordancy and its impact on the family. *AIDS Care*, **9**(5) (1997): 609–15.

Wiktor, S., Ekpini, E., Karon, J. *et al.* Short course zidovudine for prevention of mother to child transmission of HIV-1 in Abidjan Cote d'Ivoire – a randomised trial. *Lancet*, **353** (1999): 781–5.

Wilson, S. R., Lavori, P. W., Brown, N. L. and Kao, Y. M. Correlates of sexual risk for HIV infection in female members of heterosexual California Latino couples. *AIDS and Behavior*, **7**(3) (2003): 273–90.

Worth, D. Women at high risk of HIV infection. In *Behavioural Aspects of AIDS*, D. Ostrow, ed. New York: Plenum.

15

Couples

Barbara Hedge Ph.D.

Director of Clinical Psychology Training, Department of Psychology, University of Waikato, New Zealand

Introduction

The vast majority of people with HIV, whether heterosexual, bisexual, or gay, live at least some of the time with a partner. Most studies of partners of people with HIV have focused on their caregiving role. However, many people living with HIV are well for many years, and the psychological impact on partners begins before the need for physical caregiving, and can continue long after.

This chapter looks at the impact HIV infection has on couple relationships, and suggests therapeutic interventions that can improve a couple's ability to cope and their quality of life.

Case study: Impact of HIV in a serodiscordant couple

Robin and David had been partners since they were students at law school together. In the early 1980s, they became aware of AIDS and realized that their past sexual behaviors had put them at risk of HIV infection. After many years of deliberation, they decided to be tested. Robin was HIV-seropositive, but David was not infected.

Unsure how long he would remain well, Robin retired from work and both partners put much effort into enhancing their quality of life, socializing, and traveling widely. Several years later, Robin suffered several severe bouts of herpes and began feeling extremely tired. His CD4 count fell, his viral load rose rapidly, and he started taking highly active antiretroviral therapy (HAART), including a protease inhibitor (PI). Although he suffered many drug-related side effects initially, Robin persevered with the medication schedule. After 6 weeks, his viral load became undetectable, his CD4 cell count rose, and he began to put on weight and regain his energy and enthusiasm.

While David and Robin had previously enjoyed planning their social life and travel together, Robin has now decided to take over the planning role. David finds it increasingly difficult to cope with Robin's independence. He is worried when Robin goes out alone and wants him to stay in. Although Robin's health is much improved, he avoids having sex. David and Robin communicate less and less. The discussions they do have frequently

HIV and Psychiatry. A Training and Resource Manual, Second Edition, ed. Kenneth Citron, Marie-Josée Brouillette, and Alexandra Beckett. Published by Cambridge University Press. © Cambridge University Press 2005.

> lead to arguments. David is drinking more. He reports being distressed by the thought that Robin might leave him. Alcohol tends to blur his emotions.
>
> The infectious disease consultant refers the couple to the mental health unit for sex therapy.

What impact can HIV have on a relationship?

HIV is a major life transition for both partners in a couple. Each is confronted by multiple losses, including the loss of health, independence, intimacy, privacy, and possibly the death of the person with HIV and loss of their future together.

Although HAART has proved efficacious and is largely responsible for the recent decline in AIDS deaths, it is not a miracle cure. The overall prognosis for people with HIV is still uncertain. In Robin's case, both he and David had hoped a cure would be available by the time he needed one. The realization, with HAART, that he is dependent on medication raised the thought of mortality for both Robin and David.

The psychiatrist interviewed Robin and David separately, promising each that the discussion would be kept confidential.

Robin reports that David has never enjoyed using condoms and was extremely understanding when Robin felt too unwell for sex. Now that Robin's viral load is undetectable, David has suggested that they have unprotected sex. Robin is determined that he will not infect anyone, especially David whom he loves. Fearful that he will not be able to prevent David from unsafe sexual practices, he avoids sex whenever possible.

David reports that Robin shows no interest in sex, which he interprets as meaning that Robin no longer finds him attractive. He has tried to show Robin that he loves him and will do anything to keep him including having unsafe sex. However, the more he offers Robin, the more distant he becomes. This confirms David's opinion that Robin no longer cares for him. To drown his sorrows, he drinks more so sex is no longer an option.

What impact can HIV infection have on sexuality in a couple?

Sexual difficulties have been widely reported in people with HIV disease and their partners (Catalan *et al.*, 1995). People infected with HIV are usually very keen to protect their sexual partners from acquiring HIV, and partners who are HIV negative are usually keen to remain so.

Discussing safer sex can be disturbing, even with a regular partner who is aware of the infection, because it is a reminder of the risks of infection, illness, and death. Such thoughts may reduce sexual desire and induce fears of sexual expression. This can cause people to avoid any physical contact in case it leads to a sexual encounter. It is very easy for a partner's withdrawal of physical affection to be misinterpreted. Because signs of love and affection such as touching, hugging, and kissing are all boosts to a person's self-esteem, the person denied physical comfort may feel unattractive and not valued. This may lead to lowered mood and diminished quality of life, which can undermine any relationship.

Often a simple statement of sexual desires and concern is sufficient for a couple to start discussing their feelings and safer sexual options and to renew their sex life.

Assessing Robin and David's sexual difficulties reveals an underlying problem with communication. The psychiatrist suggests that Robin and David attend couple therapy.

What is the role of couple therapy in addressing communication difficulties?

Discussing difficult but important issues is never easy. Paradoxically, it is often more of a problem in couples who are very fond of each other. Neither partner wants to distress the other and so difficult issues (e.g., safer sex, planning for the future, dying, power of attorney, wills, funeral) are avoided. However, postponing difficult discussions does not ease the situation. It often increases each partner's stress as they both try to guess the other's position from their demeanour and behavior.

Couple therapy can be very useful when partners report problems that affect the relationship, particularly communication difficulties. Encouraging couples to role-play alternate ways of communicating (e.g., linking behaviors to one's own feelings rather than as a consequence of the other's behaviors) can model effective communication styles.

Other difficulties that can usefully be addressed in couple therapy are:

- dealing with conflict and disagreement
- balancing the needs of both individuals
- dealing with negative emotions such as anger and guilt
- sexual problems
- anticipating the problems that may come as the health of the partner with HIV deteriorates
- developing mutually agreeable social support for the couple and ultimately the surviving partner.

How can clinicians maintain confidentiality in couple therapy?

As individuals may have issues that they are not ready or able to discuss in front of their partner, it is important to consider individual confidential information (e.g., an episode of unfaithful behavior) before the start of therapy (Glass and Wright, 1997). Therapists are divided over whether such secrets belong to the possessor, in which case only he or she can decide to disclose them, or whether they belong to the relationship, in which case they should be shared between partners.

As collusion between the therapist and one partner can alter the dynamics of the therapeutic relationship, many therapists require the partner to either stop any ongoing extra-relationship infidelities for the duration of therapy, or share the information with the partner. If the partner violates this contract, the therapist may suspend therapy. Other therapists are prepared to work with secrets. In these cases, it is important to provide some time when each person can talk privately and confidentially with the therapist. In all cases, it is crucial to clarify the rules of confidentiality and secrecy between partners and between cotherapists (if any) early in therapy.

Robin and David agree to start couple therapy. The psychiatrist offers to see each of them alone briefly, before the start of the couple sessions in case they have any issues they feel they can't discuss in the joint session. Although this opportunity is available, neither partner uses it. During the couple session, the two men are able to communicate with each other.

ROBIN: "I love you so much that I couldn't bear to give you HIV. Even if the chances are slim, the thought of it puts me off sex. When you come and cuddle me, I worry that it will lead to unsafe sex so I make an excuse that I have other things to do."

DAVID: "So long as you want me, I am happy to be very safe in all our sex. You can trust me never to do anything unsafe."

The couple are pleased with the outcome of this session. Their sex life improves (safely) and David decreases his alcohol consumption. They agree that their other difficulties could well be consequences of their different perspectives on a situation. They ask to continue to be seen together.

When is individual therapy more appropriate?

Either partner may benefit from a private space in which to address his or her own emotional needs. Individual psychological support can bring about changes in coping strategies, increase the use of problem-solving skills, and address personal losses and grief reactions. Individual assessment is crucial to determine the full range of each person's issues and to provide separate perspectives on an issue. When a couple are comfortable discussing most issues together and see the benefit of addressing difficult issues jointly, the time for individual sessions can be minimized.

What effect can adherence to antiretroviral medications have on a couple?

Adherence to the medication schedule is essential to the success of HAART (Rabkin and Chesney, 1999), but adherence requires considerable self-discipline. Many combination therapy regimens are complex and demanding; some medications must be taken at precise time intervals under strict nutritional conditions, and some have notable toxic effects. Incorporating them into a daily routine is no mean feat.

Robin reports that his medication schedule requires him to take pills with food at regular intervals. This is very hard unless he plans his days carefully. One of the ways he ensures that he does not forget to take his medication is by taking total control of planning the couple's daily activities. When David wants to change their social plans, Robin becomes anxious and depressed. For Robin, the strain of keeping control makes him question whether his quality of life is better now than it was without the medication.

Robin and David agree to attend a HAART adherence boosting group. The group sessions cover obtaining useful information, developing good communication and assertiveness skills, taking responsibility, planning a suitable medication schedule with the physician, addressing emotional difficulties, increasing self-efficacy, developing routines, pre-planning difficult times and situations, and techniques to reduce forgetting. Robin and David enjoy the problem solving and draw up a weekly diary of events and medications that highlight potential clashes.

Robin could attend the adherence group on his own or receive individual support. However, as David is available to attend, it is useful to recognize the "couple's social life" in planning by including him. Both Robin and David report enjoying an increased quality of life.

Is group therapy useful for couples?

Groups for people with HIV and their partners can provide a useful forum for sharing information, discussing adaptive coping experiences, and obtaining support from others in similar circumstances. Groups for only one member of the couple – either the person with HIV or the partner – can also be beneficial because they provide forums where the partners can discuss their particular perspectives in a nonpersonal setting.

Case study: Partner as caregiver

Philip, a busy company director and Michael, an actor, are partners. Philip is HIV-seronegative, while Michael is seropositive. Currently available antiretroviral medications no longer offer Michael any benefit. He is becoming physically weaker and has developed cognitive difficulties.

Although the couple initially adjusted well to Michael's infection, Philip has recently approached his family doctor for sleeping pills. An initial assessment reveals that Philip is finding it difficult to provide the care Michael requires and attend to his business. He wakes intermittently worrying about Michael and how he will cope if Michael deteriorates further. The family doctor sends Philip to the mental health unit to assess his mood, coping strategies, and social support.

What impact does caregiving have on the couple?

The role of caring for people with chronic or terminal illnesses has typically fallen to older, female family members. For young gay men with HIV disease, primary caregivers are often their long-term male partners. Frequently the HIV-seronegative partner becomes the principle caregiver and family manager, particularly when the person with HIV becomes symptomatic. He or she may also become the main economic provider. If these roles do not mirror those in the relationship before HIV disease, this change can cause upset and disturbance in the couple.

What impact does caregiving have on the caregiver?

Being the partner of a person with HIV is neither a simple nor singular task. The diseases associated with advanced HIV infection are now typically managed at home, rather than in hospital. As HIV disease progresses, the responsibilities related to caring for a partner can increase. Caregivers may become physically and mentally exhausted, especially if they have not sought out or been in a position to receive support from others (e.g., friends or families).

Hays *et al.* (1994) discuss helpful behaviors identified by a group of gay men with AIDS. Most important are:

• providing love and concern
• being a confidant
• providing encouragement
• offering proactive assistance.

Partners' responsibilities can also include helping with the everyday practicalities of living with HIV, such as ensuring the partner takes the recommended medication or assisting with complex medication regimens.

The uncertainty associated with this illness can also cause practical difficulties for caregivers. It is not easy to predict when the partner with HIV will require full-time care. Even if an employer is willing to support the caregiving partner by offering long-term leave, it is difficult to organize leave when it cannot be planned in advance. Couples in which the caregiving partner is also the main financial provider may have to make the difficult decision about whether the caregiving partner continues working and leaves the care of the sick person to others, or abandons financial independence and perhaps his or her career to care for the HIV-infected partner.

With current HIV medications, people with HIV may swing a number of times from needing a large amount of care to being well and independent. Although many employers and careers can cope with one period of time spent away from work for caregiving, it is less likely that most can withstand several, unplanned, and unpredictable absences.

What is the emotional impact on caregivers?

In the midst of providing care and support, caregiving partners have to cope with physical and possible mental deterioration in people they love, the reality of their own losses, the changes in their relationships, and an uncertain future. They may also have to cope with anticipatory grief as they recognize that their partner is dying. These tasks have to be accomplished without the support they would normally have from their partner.

A number of studies have reported high levels of distress and poor physical health in caregivers (Folkman *et al.*, 1994). Despite recent advances in treatment and more therapeutic optimism, partners still experience high levels of distress. A significant number of partners of men with AIDS have definite psychiatric diagnoses. However, many caregivers derive meaning from their caregiving.

Philip reveals that Michael is becoming increasingly forgetful. He is no longer contributing to everyday household tasks nor is he reading biographies (which he previously enjoyed) but spends his time watching TV game shows (which he previously detested). Philip is diagnosed with adjustment disorder with mixed emotional features.

Does the severity of illness affect the caregiving burden?

It would be reasonable to expect that the more severe the illness, the greater the caregiving burden. Although not all studies have found a link between severity of illness and level of caregiving distress, the caregiving burden does appear to increase with specific problem behaviors, such as frequent demands for attention associated with emotional disturbance or organic brain disease.

The mental health team assesses Michael and confirms that he has cognitive deterioration, and suggests that Philip enlist social support. Although most of the couple's friends are supportive, they work long hours and are not available during the day. Michael's family lives close but, as family members have difficulty accepting the two men as a couple, they have not yet been told about his HIV status. There is no day care centre or respite care available locally. Philip realizes that he will have to disclose Michael's HIV status to his family in order to get the support the couple needs.

How important is social support?

Caring for someone who is severely disturbed can be onerous, and social support for the person with HIV and the caregiving partner is extremely important. If residential care is not available or not desired by the person with HIV or the caregiver, the caregiver should try to arrange for day care and respite care, which will make it possible to maintain the person in the community.

Support from significant others is widely believed to buffer the impact of a wide variety of stressful life events including chronic illness (Cohen and Wills, 1985; Littlefield *et al.*, 1990). Social support has been linked with improved psychological well-being and decreased depression and anxiety in homosexual men with HIV infection (Hays *et al.*, 1993). In addition to buffering the impact of stress on mental health, social support is also considered an important factor in coping with/recovering from physical illness and in increasing adherence to medication regimens (Wallston *et al.*, 1983). Satisfaction with social support is associated with low levels of distress (Gray and Hedge, 1999).

Friends or family members can only be supportive to a couple coping with HIV disease if they are aware of the issues. Disclosure can be difficult. The couple may fear that people will judge their lifestyle which resulted in acquiring HIV. They may dread the stigma and fear of contagion. They may also feel guilty about engendering negative emotions in those they tell, such as grief and anger.

HIV-seropositive gay men are more likely to seek support from their gay peers than their family members (Hays *et al.*, 1993). HIV-seropositive heterosexual men and women are more likely to disclose their serostatus to partners and friends, and less likely to disclose to immediate family members. Lack of social support is particularly marked for individuals from cultures that either do not accept homosexuality or do not openly discuss sexual matters (Petrak *et al.*, 2001).

Many couples delay disclosure until the HIV-infected partner is hospitalized or other symptoms of the illness (e.g., altered physical appearance, depression, or strange behaviors associated with organic brain disease) make some explanation inevitable. They have some justification for withholding information. In a rural area, parents of an HIV-seropositive adult reported that the stigma associated with the disease caused them more difficulties than the physical and mental care of their gay adult son (McGinn, 1996).

Assessment reveals that Michael has become the center and focus of Philip's life, at the expense of his own needs. Philip breaks down and reveals how Michael's recent deterioration makes him feel that he has already lost Michael. He has considered taking his own life to rid himself of the distress.

Are partners of individuals with HIV at increased risk of suicide?

Partners of people with HIV experience many stressors associated with increased suicide risk in the general population, such as life events, depression, social isolation, and cumulative stress. Over 50% of gay or bisexual male caregivers of partners with AIDS report suicidal ideation (Rosengard and Folkman, 1997). Suicidal ideation has been shown to be more prevalent in caregivers bereaved by HIV than in those who are not bereaved.

Thoughts of suicide just prior to and immediately following the death of the partner are related to caregiver burden, perception of poor social support, and ineffectual coping strategies such as behavioral escape-avoidance. The death of a person with AIDS is often a time when services that could provide some support to surviving partners are withdrawn.

Because of high rates of suicidal ideation in caregivers, it is important that clinicians raise the topic of suicide, provide opportunities for caregivers to discuss these thoughts and feelings, acknowledge the mental health needs associated with the death of a partner, and provide support and encourage effective coping strategies.

The therapist encourages Philip to positively reappraise the situation, actively problem solve, seek social support, and occasionally distance himself from the situation. The therapist stresses that he and Michael have made the most of their time together, and suggests that Philip contact Michael's family and maintain some of his outside interests. Philip is able to assign positive meanings to events which happen. For example, a smile or enjoying a day in the sunny garden generate positive mood states that help him cope with the terrible reality.

What are the best coping strategies for caregivers?

Coping can be conceptualized as the emotional, cognitive, and behavioral strategies that are used to manage a stressful situation. Strategies can be either problem focused (attempts to solve the stressful situation), or emotion focused (attempts to live with the emotions generated by the stressful situation). Depending on the situation, either can be adaptive (Lazarus and Folkman, 1984). Problem-focused strategies are most beneficial when the situation is controllable, whereas emotion-focused strategies are beneficial when the situation it is not controllable. Problem-focused coping strategies that have been shown to be beneficial for partners of people with HIV include active problem solving, distancing, positive reappraisal, and seeking social support (Folkman *et al.*, 1994). Those that have been linked to negative mood include avoidance or disengagement and suppression of competing activities.

The clinician encouraged Philip to increase his use of problem-focused coping strategies, specifically: to positively reappraise the situation – Michael and he had made the most of their time together; actively problem solve – assess all possible solutions to problems that arose; seek social support – contact Michael's family who live close by and occasionally distance himself from the situation by maintaining some of his outside interests – partaking in a Sunday walking group once a month in order to feel refreshed. Anticipatory bereavement (emotion-focused coping) was also addressed.

Are there specific issues for gay couples?

The vast majority of people with HIV in the western world are young gay men, and their primary caregivers are their young gay partners. In this respect, HIV disease is unlike other diseases where families carry the burden of care. There are few role models for partners of gay men with HIV disease and little societal support.

In many jurisdictions, gay relationships are not recognized legally, which can create difficulties. The couple relationship may not be recognized at work, and employers may not afford the same privileges (e.g., time off) they would to hetero-sexual couples dealing with a terminal illness. The couple may face financial and housing problems if the partner dies without a will or with inadequate insurance.

Gay couples may also have to cope with stress associated with stigma/homophobia. Many people are "out" to friends but not to families or in the workplace, which means they may face more difficulty accessing social support (including emotional support), companionship, information and advice, help with tasks, and material aid which could significantly enhance their quality of life.

Case study: HIV in a seroconcordant couple

Matthew and Martha are partners. While on work experience in Europe when she was a student, Martha had injected heroin a few times. When she learned that a friend from that group tested HIV-seropositive in a prenatal screening programme, she went for testing and learned she was infected. When Michael learned of her status, he was tested and found to be positive.

The two want to stay together and support one another. They have decided not to have children, although this deeply saddens them both.

Are there specific difficulties for couples who are both positive?

With HIV, unlike most chronic illnesses, a significant proportion of couples will both be infected and face the same uncertainties. In a US sample, 36% of caregivers of people with HIV were also HIV-seropositive. In couples where both partners are infected, it is not always clear who is the "patient" and who is the "caregiver". These roles often change over time.

Caring for a partner who has a life-threatening illness is stressful. When the caregiver has the same disease, it can become even more stressful. HIV-seropositive caregivers are no more likely than HIV-seronegative caregivers to report suicidal ideation. However, the experience of HIV-infected caregivers is somewhat different from those who are are not infected, particularly before and after the partner's death. While their partner is alive, HIV-seropositive caregivers report less distress than those who are not infected. After their partner's death, HIV-infected caregivers show more distress. This may be because infected caregivers view the experience as a model for their own death. Before death, they empathize with their partner; after death, they become more aware of their own mortality, and realize that they have to face that trauma without a partner's love or support.

Factors associated with unrelieved depressive symptoms in HIV-seropositive caregivers appear to be: long relationships, high levels of daily hassles, self-blame, and distancing. The factors that distinguish between those who report suicidal ideation and those who do not are: a perceived lack of support, a greater use of behavioral escape-avoidance coping strategies, and a high burden of caregiving (Rosengard and Folkman, 1997).

Conclusion

HIV can have a significant psychological impact on couples, their relationship, and their ability to function as individuals, even when the partner(s) with HIV are asymptomatic and well. When one partner's health deteriorates and the other partner becomes a caregiver, the dynamics of the relationship change. Support from mental health providers can help couples develop more adaptive patterns of communication, more effective coping strategies, and better social support.

REFERENCES

Catalan, J., Burgess, A. and Klimes, I. *Psychological Medicine of HIV Infection*. Oxford: Oxford Medical Publications, 1995.

Cohen, S. and Wills, T. Stress, social support and the buffering hypothesis. *Psychological Bulletin*, **98** (1985): 310–57.

Folkman, S., Chesney, M. and Christopher-Richards, T. Stress and coping in caregiving partners of men with AIDS. *Psychiatric Clinics of North America*, **17** (1994): 35–52.

Glass, S. and Wright, T. Reconstructing marriage after the trauma of infidelity. In *Clinical Handbook of Marriage and Couples Intervention*, W. K. Halford and H. J. Markman, eds., pp. 471–507. Chichester: John Wiley & Sons, 1997.

Gray, J. and Hedge, B. Psychological distress and coping in the partners of gay men with HIV-related disease. *British Journal of Health Psychology*, **4** (1999): 116–26.

Hays, R., McKusick, L., Pallack, L. *et al*. Disclosing HIV seropositivity to significant others. *AIDS*, **7** (1993): 425–31.

Hays, R., Magee, R. and Chancey, S. Identifying helpful and unhelpful behaviours of loved ones: the PWA's perspective. *AIDS Care*, **6** (1994): 379–92.

Lazarus, R. and Folkman, S. *Stress, Appraisal and Coping*. New York: Springer, 1984.

Littlefield, C., Rodin, G., Murray, M. and Craven, J. Influence of functional impairment and social support on depressive symptoms in persons with diabetes. *Health Psychology*, **9** (1990): 737–49.

McGinn, F. The plight of rural parents caring for an adult child with HIV. *Families in Society*, **77** (1996): 269–78.

Petrak, J., Doyle, A. M., Smith, A. *et al*. Factors associated with self-disclosure of HIV serostatus to significant others. *British Journal of Health Psychology*, **6** (2001): 69–79.

Rabkin, J. G. and Chesney, M. Treatment adherence to HIV medications: the Achilles heel of the new therapeutics, In *Psychosocial and Public Health Impacts of New HIV Therapies. AIDS Prevention and Mental Health,* D. Ostrow, and S. Kalichman, eds., pp. 61–82. New York: Kluwer Academic/Plenum Publishers, 1999.

Rosengard, C. and Folkman, S. Suicidal ideation, bereavement, HIV status and psycholosocial variables in partners of men with AIDS. *AIDS Care,* **9** (1997): 373–82.

Wallston, B., Alagna, S., DeVellis B. and DeVellis, R. Social support and physical health. *Health Psychology,* **2** (1983): 367–91.

HIV and cultural diversity

Cecile Rousseau, M.D. FRCP(C)

Associate Professor, Psychiatry Department, McGill University, Montreal
Director, Transcultural Child Psychiatry Team, Montreal Children's Hospital, Montreal, Canada

Introduction

Disease does not occur in a vacuum. It occurs in a specific cultural context which determines how the illness will be identified, interpreted, and managed. Culture is a social matrix that includes the ethnocultural background of both patient and clinician, as well as the knowledge and practices that each brings to understanding and treating illness (Kirmayer *et al.*, 2003). Cultures are not fixed, stable entities. They are fluid and dynamic, especially in the face of globalization which increases tension between local worlds and global trends (Bibeau, 1997).

In pluralistic societies, cultural diversity is both a source of richness and a clinical challenge. Culture-related barriers to healthcare range from language to poor adherence (which has been documented frequently but is still not well understood) (Beiser, 1988). Unfortunately, healthcare providers tend to focus on cultural differences and de-emphasize the role that specific cultural value systems, coping strategies, and solidarity networks can play in the healing process or in framing chronic illnesses.

Different countries have developed a variety of models for culturally appropriate care, which tend to reflect the historical, social, and political orientations of mainstream societies. For example, the UK model focuses on avoiding racism, the US model attempts to match patients with clinicians from the same ethnic background, while the Australian and Canadian models focus on developing culturally competent healthcare providers who are able to provide culturally responsive services (Kirmayer and Minas, 2000).

To address cultural dimensions in clinical care, clinicians will identify:
- their own personal, professional, and institutional subcultures
- how these may shape the clinician–patient interaction.

The impact of the institution's culture on service provision is often a blind spot, but clinicians who are aware of the wider context in which the clinical

HIV and Psychiatry. A Training and Resource Manual, Second Edition, ed. Kenneth Citron, Marie-Josée Brouillette, and Alexandra Beckett. Published by Cambridge University Press. © Cambridge University Press 2005.

encounter occurs are more likely to recognize and overcome any culture-related barriers.

Clinicians should approach people with HIV with the same sensitivity to culture they would use with any illness. But in HIV, the universality and strength of the evocation of Eros and Thanatos (love and death) is a particularly powerful link between the patient and the clinician. This shared humanity in the face of suffering and death should invite the clinician to discover the person's world in a very respectful way before co-constructing the medical contribution to his or her care.

How does cultural diversity affect assessment?

When working with patients from diverse cultures, clinicians should ensure that clinical assessment is seen as a process and is carefully planned. A rigid assessment process may not allow the clinician to build a strong alliance with the patient, and may hinder the chances of providing successful continuity of care. For example, pushing a patient to disclose delicate aspects of his or her life (e.g., sexuality, family dynamics, previous trauma) may have a negative impact on the clinician's ability to establish trust. To be culturally responsive, the clinician may also have to rethink concrete procedural aspects of assessment, such as appointment making, in-take process, time, and space issues.

When planning the assessment, clinicians should consider the following:

- Is an interpreter needed? When discussing life and death issues or taboo subjects like sexuality, patients who have only a basic understanding of the clinician's language may not be able to communicate their feelings, understanding of their illness, personal situation, or their reaction to the clinician's proposals. When an interpreter is needed, clinician and patient should discuss who would be acceptable. Whenever possible, the interpreter should not be someone from the patient's family. When choosing an interpreter, clinicians should also take into account factors such as gender, age, and the interpreter's specific ethnic or religious affiliation.
- Has the patient experienced discrimination? If the person belongs to a minority group, the clinician should consider the power differential within the therapeutic relationship and the impact it may have. By openly addressing the prejudices, discrimination, or blatant racism the person may face in society, the clinician may be able to relieve the sense of powerlessness in the clinical encounter and strengthen the therapeutic alliance.
- Is the patient's knowledge valued? Before investigating the person's understanding of her or his illness, the clinician should acknowledge the knowledge that he or she brings to the encounter. This will demonstrate that the clinician is interested in the patient's point of view, and will respect the information/ knowledge the person shares.

- Does the clinician have a clear understanding of the problem? Having a number of different points of view on a health problem (i.e., from the person, the family, other people from the same community) can give clinicians very useful information about the patient, and his or her network and system of values. However, clinicians should be careful not to label one of these perspectives as "the truth". Differing points of view usually reflect the complexity of the person's situation and may keep the clinician from stereotyping.

Individuals' own understanding of their symptoms and illness guide their illness behavior and responses to treatment (Good and DelVecchio-Good, 1980; Kleinman, 1980). To understand more about the patient's meaning systems, the clinician should discuss the person's perception of the cause, course, appropriate treatment, and expected outcome of his illness. However, people do not always provide a clear and coherent explanation of their illness. Sometimes they may associate their stories with similar stories, or with specific events that happened when their symptoms developed (Kirmayer *et al.*, 1994). Frequently the meaning systems will evolve with time and will vary as a function of life events and disease evolution. The degree of similarity or discrepancy between the meaning that a person attributes to his or her illness and the family's and community's understanding may indicate, to a certain extent, the level of support or rejection the person can expect from his or her family/community.

To improve cross-cultural communication, Berlin and Fowkes (1983) have suggested the mnemonic LEARN:

Listen to the patient's perception of the problem

Explain your perception of the problem

Acknowledge and discuss differences and similarities

Recommend treatment

Negotiate an agreement

How does cultural diversity affect treatment planning?

Treatment planning should take into account both the patient's and the clinician's meaning systems, and include an implicit or explicit negotiation around some components, such as the number of blood tests, the medication, disclosure to significant others, changes in sexual behavior, and sources of support.

Out of respect for professionals or fear of institutions, some people with diverse cultural backgrounds will not disagree directly with a proposed treatment plan. However, they may demonstrate their disagreement by not adhering to the plan. When faced with adherence problems, clinicians often try to overcome the person's resistance by presenting more arguments to defend or explain the treatment plan. When this strategy fails, members of the care team may become impatient or angry.

However, clinicians should interpret adherence problems as a message from the patient, listen to the person's concerns, and reopen the negotiations or discussions about the treatment plan without negating their own priorities or beliefs.

When developing a treatment plan or intervention, clinicians should consider the following:

- Does the treatment plan encourage a plurality of approaches? Clinicians may find it helpful to use a plurality of approaches to the illness, including modern medical practices, religious healing and support, traditional healing, or other alternatives. Patients should feel they can question medical assumptions and prescriptions in the same way that clinicians might question a traditional medication they think might be harmful.
- What are the person's sources of social support? In general, clinicians will find it helpful to mobilize the person's support network, including family and community resources. However, if the patient's medical condition is secret or taboo, he or she may not be able to use traditional or family supports. Mainstream community groups may be able to play a role, but often cannot replace the patient's family or cultural networks. In these cases, the clinician may have to rethink the role that the person's support system can play.
- What role will the person's cultural beliefs play? During chronic illnesses, like HIV, the person's beliefs and the way he/she seeks help can vary considerably from one phase of the disease to another. When faced with death, some very acculturated people return to traditional beliefs and practices systems, while others lose faith. Clinicians should be attentive to these shifts and keep a flexible vision of the person through the whole illness process.

REFERENCES

Beiser, M. Influences of time, ethnicity, and attachment on depression in Southeast Asian refugees. *American Journal of Psychiatry*, **145**(1) (1988): 46–51.

Berlin, E. O. and Fowkes, W. C. A teaching framework for cross-cultural health care. *Western Journal of Medicine*, **139** (1983): 130–4.

Bibeau, G. Cultural psychiatry in a creolizing world: questions for a new research agenda. *Transcultural Psychiatry*, **34**(1) (1997): 9–41.

Good, B. and DelVecchio-Good, M. J. The meaning of symptoms: a cultural hermeneutic model for clinical practice. In *The Relevance of Social Science for Medicine*, L. Eisenberg and A. Kleinman, eds., pp. 165–96. Dordrecht: D. Reidel Publishing Co., 1980.

Kirmayer, L. Minas, I. H. The furure of cultural psychiatry: an international perspective. *Canadian Journal of Psychiatry*, **45**(5) (2000): 438–46.

Kirmayer, L., Rousseau, C., Jaruis, E. G. *et al.* The cultural context of clinical assessment. In A. Tasman, J. Lieber and J. Kay, eds., *Psychiatry*. New York: John Wiley & Sons, 2003.

Kirmayer, L. J., Rousseau, C., and Santhanam, R. Models of diagnosis and treatment planning in multicultural mental health. In *Navigating Diversity: Immigration, Ethnicity and Health*, A. Rummens, M. Beiser, and S. Noh, Eds., Toronto: University of Toronto Press, 2003.

Kirmayer, L., Young, A. and Robbins, J. M. Symptom attribution in cultural perspective. *Canadian Journal of Psychiatry*, **39**(10) (1994): 584–95.

Kleinman, A. *Patients and Healers in the Context of Culture: An Exploration of the Borderland between Anthropology, Medicine, and Psychiatry*. Berkley: University of California Press.

African Americans

Kenneth Ashley, M.D.

Assistant Professor of Psychiatry and Behavioral Sciences, Albert Einstein College of Medicine, New York, NY
Attending Psychiatrist at Beth Israel Medical Center, New York, NY, USA

Introduction

Although HIV first affected mainly white men in the USA, the number of cases in African Americans has increased steadily and dramatically. By 1996 in the USA, more cases of AIDS occurred in African Americans than in any other racial/ethnic population. In 1999, almost half the AIDS cases in the USA were African American and in 2001, African Americans accounted for 21 000, or 49%, of the more than 43 000 new adult AIDS cases reported (CDC Fact Sheet). In 2001, African American women accounted for nearly 64% of HIV cases reported in women (CDC Fact Sheet). African American children represent almost two-thirds of all reported pediatric cases (CDC, 2001a). AIDS is the leading cause of death among African American men ages 35–44 and African American women ages 25–34. AIDS is among the top three causes of death for African American men ages 25–54 and African American women ages 35–44 (CDC Fact Sheet). It has become such a serious issue that, in February 2001, there was a call for a Federal State of Emergency for African American Communities and HIV/AIDS.

When working with African Americans, clinicians should remember that they are not a monolithic group. Each person is an individual with his or her own experiences and beliefs. There is no simple model or explanation of community behavior. However, the concepts discussed in this chapter may play some role in patients' life experience and development.

While African Americans with HIV face many of the same issues as others with HIV, they also have some unique issues. For many African Americans, HIV is yet one more issue on a long list of problems including poverty, unemployment, limited economic opportunities, disenfranchisement, poor education, substance use, and violence. Many African Americans also have difficulty trusting the medical establishment.

HIV and Psychiatry. A Training and Resource Manual, Second Edition, ed. Kenneth Citron, Marie-Josée Brouillette, and Alexandra Beckett. Published by Cambridge University Press. © Cambridge University Press 2005.

This chapter:

- discusses the causes of the disproportionate rates of HIV infection in the African American community
- explores the reasons why many interventions that are successful in the white gay male community are less effective among African Americans
- proposes and describes culturally sensitive/appropriate interventions to address HIV in the African American community.

Case study: An African American man with HIV and adherence issues

Robert is a 40-year-old heterosexual African American man with HIV. He has a history of polysubstance dependence, including injection drug use, and is on opioid agonist therapy. Because he was previously nonadherent to prescribed medications, his primary care provider refers him for psychiatric assessment before initiating highly active antiretroviral therapy (HAART).

The psychiatrist assesses Robert and identifies no current psychiatric disorder that would impair his ability to adhere to medication. However, Robert voices concerns that the medication is "poison", and talks about many friends who started medication (AZT) years ago and who are now dead. He is worried that the medications are experimental and does not want to be a "guinea pig". He refers to "Tuskegee" and, although he does not know the specifics of the Tuskegee Syphilis Study, he does know that, in the past, the US government conducted improper research on African Americans. Robert is also afraid of the side effects he might experience.

What are some of the historical factors that account for the difficulty many African Americans have in trusting the medical establishment?

One barrier to helping the African American community deal with HIV is its historic mistrust of the medical community. There are long-standing historical tensions in the relationship between African Americans, the US government, science, and medicine as illustrated by the "Tuskegee Study of Untreated Syphilis in the Negro Male". This study of untreated syphilis began in 1932 and lasted 40 years, ending in 1972. Approximately 400 African American sharecroppers were enrolled in the study to document the natural history of syphilis. The participants were not educated about the sexual transmission of syphilis or the vertical transmission from mother to fetus. Men in one arm of the study were excluded from treatment even when penicillin became the standard of care for syphilis in 1951. The longest nontherapeutic experiment on human beings in medical history, it involved the US Public Health Service, the Tuskegee Institute in Alabama (a historically Black college founded by Booker T. Washington, its first president), a variety of governmental health agencies, and local black churches and public schools.

When details of the study gradually became known, the African American community began to suspect that the US government, science, and the field of medicine, which were willing to experiment on African Americans, might be working together to exterminate the Black race. Although many years have passed, the distrust continues to resonate among many in the African American community. Recent findings that African Americans receive lower quality healthcare, regardless of socioeconomic status or medical coverage, have only reinforced that sense of mistrust. The Institute of Medicine (2003) has concluded that "[al]though myriad sources contribute to these disparities, some evidence suggests that bias, prejudice, and stereotyping on the part of health care providers may contribute to differences in care."

This history has made many segments of the African American community receptive to conspiracy theories about HIV (e.g., HIV was created by the government as part of a genocidal plot, HIV is not the cause of AIDS and the drugs are part of a profit-making scheme, the medications for HIV are part of an effort to experiment on people of color, the drug companies have a cure but are keeping it off the market so they can sell more medications that extend life). Unfortunately these theories have been discussed in forums sponsored by individuals who are considered leaders in the African American community, which gives them more credibility. The way African Americans view HIV is also influenced by the concerns about the connection between HIV and AIDS which was until recently being loudly debated in South Africa. Their sense of distrust is compounded by the drug companies' and the US government's resistance to the production and distribution of generic formulations of HIV medications, particularly in Africa, which reinforces for many African Americans that corporate profits are more important than saving lives.

How do racial differences affect the ability to develop a therapeutic relationship?

Because racism is an issue for many African Americans, non-African American caregivers working with this population should listen closely, especially during early sessions, for any comment on racial issues. This can provide an opportunity to discuss the issue of racial difference in the dyad – something that is usually evident, but rarely addressed.

Acknowledging that there are racial differences between the clinician and the client is often enough. However, issues of race may also have to be addressed during assessment and treatment planning. The client may question whether the caregiver can be trusted or will understand his or her particular issues or concerns. While this may be no different from the early stages of any therapeutic relationship, any problems that arise in the relationship are more likely to be attributed to ethnic differences.

To avoid this and address it early, the caregiver should inquire about cultural issues that are important to the patient. Remembering the patient may not want to be a "teacher", caregivers should have other resources they can refer to for questions about cultural differences.

How can the psychiatrist help address issues of adherence when working with African American patients?

A patient's willingness to adhere to medication can be affected by a psychiatric condition, by side effects of the medication, or by his or her belief system.

A careful patient assessment will often reveal the presence of a psychiatric or psychological issue, such as depression, substance use, or impaired cognition, which can influence adherence. The physical and psychological side effects of HIV medications may also be a factor.

When trying to improve adherence, clinicians should assess the role that the patient's belief system may be playing. Patients are more likely to adhere to medication if:

- they believe they have HIV (and that AIDS is caused by HIV)
- they believe the medications will be helpful.

Some African American individuals may distrust caregivers simply because they are part of a larger healthcare system that, in their view, is not concerned about patients. In these cases, it will take time for the caregiver to prove him or herself and to develop a trusting relationship. Strategies clinicians can use to build trust and an effective alliance include:

- being on time and respectful (i.e., if late, apologize)
- taking an interest in the person's life
- ensuring patients feel they are being listened to and taken seriously
- acknowledging some of the history and community distrust, when appropriate
- working with the patient's primary care provider
- answering the person's questions openly and honestly
- fulfilling promises (e.g., calling with test results)
- providing resources from the community literature
- referring the person to peer support groups addressing medication issues.

One conversation will not necessarily convince the patient to begin taking HAART. The first session is often the beginning of a process of developing a trusting relationship, which may increase the likelihood that the patient will take the medication.

Over time, the psychiatrist develops a trusting relationship with Robert and determines that Robert's reluctance to take HIV medication is due to his fear of the side effects. Because Robert is not feeling ill, he worries that the medication will make him feel worse and continues to refuse antiretroviral therapy. Although he trusts his healthcare providers and feels they are doing the best job they can, he continues to distrust the healthcare system. Despite the psychiatrist's efforts, Robert continues to refuse medication.

Case study: An African American woman with HIV

Marie is a 38-year-old woman who was infected with HIV many years ago through sexual intercourse with her husband, who injects drugs. She lives alone with three of her children (the other ones recently moved out). The children's father visits irregularly. Marie is generally healthy and is not on any HIV medications.

Unemployed and the primary caregiver for her younger children and her elderly parents, she reports a long history of depression and anxiety. She claims that all she wants to do is to live long enough to see her youngest daughter graduate from high school. She says she has no interest in developing a loving, intimate relationship with anyone.

Marie is relatively stable on sertraline for depression and anxiety. She keeps most of her appointments and, when she misses one, it is usually because another family member has a need she feels is more important than her own. She is somewhat isolated. Her only close relationships are with family members, none of whom know about her HIV. Marie spends most of her time caring for her ill parents, visiting her mother who is in a nursing home every day. She socializes regularly with her sister.

The psychiatrist works with her to help her achieve some balance between taking care of others and taking care of herself (i.e., keeping her appointments, taking her psychotropic medications) and to tell her family that she has HIV. The therapist works with her on family issues, on issues of dependence and independence, and on goal-setting.

What additional issues need to be considered when working with African American women with HIV?

African American women with HIV are dealing with the same issues as other women (e.g., caring for children, partners and parents, putting the needs of others before their own, neglecting their own care, power imbalances in relationships). The fact that they are African American simply adds another layer.

Some data suggest that African American women are more likely than white women to be poor, single, underemployed mothers. Given the large number of African American men who are incarcerated, there are fewer men "available" so many African American women feel pressured to maintain their relationships with men, even when the men are unwilling to engage in safer sex.

Clinicians should routinely discuss strategies the woman can use to balance her own needs with those of others. They should also discuss relationship issues and safer sex, and explore whether there is a history of sexual abuse or domestic violence.

If the woman's partner is unwilling to wear a condom, the clinician should discuss ways of having sex that do not involve penetration. When encouraging an

African American woman to take more care of herself or be more assertive in her relationships, the clinician must be careful to avoid alienating the woman by pushing concepts that she may view as culturally foreign or unacceptable. Some women may find it helpful to participate in group therapy with other African American women, and be more accepting of strategies and ideas that come from women in the same situation. Others may find groups too anxiety provoking and prefer individual therapy. Some women, particularly those with a history of abuse, may respond better to a female clinician. If abuse or violence is an issue, the clinician should make appropriate referrals.

When working with African American women, clinicians should also be aware that this population has high rates of high-risk behaviors. As of December 1999, 42% of AIDS cases in African American women were associated with injection drug use, while 38% were due to heterosexual contact. The clinicians should discuss drug and alcohol use in an open, nonjudgmental way, and suggest strategies that may help the patient remain drug free (e.g., getting the woman's consent to request random toxicology screens). Clinicians working with African American women with a history of drug use should have a high index of suspicion for relapse in patients who exhibit a sudden change in behavior (e.g., the woman appears intoxicated or stops keeping regular appointments, or reports greater family or environmental stress).

What is the significance of child bearing and child raising in the African American community?

For many African American women, and the African American community in general, motherhood confers status and respect. To help ensure African American women with children keep their appointments, the treatment facility should provide childcare services and, if possible, treatment for both infected and affected children. If appointments for both mother and children can be scheduled on the same day, the mother can ensure her children's needs are met without neglecting her own.

With antiretroviral therapy, people with HIV are living longer, entering into new relationships, and may be interested in having children. Women with HIV are now able to give birth with a relatively low risk of infecting the child. When the issue of pregnancy and childbirth arises, it should be addressed with various members of the healthcare team:

- the psychiatrist can discuss with the woman her desire to have a child and, at some point, include her partner in the discussion
- the primary care provider should address the woman's and her partner's medical condition
- a member of the high-risk obstetrics team can discuss the risks and benefits of pregnancy and childbirth.

It may also be helpful for the woman to talk with other HIV-infected women who have had children to fully appreciate the issues involved so the woman can make an informed decision.

Marie continues in treatment, but is preoccupied with taking care of her father who is terminally ill with end-stage metastatic lung cancer. Shortly before his diagnosis, she had planned to begin group therapy as a way to reduce her isolation and discuss living with HIV. She has postponed group therapy and recently is missing more appointments.

> ## Case study: An African American man who has sex with men
>
> Jordan is a 25-year-old man who was recently infected with HIV through unprotected sex with another man. After his diagnosis Jordan began to feel physically weak and somewhat depressed, and he quit his job. Since then, he has been isolated, spending most of his time at home where he lives with his mother. He says that he has been feeling anxious for several years, ever since he began to go out to clubs and have sex with men. He fears that the people around him perceive him as gay.
>
> His primary care provider would like Jordan to begin taking HAART but he refuses to do so until he can move out on his own. Jordan is afraid his mother will find out that he has HIV, either by finding the medication or noticing some change in his behavior due to medication side effects.
>
> Jordan considers himself an unfortunate victim of a potent sex drive and low self-esteem, which led him to engage in unsafe sex. He is taking paroxetine and clonazepam for anxiety and depression, and is dealing with his relationship with his mother and his self-esteem issues.

What are the issues facing African American men who have sex with men?

Although many African American men who have sex with men identify themselves as gay, many do not. As a result, many men of color tend to ignore education and care focused on gay men. In some communities, to be gay is to be white or effeminate or the receptive partner. If a man does not see himself as any of these things, he may not consider himself gay. Although there is an increasing amount of literature on internalized homophobia (i.e., self-hate and other negative internalizations about one's homosexual orientation), an African American man's decision not to identify as gay may have other meanings than internalized homophobia.

Many African American men who have sex with other men also have sex with women. Many are married and have children. When working with an African American man who has sex with men, clinicians should explore:

- the man's sexual behavior
- how he self identifies (i.e., gay, heterosexual, bisexual)

- how strongly he does or does not identify with the gay community
- whether the man's family and friends know he has sex with men.

This information will be important in determining the patient's sense of isolation, his support system, and his ability to adhere to treatment (i.e., some patients will skip doses to keep their condition secret). This information can also guide treatment interventions, which may include referrals to a community-based organization.

During discussions about sexual behavior, the clinician may learn that the person with HIV is engaging in unprotected sex with his partner(s). In these cases, it is important to understand why. Is it a desire for children? Fear that using a condom will make partners think that he is infected? Lack of access to condoms? Concerns about diminished sensation with the use of condoms? Men who have been having unprotected sex may be reluctant to inform partners, and clinicians may have to work with them to look at the barriers to disclosure. In some cases, psychotherapeutic interventions may be appropriate and helpful. Clinicians should encourage any known sexual partners to be tested for HIV. (For more information on partner notification, see Chapter 18 on Legal and ethical issues.)

In an effort to deal with HIV, the African American community has developed community-based organizations, and the black churches have generally ended their silence on HIV. In addition, larger HIV/AIDS facilities have developed outreach programs or established satellite clinics in communities of color, and people from the disenfranchised communities have been involved in developing appropriate education materials. As a result of these efforts, an increasing number of African Americans are receiving education and care. However, in spite of the progress that has been made, data from a recent, large, multisite study indicate that young men who have sex with men of all races are still engaging in high-risk behaviors (i.e., having five or more male sex partners during the preceding 6 months, having unprotected anal sex with men, or injecting drugs) (CDC, 2001b). This highlights the need for everyone who has contact with African American males to reinforce safer sex and drug use practices, and for mental health professionals to explore and address the root causes of this risk-taking behavior.

Jordan has moved into his own apartment and is taking HAART and adhering to treatment. He is stable on his psychotropic medications, but is resistant to individual psychotherapy. He continues to have difficulty addressing the issues of low self-esteem, social isolation, and poor relationships.

Conclusion

HIV/AIDS is ravaging the African American community. Those living with HIV are often in need of mental health services to address underlying psychiatric conditions, to help them deal with mental health issues related to HIV (e.g., anxiety, depression), or to help them adhere to complicated medication regimens.

While African Americans with HIV face the same issues as others living with HIV, they also face some unique cultural issues that may have an impact on their treatment. Clinicians must keep in mind the potential impact of African Americans' historical distrust of the healthcare system, as well as their attitudes towards sexuality and relationships.

REFERENCES

Centers for Disease Control. HIV and AIDS – United States, 1981–2000. *Morbidity and Mortality Weekly Report,* **50** (2001a): 430–4.

The Institute of Medicine. *Unequal Treatment: Confronting Racial and Ethnic Disparities in Healthcare.* Washington, DC: National Academies Press, 2003 (Available as a living document at www.iom.edu or www.nap.edu).

Centers for Disease Control. HIV incidence among young men who have sex with men – seven U.S. cities, 1994–2000. *Morbidity and Mortality Weekly Report,* **50** (2001b): 440–4.

SUGGESTED FURTHER READING

Centers for Disease Control and Prevention (CDC). Fact Sheet – HIV/AIDS Among African Americans.

Fernandez, F., Ruiz, R. and Bing, E. The mental health impact of AIDS on ethnic minorities. In *Culture, Ethnicity, and Mental Illness,* A. Gaw, ed., pp. 573–86. Washington, DC: American Psychiatric Press, 1993.

Griffith, E. E. H. and Baker, F. M. Psychiatric care of African Americans. In *Culture, Ethnicity, and Mental Illness,* A. Gaw, ed., pp. 147–73. Washington, DC: American Psychiatric Press, 1993.

Smith, C. African Americans and the Medical Establishment. *Mount Sinai Journal of Medicine,* **66** (1999): 280–1.

WEBSITES

African American AIDS Institute:
    www.aaainstitute.org(or www.blackaids.org)
Gay Men of African Descent:
    www.gmad.org

The Balm in Gilead: (Supports and educates Black churches about HIV)
  www.balmingilead.org
National Black Leadership Commission on AIDS:
  www.blca.org (under construction)
National Minority AIDS Council:
  www.nmac.org
  CDC. Fact Sheet – HIV/AIDS Among African Americans, www.cdc.gov/hiv/
  pubs/facts/afam.htm

Latinos and HIV disease

Frank Hector Galvan, Ph.D., L.C.S.W.

Assistant Professor, Department of Psychiatry and Human Behavior, Charles R. Drew University of Medicine and Science, Los Angeles, CA, USA

Introduction

Latinos (Hispanics) living in the USA have been disproportionately affected by HIV/AIDS. Although Latinos comprise only 12.5% of the US population (US Census Bureau, 2001), they accounted for 19.7% of people diagnosed with AIDS between 1996 and 2000 (CDC, 2001a). Through June 2000, men accounted for 82% of all AIDS cases among Latinos (CDC, 2000), and the main routes for HIV transmission in Latino men were male-to-male sexual contact (42%), injection drug use (35%), heterosexual contact (6%), and both male-to-male sexual contact and injection drug use (7%). Among Latina women with AIDS, 47% contracted the illness through heterosexual contact and 40% via injection drug use.

The primary risk for exposure to HIV varies among Latino groups. For example, male-to-male sexual contact is the primary risk factor for both Mexican- and American-born Latinos (CDC, 2001b). In contrast, intravenous drug use is the primary HIV risk factor among Latinos born in Puerto Rico.

The clinician working with HIV-seropositive Latinos must recognize the diversity that exists within the Latino community. Age, gender, nationality, social class, educational level, migratory experience, and degree of acculturation each have a profound impact on the individual's experience. Furthermore, cultures are themselves dynamic, changing with time and circumstance. Nevertheless, certain common cultural characteristics can be identified among Latinos of different backgrounds. Clinicians who understand these cultural factors will be able to work more effectively with Latinos with HIV.

To provide culturally competent mental healthcare, clinicians must contend with language. When possible, it is best for a Spanish-speaking patient to receive services in his native language from a Spanish-speaking provider. Clinicians who

This work was supported by the National Institute of Mental Health (5P30-MH58107–03/PO#2000-G-AJ057) and the Universitywide AIDS Research Program of the Regents of the University of California (IS99-DREW-203). Appreciation is extended to Dr. Eric Bing, Dr. Ricky Bluthenthal and Norma Guzman-Becerra who reviewed the manuscript and provided valuable recommendations.

HIV and Psychiatry. A Training and Resource Manual, Second Edition, ed. Kenneth Citron, Marie-Josée Brouillette, and Alexandra Beckett. Published by Cambridge University Press. © Cambridge University Press 2005.

use a translator, even one who speaks perfect Spanish, run the risk of not picking up some of the nuances that could be conveyed by certain words or phrases and could be lost during the translation process. However, if an interpreter is required, clinicians should avoid using a patient's family member, friend or significant other, because the patient may not be fully forthcoming with information (e.g., sexual activities or drug use) in front of family or friends. Whenever possible, clinicians should try to match a patient with interpreters of the same background and gender. For example, a patient who is a Mexican national should ideally be matched with an interpreter who is also a Mexican national (rather than a Mexican American born in the USA) who will be familiar with specific colloquialisms or the fine nuances of certain words or phrases the patient may use. Every effort should also be made to match patients with interpreters of the same gender. Some Latino immigrants, particularly those who are more traditional, may be uncomfortable talking about medical conditions, especially those that are sexually related, in front of an interpreter of the opposite sex. If this is not possible, the clinician should be aware that the patient may not disclose some information or ask certain questions.

Case study: A Latino gay man with HIV

Benito, a 34-year-old, bilingual immigrant from México, has been living in the USA for eight years. All his family, except one sister who lives nearby, is in México. He lives alone and works as a car mechanic. He was diagnosed with HIV about a year ago, but has only recently begun medical treatment for the disease. He was referred by his HIV specialist to a psychiatrist for treatment of depression.

   Benito describes himself as gay but does not seem at ease with his sexual orientation. He has not discussed his sexuality or his HIV status with his family. Benito reports feeling guilty about his sexual contacts with men. He worries about how his family would respond to learning that he has HIV. Although he feels certain his family would not reject him, he does not want to cause them worry about his medical condition.

How important is the family for HIV-positive Latinos?

The family plays a very important role for Latinos (Gaines *et al.*, 1997), including those with HIV infection (Galvan, 1999). *Familism* is a strong cultural value among Latinos and is reflected in family relationships by a powerful sense of loyalty and reciprocity (Gaines *et al.*, 1997). These relationships extend beyond the immediate nuclear family and include extended family members and *compadres/ comadres* (the godparents of one's child).

   The clinician should explore the patient's relationship with his family and the role this relationship plays in his life. While the family may be a source of strength for some, it can cause significant stress for others. The clinician may want to help the patient weigh the pros and cons of disclosing his HIV status to his family. With patients whose family may not be supportive, the clinician should explore alternative sources of support.

How is homosexuality perceived in Latino cultures?

Many Latino gay men grow up in a context that views homosexuality as something to be scorned and ashamed of (Diaz, 1998). This view of homosexuality places a high value on *machismo* or "hypermasculinity", an exaggeration of masculine traits (Diaz, 1998). This conceptualization of masculinity is not unique to Latinos, nor is it shared by all Latinos (Gaines *et al.*, 1997). Nevertheless, an overemphasis on "hypermasculine" traits can result in low self-esteem among Latino gay men (Diaz, 1998).

The clinician working with a gay HIV-seropositive Latino man should explore how he integrates his sexuality into his life. If the patient experiences low self-esteem because of failing to achieve a "hypermasculine" ideal, he may benefit from a referral to a support group (Diaz, 1998). The group provides a forum in which these stereotypes and beliefs about masculinity may be examined and challenged.

Support groups can break down the sense of isolation such patients may feel and promote a sense of camaraderie. They are also a good source of information for individuals coping with different aspects of HIV, such as disclosing one's HIV status to family, friends, and sexual partners, and dealing with complex treatment regimens.

For some individuals, disclosing their HIV status to family members may also involve informing them for the first time of their gay or bisexual orientation. Referring these patients to a support group of other Latino gay or bisexual men may provide additional support as well as the opportunity to learn from others who have gone through similar experiences with their own family members.

Patients who may not feel comfortable attending a support group or who live in places with no support groups might find support and information on the internet (see list of websites at the end of this chapter).

How would the situation be different for Benito if he were heterosexual?

Benito would probably still experience the stigma and discrimination associated with having HIV because of the disease's association with other behaviors (e.g., injection drug use) that are not morally sanctioned. Some people may believe that he is bisexual or homosexual. Others may react with judgmental attitudes because of their perception that acquiring HIV is due to a deficit in character.

A clinician working with an HIV-seropositive Latino heterosexual male should explore any negative interactions the patient may have had with others because of his HIV status. The patient may need assistance in developing adaptive coping skills that he can use to manage similar situations in the future.

During the course of his therapy sessions, Benito admits to taking his HIV medications irregularly and not adhering to other aspects of his HIV care. There are several reasons associated with his nonadherence. Benito appears to have a limited understanding of the importance of complying with all aspects of his HIV care. His nonadherence also appears to be related to his depression and subsequent diminished interest in several aspects of his life. In addition, Benito experiences powerlessness over his HIV. His comments during therapy suggest that he believes that fundamentally there is nothing he can do to alter the course of his infection.

What can the clinician do to increase adherence?

It is important to address the issues that may be affecting an individual's adherence to his or her medical regimen for HIV. In Benito's case, the focus can be on increasing his basic knowledge of HIV medical care as well as addressing his depression. The former can be done through referrals to AIDS service organizations that offer a multitude of services for HIV-seropositive patients, including basic knowledge of HIV care and the importance of adherence to medical guidelines. To address his depression, some alternatives include individual psychotherapy, referrals to support groups, and psychotropic medications if indicated.

Diaz (1998) has observed that for many HIV-seropositive Latino men, living with HIV is only one of several life adversities that they may face, including experiences of poverty and racism. He adds that one effect of such experiences, over which these men feel they have little control, is that these individuals then generalize their sense of powerlessness to other areas of their life where they could exercise some control. It is possible that this is the case with Benito, who believes he is powerless to alter the course of his HIV.

The clinician should be aware of experiences such as poverty and racism in an individual's life history that could influence how that person approaches his HIV. Some Latinos are also more likely to experience discrimination than others. For example, Finch et al. (2000) showed that Latino immigrants who are highly acculturated are more likely to perceive discrimination than less acculturated immigrants. This is in contrast to highly acculturated US-born Latinos who are less likely to experience discrimination than their less acculturated US-born counterparts (Finch et al., 2000).

Knowing about a patient's place of birth, acculturation level, and experiences with racism, discrimination, and poverty can be useful in assessing how that person may cope with HIV and providing guidance to the clinician about the need to intervene. One possible intervention is to educate the person about the direct benefits of adherence to his HIV medical regimen. Another potential intervention is to refer the individual to support groups that attempt to empower HIV-seropositive Latino gay and bisexual men to take greater control over their lives. Such groups provide the opportunity for participants to critically examine the factors contributing to their behaviors (Diaz, 1998). This is done in a supportive context of other individuals who have had similar experiences.

Benito's psychiatrist explores with him his ambivalence about his same-gender feelings and sexual activities. Benito reports experiencing conflict between his beliefs about masculinity and his same-sex sexual behavior. His psychiatrist recommends that, in addition to individual therapy, he participate in a support group for HIV-seropositive Latino gay men to address such concerns. Benito begins to attend the group.

The psychiatrist also examines with Benito the pros and cons of revealing his HIV status to his family. It appears to the clinician that Benito's lack of disclosure to family members could be depriving him of the support that he needs and contributing to his depression. After several weeks, Benito informs his sister of both his HIV status and sexual orientation. Her response is very supportive. With her assistance, he appears to be making a better adjustment to having HIV and being gay.

Benito also starts attending informational workshops about HIV and learns the importance of adherence to his HIV medications and other medical guidelines. He becomes more adherent to his medical regimen. His emotional state also improves through a combination of individual therapy, antidepressant medications, and participation in a support group. His support group meetings include discussions on the powerlessness experienced by many Latino gay men with HIV, as well as ways to counter this by taking an active involvement in one's medical care.

Case study: A Latina woman with HIV

Lupe, a 28-year-old Puerto Rican single mother of a 3-year-old girl, was diagnosed with HIV 2 years ago and has been receiving medical treatment ever since. She was referred by her doctor to a psychiatrist because of symptoms of depression.

Prior to her diagnosis with HIV, Lupe had a relationship with a man who had a history of injection drug use and has also been diagnosed with HIV. She herself has never used any drugs.

Lupe lives with her daughter, who is HIV-seronegative. She reports having no contact with her daughter's natural father. Lupe has a high school education and works as a receptionist for a business firm. Although she describes herself as being in good health, she admits she does not always attend her medical appointments. This is because she occasionally has difficulty finding childcare for her daughter.

How do the personal responsibilities of Latinas with HIV affect their medical care?

Lupe occasionally misses her medical appointments to take care of her daughter. Her experience is very similar to that of other HIV-seropositive women whose care-giving responsibilities (for children or others) may compromise their medical care (Stein *et al.*, 2000).

For the clinician working with a Latina in this situation, it is important to discuss the patient's practical needs and barriers to healthcare, and explore options for providing some relief or support with caregiving responsibilities. For example, the clinician could make a referral to an HIV case manager who could link the woman with social services and other resources that can provide assistance. By responding to a patient's concrete needs, the clinician can help her to prevent deterioration in both her physical health and psychological well-being.

Lupe reports feeling overwhelmed by her situation. She worries about what the future may hold. Although she reports having a close relationship with her family, they all live very far away, and she feels isolated from them. Although she describes herself as religious, she does not attend any particular church.

What coping resources can Latinas with HIV draw on to help them live with their diagnosis and concomitant stressors?

The value of *familism* described earlier extends also to Latinas (Gaines *et al.*, 1997). It is important for clinicians working with Latinas to examine the extent of emotional and other support from family members. If a patient has limited contact with family members, the clinician may want to explore with her whether she should increase her contact with them and/or seek other sources of social support.

Another cultural resource available to Latinas with HIV is spirituality/religiosity, which has been described as a great source of strength by both Latinas (Simoni and Cooperman, 2000; Valdez, 2001) and Latinos (Galvan, 1999) with HIV. A clinician should explore the extent to which spirituality can help the patient cope with the stresses of living with HIV. If a patient identifies spirituality as an available coping resource, the clinician can encourage the person to find the most appropriate way to express this.

Clinicians should also help Latinas with HIV find ways to develop a sense of mastery over their situation. According to research with this population, a sense of mastery is associated with less depression and better physical well-being (Simoni and Cooperman, 2000). One way of doing this is to help a patient reflect on occasions in her past when she successfully overcame a particular challenge and then apply that same capacity to her present situation.

Lupe admits having recently met a man in whom she is interested and who is also infected with HIV. Although she reports not yet having engaged in sexual relations with him, she worries about the possibility of re-infecting herself. She is also concerned about how he might react if she suggests they use condoms.

How can a Latina with HIV be empowered to negotiate safer sexual practices with her sexual partner?

To prevent the risk of re-infection with HIV or exposure to other infections, an HIV-seropositive Latina needs to be empowered to take the necessary steps to protect herself. She should be aware of how to negotiate sexual activity between her and her partner, and of any power differences that may exist between them. For some, this may require information on conflict resolution and negotiation skills (Ortiz-Torres *et al.*, 2000).

A clinician who works with a Latina who has difficulty negotiating safer sex practices should consider referring her to a group or workshop specifically on this topic. These groups focus on teaching women empowering skills that increase their ability to negotiate safer sexual practices. These groups examine the social construction of sexuality and gender roles, how unequal power gender relationships contribute to the practice of risky sexual behaviors, and the role of social networks in reinforcing the practice of safer sex (Ortiz-Torres *et al.*, 2000).

Clinicians should be vigilant for any signs of possible abuse by the woman's partner that may be associated with the woman's attempt to be more assertive. In such cases, it may be appropriate to involve the legal system and refer the woman to a shelter.

During the course of her therapy, Lupe begins to consider various ways to improve her situation. She becomes more open with her family about the stress that she has been experiencing. As a result, her 24-year-old sister moves in with her. This provides additional emotional support to Lupe as well as someone to look after her daughter. Lupe no longer misses any of her medical appointments.

Lupe also reports making greater use of her religious faith to help her cope, having a greater sense of mastery over her situation, and experiencing less depression. She starts attending a women's support group where members discuss techniques for negotiating safer sex practices with sexual partners. However, when she tries out these new skills with her new partner, he is not receptive. As a result, she decides to end the relationship.

Lupe reports experiencing better mental health. She indicates that she feels less overwhelmed by her situation and less worried about her future. She reports feeling more optimistic in general and better able to cope with her HIV.

Conclusion

Clinicians caring for Latinos with HIV should be familiar with their patients' cultures. Providing culturally competent mental health services to this population requires more than offering services in the patients' language. Clinicians must also be aware of the differences and similarities among various Latino populations and the resources these cultures provide that can help Latinos cope with HIV. The benefits for patients who receive effective culturally relevant services include improved mental health and greater trust of mental health providers.

REFERENCES

Centers for Disease Control and Prevention (CDC). National Center for HIV, STD and TB Prevention. Surveillance Report, **12**(1) (2000). (Available as a living document at http://www.cdc.gov/hiv/stats/hasr1201/table9.htm and http://www.cdc.gov/hiv/stats/hasr1201/table11.htm).

Centers for Disease Control and Prevention (CDC). HIV and AIDS – United States, 1981–2000. *Morbidity and Mortality Weekly Report*, **50**(21) (2001a). (Available as a living document at http://www.cdc.gov/nchstp/od/20years.htm).

Centers for Disease Control and Prevention (CDC). *HIV/AIDS among Hispanics in the United States* (2001b). (Available as a living document at http://www.cdc.gov/hiv/pubs/facts/hispanic.htm).

Diaz, R. M. *Latino Gay Men and HIV: Culture, Sexuality, and Risk Behavior*. Routledge: New York, 1998.

Finch, B. K., Kolody, B. and Vega, W. A. Perceived discrimination and depression among Mexican-origin adults in California. *Journal of Health and Social Behavior*, **41** (2000): 295–313.

Gaines, S. O., Rios, D. I. and Buriel, R. Familism and personal relationship processes among Latina/Latino couples. In *Culture, Ethnicity, and Personal Relationship Processes*, S. O. Gaines, R. Buriel, J. H. Liu and D. I. Rios, eds., pp. 41–66. New York: Routledge, 1997.

Galvan, F. H. Sources of personal meaning among Mexican and Mexican American men with HIV/AIDS. *Journal of Multicultural Social Work*, **7**(3/4) (1999): 45–67.

Ortiz-Torres, B., Serrano-Garcia, I. and Torres-Burgos, N. Subverting culture: promoting HIV/AIDS prevention among Puerto Rican and Dominican women. *American Journal of Community Psychology*, **28**(6) (2000): 859–81.

Simoni, J. M. and Cooperman, N. A. Stressors and strengths among women living with HIV/AIDS in New York City. *AIDS Care*, **12**(3) (2000): 291–7.

Stein, M. D., Crystal, S., Cunningham, W. E. *et al.* Delays in seeking HIV care due to competing caregiver responsibilities. *American Journal of Public Health*, **90**(7) (2000): 1138–40.

U.S. Census Bureau. *The Hispanic Population: Census 2000 Brief*. (May 2001). (Available as a living document at http://www.census.gov/prod/2001pubs/c2kbr01–3.pdf).

Valdez, M. A metaphor for HIV-positive Mexican and Puerto Rican women. *Western Journal of Nursing Research*, **23**(5) (2001): 517–35.

WEB SITES

www.altamed.org. This is the website of AltaMed Health Services whose headquarters is in Los Angeles, California. It is a Latino agency offering a variety of medical, mental health and social services in Spanish and English to HIV-positive Latinos and Latinas.

www.bienestar.org. This is the website of Bienestar Human Services, Inc., whose headquarters is in Los Angeles, California. It is a Latino agency offering a variety of mental health and social services in Spanish and English to HIV-positive Latinos and Latinas.

www.caps.ucsf.edu/projects/hlsindex.html. This is the website of Hermanos de Luna y Sol, which describes itself as an empowerment HIV prevention program for Spanish-speaking Latino gay/bisexual men. Its headquarters is in San Francisco, California. It is primarily a support group for Spanish-speaking Latino gay/bisexual men. It does not offer any other services, but would be able to refer HIV-positive Latinos to any needed services. This program is also affiliated with the Center for AIDS Prevention Studies of the University of California, San Francisco, which conducts research with this population.

www.critpath.org/galaei. This is the website of the Gay and Lesbian Latino AIDS Education Initiative whose headquarters is in Philadelphia, Pennsylvania.

www.latinoaids.org. This is the website of the Latino Commission on AIDS whose headquarters is in New York City.

One heart, two spirit, and beyond: HIV and the people of the First Nations

Terry Tafoya, Ph.D.

Executive Director,, Tamanawit, Unltd., Seattle, WA, USA

Introduction

There are approximately two million Native Americans in the USA. Well over half (more than 60%) live in urban areas, and the rest on or near a reservation. Defining who is and who is not Native American is so complicated (see Box 16D.1) that it was not until the late 1980s that the US Centers for Disease Control began to distinguish American Indian/Alaskan Natives as a separate AIDS reporting category (Tafoya, Personal Files, 1987).

Official Centers for Disease Control and Prevention (CDC) records list two AIDS cases in American Indians and Alaskan Natives in 1984 and 2301 cases in 2003 (Figure 16D.1). In the early years of the epidemic, reporting likely underestimated the actual impact of the disease on this population.

American Indian/Alaskan Native males account for the majority of AIDS cases in this population (82.6%) while women account for only 17.4% (Table 16D.1). In terms of risk factors for acquiring HIV, most men are infected through sex with men, while the majority of women are infected through intravenous drug use and heterosexual contacts.

Box 16D.1. Who is Native American? The problem of defining a Native identity

There are at least nine different legal definitions of Native American (Tafoya 1989, p. 282). American Indians and Alaskan Natives are the only ethnic group still tracked by blood quantum by the US federal government. In this context, to be an American Indian individuals have to be one-quarter blood of a formally recognized tribe.

Until Constitutional revisions in the late twentieth century, people of the First Nations in Canada operated under a different system of identity. If a

---

HIV and Psychiatry. A Training and Resource Manual, Second Edition, ed. Kenneth Citron, Marie-Josée Brouillette, and Alexandra Beckett. Published by Cambridge University Press. © Cambridge University Press 2005.

woman with recognized "Native status" married a husband who was "non-status", she lost her status by "marrying out" and their children were considered "non-status". This led to a number of generations of "illegitimate" children so the woman and her children could maintain "status."

American Indians, Alaskan Natives, and people of the First Nations in Canada also share the political reality of being the only North American ethnic groups who have treaties with their federal governments. In exchange for a number of different rights, (including land use and water rights), these groups were promised support for, among other things, healthcare and education. Eligibility for these rights is one reason why status is so important.

Table 16D.1. Risk factors for HIV infection in American Indians and Alaskan Natives

Risk factor for HIV infection	Men 82.6% of cases	Women 17.4% of cases
MSM	60.9 %	
MSM/IDU	17.4%	
IDU	14.6%	53%
Heterosexual	6.5%	41%
Transfusions	0.04%	5%
Hemophiliac	0.2%	1%

MSM, men having sex with men; IDU, intravenous drug use.

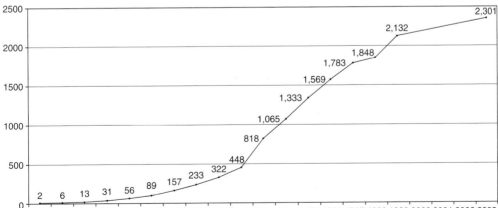
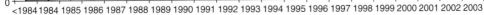

Figure 16D.1: Cumulative growth in AIDS cases in American Indians/Alaskan Natives 1984–1999

In Canada, the People of the First Nations constitute only 2.8% of the Canadian population, but accounted for 12.9% of reported AIDS cases in 2002. Their risk factors for infection are similar to those of American Indians and Alaskan Natives, although the number of cases attributed to intravenous drug use increased from 2% before 1991 to 15% between 1991 and 1995, and up to 34% between 1996 and 2000. Native women in Canada show a much higher rate of IDU as an exposure risk compared with non-Native AIDS cases (34.3% to 5.9%). Vertical transmission from mother to child is a concern in the Native population, as is the large proportion of Native street youth.

According to the Canadian Center for Infectious Disease Control and Prevention, "... available evidence suggests that Aboriginal persons are infected at a younger age than non-Aboriginal persons; that injecting drug use is the most important mode of transmission, and that the HIV epidemic among the Aboriginal community shows no sign of abating. Furthermore, the mobility of Aboriginal persons between inner cities and rural areas may bring the risk of HIV to even the most remote Aboriginal community" (Center for Infectious Disease Prevention and Control, 2001).

What impact has HIV infection had on Native communities?

As Native people began feeling the impact of their HIV status, many chose to return to their own communities as a way of dealing with the disease. People who had moved away from their communities to explore their sexuality became infected in the "city," and then moved back "home." This "returning migration" is problematic because:

- clinics in the often remote communities often have little experience of dealing with HIV
- confidentiality is an issue in small, rurally based reservations and reserves
- if the "returnees" engage in unprotected sex or share needles, this can create a vector of infection within the Native community.

Case study: Spiritual possibilities and HIV

Luke is a 52-year-old American Indian of the Lakota Nation. One of several children, he grew up, like many American Indians of his generation, with a combination of urban and extremely rural reservation experiences. He reports childhood memories of a home without electricity or running water. He was raised with a combination of Native traditional spirituality and Catholicism (a common mix for many Natives), and Lakota and English. From an early age, Luke recalls being attracted to a spiritual path, inspired by a grandmother identified as a Medicine Woman (traditional healer), as well as a more fundamentalist church. His dreams of becoming an ordained minister were shattered when he was "outed" as a gay man. He reports being demonized and prayed for before being ultimately rejected by the church members.

Luke moved to a major urban area where he completed his higher education and started exploring life in the gay community. At that time, he was involved in a number of episodes of high alcohol use. When he returned to the reservation, he had a number of jobs involving social services.

He was diagnosed with HIV at the local Indian Health Clinic in the late 1980s. A breach of confidentiality resulted in Luke being "outed" once again – this time as someone with HIV. His Tribal Nation responded out of fear and ignorance, firing him from his position as Tribal Planner. His firing was directly related to HIV and not to his sexual orientation. His physician realizes that Luke is experiencing significant distress and offers to refer him to a therapist but Luke refuses. He mentions that he may explore traditional ceremonies that might promote healing, and the physician encourages him to explore that path. They both agree that the traditional approach would complement, rather than replace Western approaches. The physician's interest in traditional ceremonies fosters the development of a trusting relationship.

What is the Native concept of sexuality and gender?

Data indicate a higher level of bisexual behavior among Native Americans than any other ethnic group studied (Tafoya, 1989). This may demonstrate a consistently more fluid concept of sexuality. Of the nearly 200 Native languages still spoken in North America, more than two-thirds have terms for more than two genders (Tafoya and Rowell, 1988; Tafoya and Writh, 1996). In more recent times, a number of Native people have coined the term "Two Spirit" as a term to describe a third gender. In 1987, this term was formally accepted by an international gathering of Native peoples from Gay, Lesbian, Bisexual, Transgender, and Queer (GLBTQ) communities. This group shared the feelings of other Natives that the more "standard" GLBTQ terminology was too "Euro-centric" and missed the elements of gender role and spirituality that were part of the Native traditions. The term also incorporates the idea that many Natives hold: that we have both male and female "energies" or "spirits" within. This is one of the traditional explanations of why so many American Indians and people of the First Nations historically wore their hair in two braids: to concretely represent the balance between the male and female for which we should strive.

For many Two-Spirit people, that balance seems to be something they "are" as opposed to something they "do." Some of the traditional roles of the Two Spirit include teaching, keeping the knowledge of the elders, healing, child care, spiritual leadership and participation, herbal wisdom, interpretation, mediation, and all forms of artistic expression (Tafoya, 1992).

The more traditional a Native community is, the more accepting it is of variations in sexual and gender orientation. The more Christianized a Native community becomes, the more it tends to reflect the values of fundamentalist Christianity, and be judgmental of homosexual behavior.

What is the basis for Native mistrust of non-Natives?

Historically, the experience of Native children in residential boarding schools and the social service interventions in Native families have been particularly significant. Native children were not originally allowed to attend public schools. In the nineteenth century, the USA and Canada established federal boarding schools for Native children. With the founding of these schools, "the rights of parents ceased to exist ... native children were removed as far from their parents as possible and frequently were not even allowed to return home on vacation." The theory behind this treatment was "to civilize the Indian, put him in the midst of civilization." Everything native had to be destroyed, even if the process sometimes meant destroying the native himself (Forbes, 1964).

The suppression of Indian languages, religion, and lifestyles, and the forced removal of children from their families were standard practices. Discipline was strict, punishment severe, and the schools suffered from overcrowding, which created health problems (e.g., tuberculosis, trachoma) (Colmant, 2000).

Today, there are fewer than 70 Indian boarding schools operating in the USA, but in the 1970s there were over 200 (Colmant, 2000). It wasn't until the close of the twentieth century that the extent of physical, emotional, and sexual abuse related to Native education was publicly acknowledged. *The Indian Residential School Study* by the Nuu-Cha-Nulth Tribal Council of Canada (1996) reported three main themes from its research (Colmant, 2000)

- great loneliness (93%) and often a sense of abandonment by their parents
- loss or repression of native culture and language (91%)
- the witnessing (92%) or experiencing (90%) of various types of abuse in residential schools.

Given the experience of education in Native lives, it should hardly come as a surprise that Native people often place less importance on education, than many other minority groups, and are less trusting of non-Natives.

In addition to providing opportunities for sexual abuse, the residential schools, with their single-sex dormitories, may have created an environment where young Native people's first sexual experiences were with someone of the same sex, regardless of their ultimate sexual orientation. For Native people who identify as gay, bisexual, lesbian or queer and who were sexually abused, there may be some clinical question (as there is with non-Natives) about the impact abuse may have had on their sexual orientation.

Another experience that has left Natives mistrustful of non-Natives is their interactions with social services. Before the passage of the Indian Child Welfare Act of 1978, up to one out of every four American Indian children were being reared in non-Native homes (Kelso and Attneave, 1981; Manson, 1982; Tafoya, 1989; Tafoya and Wirth, 1996). The statistics are very similar for Canadian People of the First Nations. Over 90% of these children were removed from their homes for "neglect" as opposed to "abuse," and the definition of neglect was based on the standards of the White community. For example, before the revision of the Washington State activity codes, a child could be removed if he or she didn't have a separate bedroom, and the adoption rates for Indian children in Washington State were 19 times higher than those for non-Indian children (Swinomish Tribal Community, 1991). Many Native Americans and people of the First Nations refer to these children, who are now adults, as "Lost Birds." Because of the "sealed" adoption records in many states, individuals may know they are American Indian or Native, but will not be able to discover the Nation to which they belong or identify biological family members.

From a clinical perspective, this means it would not be unusual to encounter someone who is "ethnically Native," but not "culturally Native." These clients may have few Native resources or points of reference.

What kind of traditional ceremony can be helpful to Native patients?

The Lakota Sundance is a central feature of Lakota Spirituality. The ceremony is, among other things, a socially sanctioned rite of purification and rebirth, which incorporates extreme physical pain with the expectation of blessing and renewal.

The Sundance involves fasting for 4 days and, in some cases, requires the Sundancer to be pierced through the muscles of the chest and then literally attached to a large wooden pole in the central dance area. The Dancers will dance until the participants are torn free. This leaves distinctive scars that are easily recognizable when seen by many other Native people and conveys a respect and status for someone who has shown bravery in enduring the pain as a way to gain strength and purification for the People.

For many American Indians and People of the First Nations, the Sundance is understood as a model of their historical experiences of surviving an armed invasion and the occupation of a hostile force. The suffering the Sundancer must go through in order to restore harmony in the future represents the subjugation and systematic attempts to destroy Native cultures, languages, and lifestyles, the removal of Native children due to non-Native governmental inter-ference, and the devastation of alcohol.

Luke decides to concentrate more on his spiritual development and his 3-year relationship with another HIV positive man he met during their medical treatments. He is completing an autobiography. He has also returned to painting, and is gaining growing recognition for his artistic talent. Luke has managed to survive for a very long time, in a way that integrates both Western and non-Western approaches in a respectful manner. He has consistently provided for his extended family, just as a heterosexual man would, and his extended family provides support, concern, and love for him. His sexuality is acknowledged, but not as the center of his existence. His male partner is treated in much the same manner as his siblings' significant others.

Case study: A heterosexual Native single mother

Marie is a 26-year-old Native heterosexual urban woman with HIV. Originally from an isolated coastal reservation in the US Pacific Northwest, she moved to the city to go to college and is employed in an office where she has worked since graduation. She has a 4-year-old daughter, who is also HIV-positive. Marie believes herself to have been infected during her relationship with her daughter's biological father, a Euro-American from a community bordering the reservation who uses injection drugs. She had a relationship with him during a summer she visited her family. He was apparently aware of his HIV infection but did not disclose this information to her.

Marie has sought help because of situational depression. The state in which the reservation is located has laws concerning people who know their HIV status and infect others, and is now suing the man who infected her. There has been a preliminary hearing regarding the case. Because it is difficult to keep anything secret in isolated rural communities, most of the people in her reservation as well as people in the adjoining town now know that she has HIV. Members of the reservation are anxious that other tribal members may also be infected, and have been trying to retrace Marie's sexual history (and that of her former lover).

Marie is the youngest of six siblings. Her father is deceased. She reports being close to her family, but does not get to spend as much time with them as she would like, since they all live on the reservation, more than a 5-hour drive from the major metropolitan area where Marie and her daughter live. Her direct contact is usually limited to various ceremonial events and holidays, when she returns to her original home, or when her nieces, nephews, and their parents attend sports activities or powwows in the "City" and stay with her.

Marie has been very forward about not wanting to use Indian Health Services resources, and has stated she feels supported by her company and its generous healthcare benefits, which give her access to "state of the art" care she would not be able to obtain on the reservation. The company also provides a daycare program for her daughter. The administration knows about her diagnosis, but her fellow workers remain unaware of her condition. Although she would like to have many children, she has decided against it for fear of infecting them.

What is the place of parenting in the Native culture?

Native culture highly values children, and associates parenting with responsible adulthood. Adults who do not have a biological child may take over primary parenting of a nephew, niece, or orphan, in order to gain the parenting experience, and to provide for the child. Adults are also traditionally expected to care for their parents in their old age.

Many Native women who identify as lesbian, bisexual, or Two Spirit are biological mothers. Some become pregnant in their early years to "prove" their heterosexuality in environments that are heterosexist and homophobic. Some become pregnant to have a child they feel will love them (particularly if they come from a dysfunctional family that has difficulty expressing love), while others make a conscious decision to have a biological child.

Are there traditional ceremonies that could be useful to Marie and her daughter?

In trying to help Marie during this stressful period, the family decides to focus on two specific ceremonies: a "Blessing/Healing" ceremony that formally asks the community to support Marie and her daughter, and make them feel more integrated; and a "Naming Ceremony" for the daughter.

Naming Ceremonies are significant in many Native Nations. Some cultures believe that the special Indian name one receives in the ceremony is the name the Creator will use to call the person to the Spirit World when one dies. A person who doesn't have an Indian name may not be able to join loved ones in the Spirit World. High status is associated with having an Indian name, and it is the way one is addressed in ceremonies and on special occasions.

Because the daughter's biological father has "diluted" her blood to below the require-ments for a Native American, she does not qualify for treaty access to healthcare and education. However, receiving an Indian name allows the community to formally acknowl-edge the daughter, and it reinforces her undisputed membership in her Nation, regardless of issues of blood quantum.

At this time, Marie has had no serious HIV-related health problems. She is adherent to her prescribed medication. Although none of her coworkers have heard of the controversial legal action taking place in her home community, she is very concerned that the news media might pick up the case and expose her and her daughter to unwanted publicity. She fears this could cost her the job she values (although she has no evidence that this would happen). She prefers to have no further contact with her daughter's father, who is abusive when he is on drugs.

Marie is also exploring having her daughter spend part of the summer on the reservation, in order to have more extended contact with the other members of her family and her peers, thereby strengthening her own status in the community.

When are Natives better served by a culturally specific service?

In some cases, Native people will deliberately seek non-Native clinical care. This may be because non-Native settings are more anonymous or because they may provide better quality care than federally funded Native health services. The extremely rural environments of most Native reserves and reservations are not conducive to keeping primary care providers abreast of the latest developments in HIV treatments.

The most important resource in working effectively with Native people is the same as working with any group of people: respect. Clinicians should allow the client to set the pace in terms of "labels" to be used, and to explain their under-standing of sexuality, gender, and identity. Be aware that these terms may change as clients go through developmental shifts and are exposed to alternative ways of thinking about themselves and HIV. Native people may also be reluctant to bring up information that non-Native people find to be unusual, such as the idea of more than two genders. As a survival technique, some Natives will deliberately withhold information if they feel a provider will laugh at them for their beliefs, or tell them to stop traditional practices.

A common problem with non-Native providers involves a difference in what is called "pausetime" in sociolinguistics. Pausetime is the duration of silence that regulates turn-taking in conversation. In other words, "I stop talking … and then you realize that you can now say something without interrupting me." Bilingual research has shown that the influence of another language can be traced over at least three generations. In other words, if a patient's parents or grandparents spoke a language other than English, then the patient will not tend to process English like a native speaker of English, even if the patient only uses English for communication. This is particularly an issue with Native patients, whose pausetime is often longer than the pause time of native English speakers. This can result in Native clients being labeled passive-aggressive, withdrawn, and noncommunicative, when in reality they are waiting for a longer pause from the clinician. That longer pause doesn't come, because when clinicians don't hear a response in their anticipated time, they repeat the question, move on to another question, or simply answer the question themselves.

What are some strategies for working with Native patients?

Trust is critical to establishing initial rapport. To help build trust, consider the following:

- Are there any visual images of People of the First Nations on the walls of your reception area or your office/examination room?
- Do posters, prints, or art convey a nonverbal message that a particular group (e.g., Native/GBLTQ/Two-Spirit) is welcome? If there is, then a "hidden" Native patient may be much more willing to "disclose" his or her actual ethnicity.

(Many clinicians are probably already treating Native patients but assuming they are members of other ethnic groups.)

- What have other Native people with HIV done? With HIV specific issues, offer Native clients examples of what others have done in their situation. For many Native people, the past is often used to provide guidelines for future conduct. Some may feel uncomfortable with a "pioneer" responsibility of proceeding into unknown territory. Explaining how other Natives in the same situation have integrated traditional ceremonies to supplement Western Medicine can be helpful. However, if the concept strikes a particular patient as odd or threatening, do not pursue it. The patient may not be actively involved in that aspect of his/her culture, or may be a "Lost Bird."

- Can you refer your patient to a Native support group? Native culture traditionally focuses on directive interaction (i.e., "here are some things you can do . . . ") versus an emphasis on emotional insight (i.e., "how do you feel about this?") For this reason, Native patients who identify with their own spiritual traditions often talk about feeling alienated from predominantly Christian support groups. If your community doesn't have a large enough group of HIV-seropositive Native patients to maintain a Native group, is there another, more appropriate alternative?

- Is the group respectful of members' different pausetime? The difference in pausetime can often cause difficulty with Native patients in support groups. Those with the shortest pausetimes tend to dominate all conversations, while those with the longest pausetimes never have an opportunity to speak. When facilitating a group, clinicians should make every effort to give each member the pausetime required to encourage participation.

Conclusion

Because there are over 500 federally recognized tribal entities in the USA, as well as many in Canada, there is no way of talking about Native issues that will not generalize their complex diversity.

Many Native people involved in public healthcare continue to be concerned about how closely Native communities mirror the African communities most devastated by AIDS. They share the following characteristics:

- relatively poor communities
- limited access to healthcare
- populations with a large percentage in the most "sexually active" age group
- substance abuse
- high incidence of other sexually transmitted diseases.

Since the beginning of the epidemic, the response of Native communities has moved from fear to better understanding. As a result, these communities are often available to provide support to their HIV-infected members, including those who return to the reservation after years of absence. This means that individual patients can draw on the rich spiritual tradition of their people, and integrate both Western and non-Western approaches in a respectful manner.

References

Center for Infectious Disease Prevention and Control. Bureau of HIV/AIDS, STD and TB Update Series. Ottawa, Ontario: CDC, 2001.

Colmant, S. U.S. and Canadian Boarding Schools: A Review, Past and Present. *Native Americas Journal*, **17** (4)(2000): 24–30.

Kelso, D. and Attneave, C. *Bibliography of Native American Indian Mental Health*. Westport, CT: Greenwood Press, 1981.

Manson, S. (ed.) *New Directions in Prevention Among American Indian and Alaskan Native Communities*. Portland, OR: Oregon Health Services University, 1982.

Nu-Cha-Nulth Tribal Council. *Indian Residential Schools: The Nuu-chah-nulth Experience*. Canada: Nuu-Chah-Nulth Tribal Council, 1996.

Salmoral, M. *America 1492: Portrait of a Continent 500 Years Ago*. Swinomish Tribal Mental Health Project. New York, NY: Facts on File Press, 1990.

Swinomish Tribal Community. *A Gathering of Wisdom: Tribal Mental Health – A Cultural Perspective*. Mt. Vernon, WA: Veda Vangarde, 1991.

Tafoya, T. Pulling Coyote's Tale: Native American Sexuality and AIDS. In *Primary Prevention of AIDS: Psychological Approaches*, V. Mays, G. Albee, and S. Schneider, eds. Newbury Park, CA: Sage Publications, 1989.

Native Gay and Lesbian Issues: The Two Spirited. In *Positively Gay*, B. Brazon, ed. Berkeley: Fine Celestial Arts Printing, 1992.

Tafoya, T. and Rowell, A. Counseling gay and lesbian Native Americans. In *The Sourcebook on Lesbian and Gay Health Care*, M. Shernoff, W. Scott, eds. Washington, DC: National Lesbian and Gay Health Foundation, 1988.

Tafoya, T. and Wirth, D. Native American Two-Spirit Men. In *Men of Color: A Context for Service to Homosexually Active Men*, J. Longres, ed. New York NY: Harrington Park Press, 1996.

SUGGESTED FURTHER READING

Bureau of Indian Affairs. *Relocation Services*. Washington, DC: Bureau of Indian Affairs, 1957.

Demer, L. Natives Receive Apology for 1950s Racial Adoptions. In *Pathways*, pp. 1–2. Portland, OR: National Indian Child Welfare Association, 2001.

Forbes, J. *The Indian in America's Past*. Englewood Cliffs, NJ: Prentice-Hall, 1964.

Goldberg, J. *Sodometries*. Palo Alto, CA: Stanford University Press, 1992.

Hampden-Turner, C. *Maps of the Mind*. NewYork, NY: Collier Books, 1981.

17

HIV in prison populations

Cassandra F. Newkirk, M.D., CCHP[1], Kimberly R. Jacob Arriola, M.P.H., Ph.D.[2] and Ronald L. Braithwaite, Ph.D.[3]

[1] Mental Health Director at Riker's Island Penitentiary, Prison Health Services, Inc. East Elmhurst, NY, USA
[2] Assistant Professor, Rollins School of Public Health of Emory University, Atlanta, GA, USA
[3] Professor, Department of Community Health and Preventive Medicine, Morehouse School of Medicine, Atlanta, GA, USA

Introduction

Although the prevalence of HIV/AIDS in prison populations varies greatly in different countries (see Table 17.1), it is significantly higher than in the general population. For example:

- in the USA, the AIDS case rate in prisons is more than five times the rate in the general population (Maruschak, 2004)
- in Canada, the prevalence of HIV in prisons is 10 times the rate in the general population (Canadian HIV/AIDS Legal Network, 2002).

In countries in sub-Saharan Africa, Latin America, Europe, and North America, HIV prevalence among prisoners ranges from 3% based on a cross-sectional seroprevalence study in Senegal to 47% among a subpopulation of injecting drug-using prisoners in Spain (Stubblefield and Wohl, 2000).

The disproportionate burden of HIV disease in prison inmates is largely due to high-risk behaviors that individuals engaged in before being incarcerated. Most inmates with HIV became infected before coming to prison (DeCarlo and Zack, 1996). However, once in prison, inmates engage in high-risk behaviors such as unprotected sex, injecting drugs, and tattooing without sterile instruments, which promote the spread of the disease within correctional institutions (Braithwaite *et al.*, 1996). This means that inmates require effective treatment for HIV as well as access to harm-reduction strategies that could reduce the risk of transmission. According to Braithwaite *et al.* (1996), prison officials in many European countries, Canada, Australia, and Brazil have begun to endorse harm-reduction strategies, such as condom and bleach distribution, and the

HIV and Psychiatry. A Training and Resource Manual, Second Edition, ed. Kenneth Citron, Marie-Josée Brouillette, and Alexandra Beckett. Published by Cambridge University Press. © Cambridge University Press 2005.

Table 17.1. Prevalence of HIV in prison systems in select countries.

Country	Prevalence of HIV in prisons
Australia	<1%
Canada	2–20%
France	<1–2%
Germany	1–8%
Netherlands	6–8%
Norway	13%
Portugal	20%
Scotland	2–9%
Switzerland	4–12%
Ukraine	6%
United States	<1–20%

Source: Canadian HIV/AIDS Legal Network, 2001; Nelles, *et al.*, (n.d.).

provision of syringes, that could potentially reduce the spread of HIV among inmates.

In addition to HIV, inmates often have serious mental health needs. A large number of inmates have dual diagnoses of mental illness and HIV/AIDS. This is not surprising considering that there is a disproportionately higher burden of mental illness in correctional facilities than in the general population: approximately 16% of US jail and prison inmates are identified as mentally ill and report either an overnight stay in a mental hospital or having a mental condition (Ditton, 1999).

The prevalence of HIV infection is also high in certain subpopulations of psychiatric patients. For example, the prevalence of HIV among psychiatric inpatients in the USA is as high as 23% in certain facilities (see Grassi, 1996 for a review of the literature). The risk of HIV transmission among inmates with psychiatric problems is also high: the fact that psychiatrically ill patients commonly engage in HIV-risk behaviors is well documented (Grassi, 1996; Stefan and Catalan, 1995) (see Chapter 8).

Caring for inmates with both HIV and a mental illness creates special challenges, including diagnosing and treating both conditions, avoiding possible drug interactions, protecting confidentiality, and ensuring that inmates with dual diagnoses continue to receive the services they need when they are released. Because of the complex needs of inmates with HIV and comorbid mental illness, and the high risk of HIV transmission, it is crucial for medical and mental health service providers in correctional settings to work collaboratively to ensure the best possible treatment and care.

Case study: An incarcerated pregnant woman with HIV

Juanita, a 23-year-old Hispanic woman, was convicted of aggravated assault for stabbing her boyfriend who had a history of beating her. She has two children, ages 3 and 4, by her boyfriend.

During medical screening and evaluation in jail, Juanita reports using marijuana and alcohol regularly for the last 8 years, and cocaine occasionally during the last 2 years – although she denies having experienced alcohol or other drug-withdrawal symptoms. She admits that her boyfriend has injected heroin and cocaine. She reports that she has not had a menstrual period for 2 months.

Juanita also reports that she was sexually abused as an adolescent by a male family member. She has had thoughts of killing herself at times during the last 3–4 years, but has made no suicide attempts and she has not sought mental health treatment. She denies feeling suicidal at the time of intake into the prison.

On physical exam, the physician notices a vaginal discharge and diagnoses candidiasis. He orders a pregnancy test, recommends an HIV test, and does a tuberculin skin test. The pregnancy test is positive.

What should be included in the initial medical assessment of an inmate?

Medical screening is often considered the first step in an integrated continuum of care for the multiple medical and mental health problems that many inmates face (Hammett and Harmon, 1999). The majority of intake facilities in the US and many facilities worldwide have some type of medical processing system to assess the health status of the offender entering the system. This screening may include assessment for infectious diseases, chronic noninfectious diseases, history of mental illness, and suicidal thoughts and/or attempts. Women are usually screened for pregnancy and other reproductive and gynecological health problems.

Prison healthcare staff should thoroughly assess behaviors that may put inmates at risk of HIV, including injecting and noninjecting drug use, sexual history, and current sexual practices. For example, the Forensic AIDS Project of the San Francisco Department of Health provides an HIV risk assessment along with counseling on behavioral risk reduction (Hammett and Harmon, 1999). This type of comprehensive HIV risk analysis helps prison healthcare staff deliver HIV prevention messages, detect disease, and initiate treatment regimens. To conduct detailed sexual histories and elicit other information, staff often need training to help them overcome any discomfort talking about sexual behaviors.

Juanita's HIV pretest counseling is done by a nurse who works with the infectious disease specialist for the prison. Juanita does not want to be tested for HIV because she fears the reaction from her family and boyfriend if she is positive. The nurse agrees to see her again in a few days to try to persuade her to be tested for HIV.

Eight days later, Juanita is seen by a psychiatric social worker for a mental health evaluation as required under institution policy. The social worker reviews the intake screening and results of the physical exam, and Juanita shares her concerns about being tested for HIV. Because of Juanita's symptoms of depression, history of suicidal thoughts, and indecision about HIV testing, the social worker refers her to the psychiatrist, who sees her the following day and diagnoses her as depressed but not suicidal. Two days later, Juanita sees the infectious disease nurse and gives her informed consent to be tested for HIV.

Three days later, she learns the result is positive. She is extremely upset during posttest counseling and makes veiled threats about wanting to kill herself. She is referred to the prison's mental health services as an emergency.

When seen by the psychiatrist, she says that she wants to die because she does not want to tell anyone about her HIV status, especially her family – for fear of the stigma and embarrassment. She is aware that she needs to begin medications immediately to prevent transmitting the virus to her unborn child. She reports feeling overwhelmed by the thought of taking care of three children with little financial or emotional support from their father. The psychiatrist does not feel comfortable sending her back to her general population living quarters and requests that she be housed on the women's special treatment unit and placed on suicide watch.

How should correctional institutions approach HIV testing?

Both the World Health Organization and the United States Department of Justice oppose mandatory HIV testing of inmates on the basis that it is unethical, ineffective, and an invasion of privacy (AIDS Action, 2001). In the USA, prison systems vary greatly in terms of their HIV testing policies. In 19 state departments of correction, HIV counseling and testing at intake is mandatory. In the other 31 states, inmates are offered voluntary counseling and testing, but the availability of testing varies as does the degree to which medical staff encourage testing (Maruschak, 2004). In correctional institutions in Canada, England, Wales, Germany, and Israel, inmates are offered voluntary HIV testing – although the extent to which the testing in any prison setting is truly voluntary is questionable (Braithwaite *et al.*, 1996). Given the power structure of most prison systems worldwide, inmates may easily be coerced into being tested by the perceived threat of restrictions and isolation. Care must be taken to offer HIV testing in a manner that is not coercive.

Mental health service providers play an important role in inmates' decisions to be tested and in the treatment process. They often work closely with medical providers to convince inmates of the importance of being tested and are typically certified to conduct the pre- and posttest counseling. They may also work with the inmate on issues such as disclosing his or her status, permanency planning for dependent children, coping with bereavement and loss, and treatment adherence (American Psychiatric Association, 2000). Mental health professionals will also play a key role in helping inmates with HIV and a comorbid condition cope with the dual stigma.

When the psychiatrist sees Juanita the next day, she orders a low dose of lorazepam twice a day for 5 days, requests that Juanita be seen by a social worker at least once a day for the next week, and plans to evaluate her the following day for suicidality. The psychiatrist relays this clinical information to the referring physician in the medical division. The physician wants to begin HIV treatment as soon as possible to reduce the risk of transmission to the fetus, but is concerned about Juanita's ability to discuss HIV medication while in crisis.

The two physicians decide to schedule a joint treatment planning conference within the week and ask the social workers on both teams to talk to Juanita and, if the patient agrees, to solicit family support. The care team also counsels her about the risks of maternal–fetal transmission if she does not adhere strictly to her HIV medications.

How is treating psychiatric illness different in the presence of HIV?

The practice of treating HIV and mental illness in prison varies considerably around the world. In the United States, inmates are offered a full regime of highly active antiretroviral therapy (HAART) and psychotropic medications, but this is not necessarily the case in other countries. HAART regimens are often complex and difficult to adhere to, and the medications can interact with the psychotropic drugs used to treat mental illness.

In most cases of dual diagnosis, clinicians would gradually begin treatment of the psychiatric condition at low doses with the least complex treatment regimen until the patient was stable before introducing HAART. However, with a pregnant inmate, it is urgent to stabilize the women's psychiatric condition quickly in order to begin appropriate HIV treatment to protect the fetus.

At the treatment planning conference, Juanita asks questions about taking HIV and psychotropic medications. She is very concerned about going to the pill call lines and having other inmates know what medications she is taking. The care team explains that, with the prison's "keep-on-person" program, she can self-administer the medication and no one has to know what medications she is taking.

The care team also educates Juanita about the importance of adhering to her medication as a way to prevent transmission to her unborn child.

How can healthcare providers influence an inmate's behavior?

The care team can encourage inmates to adopt healthy behaviors by:

- providing education about HIV
- focusing on the importance of adherence with treatment regimens
- developing programs that make it easier for inmates to adhere to treatment and still protect their confidentiality (i.e., "keep-on-person" program).

Any integrated form of psychotherapy aimed at addressing the person's bio-psychosocial milieu is likely to help the inmate adjust to the prison environment and adhere to medication.

Juanita takes her HIV medications as prescribed most of the time. She starts on paroxetine for depression but discontinues it because of side effects and asks to deal with her issues without psychotropic medication. Every 2 weeks she is followed by psychiatric social workers. She finds these sessions helpful and is able to start working on her issues of trust in relationships. She is able to tell the family member she trusts most about her HIV status and ask for support. After 5 months, she is released from jail with a referral to a specialized clinic for high-risk pregnancies. She is also encouraged to seek therapy to continue to work on these issues. At the time of her release, she had not decided whether to remain with her boyfriend.

Case study: An inmate with HIV and bipolar disorder

Victor, a 30-year-old man, was diagnosed with bipolar disorder 3 years ago. He started injecting cocaine and heroin 9 years ago and is clean only when in a hospital or prison. He has had several arrests over the years for offenses that occur while he is either using drugs or experiencing a manic episode. He is currently incarcerated for illegal drug possession.

On intake into the correctional institution, Victor discloses that he was diagnosed with HIV 8 months ago, but has not seen a medical provider. He admits to engaging in unprotected sex quite often, especially during manic episodes. He is also unconcerned whether the needles he uses to inject drugs are clean.

Before medical staff start treating his HIV, they ask the psychiatrist to explore the possibility of prescribing psychotropic medication as a way to manage the bipolar disorder and reduce Victor's high-risk behavior. Victor agrees to take valproic acid, a drug that he tolerates well and which alleviates all of his symptoms.

Based on the results of his viral load test, medical staff recommend a HAART regimen, but Victor refuses. He has heard that other inmates with HIV are isolated in a particular housing unit, attend an HIV clinic, and see a particular physician. He is concerned that other inmates will guess that he has HIV.

The social workers from medicine and psychiatry discuss the procedures in place in the institution to protect confidentiality. They reassure Victor that inmates living with HIV are housed in general population units with everyone else, the HIV clinic is held at the same time and place as several other chronic care clinics, and the infectious disease specialist deals with other infectious diseases during the clinic as well as HIV so other inmates do not know the reason for a visit.

Staff also explain that inmates living with HIV are given a supply of medication and taught the correct times and dosages, so they don't have to go to a pill call window several

> times a day. Victor is also told that correctional officers are not informed if an inmate is on HIV medications and medical staff cannot share his HIV status with anyone else in the institution without his permission. After several sessions with the social workers, Victor agrees to take the HIV medications.

How can correctional institutions keep an inmate's HIV status confidential?

Confidentiality of medical information is critically important in a closed environment such as a prison – yet the ease with which information is shared makes confidentiality difficult to maintain. Because of the stigma associated with HIV, special steps should be taken to protect the confidentiality of an infected inmate.

Many prisons have taken measures like those described in the case study to protect the confidentiality of patients with HIV. Multiple layers of protection help build trust in the healthcare system within the prison. However, complete confidentiality cannot be guaranteed. For example, some inmates and correctional officers have gained access to an inmate's medical records based on the argument that they are entitled to know if they are at risk (MacDougall, 1998).

Perhaps the most effective way to calm patient concern about confidentiality is to create an accepting environment where inmates feel comfortable disclosing their HIV status. This is difficult to do and requires commitment from prison administration.

Are there any circumstances where an inmate's HIV status should be disclosed to prison staff?

For mental health professionals, deciding when it is appropriate to disclose information about a psychiatric inmate's HIV status to prison staff can raise formidable legal and ethical issues. Many agree that "disclosure of a patient's serological status is admissible if appropriate for diagnosis, management and treatment, but it should be limited to the staff directly involved in the patient's care" (Grassi, 1996), Some argue that, in certain circumstances (e.g., potential harm to others), this information should be shared with others. In many jurisdictions, public health law requires healthcare providers to contact public health if someone with an infectious disease poses a threat to others. Mental health providers should be aware of both the legal requirements in their jurisdiction, and the disclosure policies and procedures within their institution.

> While in prison, Victor adheres to his HIV and psychotropic medications. He also attends peer-led support groups for inmates with HIV, supportive therapy groups, and Narcotics Anonymous (NA). Every 30 days, he is seen by a psychiatrist. Within the structured environment of the prison, Victor finds it much easier to adhere to both his psychiatric and medical treatment regimens. After 18 months, he is eligible for parole and he and his counselors begin making plans for his release and the follow-up care he needs.

How can providers ensure continuity of care when inmates are released into the community?

Most prisons offer very little in terms of programs that link inmates with medical and support services once they are released back into the community. However, select prison systems in the USA have been proactive in working with community-based organizations to provide discharge planning services and link HIV-infected inmates with medical and social support services outside prison (Flanigan *et al.*, 1996; Arriola, 2001). For example, the Centers for Disease Control and Prevention and the Health Resources and Services Administration jointly fund collaborations among health departments, correctional facilities, and community-based organizations in seven states, which are designed to improve services for HIV-infected inmates, particularly when they are released. These services connect patients to community-based case management, medical care, mental healthcare, substance abuse treatment, benefits, housing, and employment. Under this initiative, four of the states offer discharge planning to HIV-infected inmates who are being released, while the others primarily offer these services in county jails. Prison-based mental health service providers play an important role in the discharge planning process. They work closely with discharge planners to identify the mental health needs of soon-to-be-released inmates. For those who need medical treatment services, the in-facility providers identify places in the community where clients can receive services, and the discharge planners provide referrals and, whenever possible, set up appointments for the inmate after he or she is released. Depending on the severity of the inmate's mental illness, many systems also provide case managers who make contact with the inmate in prison and maintain contact after the inmate has been released.

What impact does the prison environment/culture have on healthcare?

Medical and mental health providers in jail and prison settings work in an environment in which safety and security (of inmates, staff, and visitors) is the primary concern. Correctional culture is very different from the culture of most healthcare settings where the priority is to improve length and quality of life through prevention, treatment, and care. Between correctional staff and healthcare staff, there is often a cultural divide that requires both parties to respect and appreciate the other's rules and regulations.

In a sense, healthcare providers are "guests" in correctional facilities, and are expected to deliver care in a manner that does not jeopardize the safety and security of the institution. Healthcare providers must often adhere to policies that they find inconvenient, such as having a correctional officer escort to dispense medication on the floor, providing directly observed therapy, and not allowing inmates to keep medications in their possession. Within prisons, dosing schedules must take into account regularly scheduled events, such as head counts, as well as unscheduled events, such as lockdowns. Because of situations that can arise in prison, entire doses can be delayed or appointments missed. Inmates may not be able to adhere to dietary requirements because they don't have access to appropriate food. When it comes to medications, inmates may not have access to tools that can improve adherence, such as pill boxes, or to advanced treatment options that are not available on the institution's restricted medication formulary.

When providing care, medical and mental health staff must work very closely with correctional staff. This means that correctional officers' attitudes and beliefs about HIV/AIDS and mental illness can have profound implications for how inmates with dual diagnoses are treated, what programs and services are offered, and how comfortable inmates feel disclosing their status. Although there have been no confirmed cases of correctional staff being infected through routine contact with infected inmates, prison personnel are concerned about the risk of HIV transmission (Braithwaite *et al.*, 1996; Kantor 1998), and this fear can affect their attitudes towards the inmates as well as the way inmates are treated. There is a need for prison personnel to have access to education about HIV/AIDS, which some prisons, both in the USA and internationally, already provide.

Victor was discharged on parole and kept his initial appointments at an HIV clinic and the mental health center. In spite of the efforts of the treatment team at the mental health center, he would not agree to substance abuse counseling. After 3 months, he was lost to follow-up.

Conclusion

Mental health staff who treat inmates with HIV and a psychiatric illness face complex challenges. To provide more effective care and treatment for inmates with dual diagnoses, mental health workers must collaborate with medical and public health practitioners to generate new knowledge that can be shared with prison officials in an effort to improve the quality of care provided in correctional institutions.

REFERENCES

AIDS Action. *Policy facts: HIV/AIDS in correctional facilities.* (2001) (Available at http://www.aidsaction.org/)

American Psychiatric Association. American Psychiatric Association practice guidelines for the treatment of patients with HIV/AIDS. *American Journal of Psychiatry*, **157**(Suppl. 11) (2000): S2–S62. (Available as a live document at http://www.psych.org/psych_pract/treatg/pg/hivaids_revisebook_index.cfm)

Arriola, K. R. J. *CDC/HRSA Corrections Demonstration Project: An overview.* Oral presentation at the semi-annual meeting of the American Correctional Association, Philadelphia, PA, 2001.

Braithwaite, R. L., Hammett, T. M. and Mayberry, R. M. *Prisons and AIDS: A Public Health Challenge*. San Francisco: Jossey-Bass, 1996.

Canadian HIV/AIDS Legal Network. *HIV/AIDS and Hepatitis C in Prisons; the Facts*. (2001) (Available as a live document at http://www.aidslaw.ca/Maincontent/issues/prisons/e-info-pa1.htm).

Canadian HIV/AIDS Legal Network. Prison needle exchange: lessons from a comprehensive review of international evidence and experience. (n.d.) (Available as a live document at www.aidslaw.ca/maincontent/issues/prisons/pnep/toc.htm).

DeCarlo, P. and Zack, B. *What are inmates' HIV prevention needs*? Center for AIDS Prevention studies at the University of California San Francisco. (1996). (Available as a live document at www.caps.ucsf.edu/capsweb/inmatetext.html.).

Ditton, P. M. Mental health and treatment of inmates and probationers. Bureau of Justice Statistics Special Report. (1999). (Available as a live document at www.ojp.usdoj.gov/bjs/.).

Flanigan, T. P., Kim, J. Y., Zierler, S. *et al.* A prison release program for HIV-positive women: linking them to health services and community follow-up. *American Journal of Public Health*, **86** (1996): 886–7.

Grassi, L. Risk of HIV infection in psychiatrically ill patients. *AIDS Care*, **8**(1) (1996): 103–16.

Hammett, T. and Harmon, P. Medical treatment and a continuum of care. In *1996–1997 update: HIV/AIDS, STDs, and TB in correctional facilities*. T. M. Hammett, P. Harmon, and L. M. Maruschak, eds., pp. 69–84. Washington, DC: National Institute of Justice, US Department of Justice, 1999.

Kantor, E. AIDS and HIV infection in prisoners. *AIDS Knowledge Base*. (1998). (Available as a live document at www.hivinsie.ucsf.eduakb/current/01pris/index.html).

MacDougall, D. S. HIV/AIDS behind bars. *Journal of the International Association of Physicians in AIDS Care*, **4**(4) (1998): 8–13.

Maruschak, L. M. HIV in prisons, 2001. *Bureau of Justice Statistics Bulletin*. (2004). (Available as a live document at www.ojp.usdoj.gov/bjs)

Nelles, J., Bernasconi, S. and Mikola, A. D. *Provision of Syringes and Prescription of Heroin in Prison: The Swiss Experience in the Prisons of Hindelbank and Oberschongron*. (n.d.) (Available as a live document at www.drugtext.org).

Stefan, M. D. and Catalan, J. Psychiatric patients and HIV infection: a new population at risk? *British Journal of Psychiatry*, **167** (1995): 721–7.

Stubblefield, E. and Wohl, D. Prisons and jails worldwide: Update from the 13th International Conference on AIDS. *HIV Education Prison Project News*, **3**(7/8) (2000): 1–5.

18

Legal and ethical issues

Marie-Josée Brouillette, M.D.[1] and David J. Roy, O.C., O.Q., LL.D. (H.C.), S.T.L, Ph.L., Dr. Theol.[2]

[1] Assistant Professor of Psychiatry, McGill University, Montréal,
  Consulting Psychiatrist, Immunodeficiency Program, McGill University Health Center, Montréal, Canada
[2] Director, Centre for Bioethics, Institute de Recherche Clinique de Montréal, Canada
  Research Professor, Faculty of Medicine, Université de Montréal, Montréal, Canada

Introduction

The management of people with HIV raises many difficult legal and ethical issues. Some are due to the nature of the illness: an infectious disease that potentially poses a risk to others. Some are due to the stigmatization and discrimination that has accompanied this illness and the marginalization of the people affected by it. Others can arise in treating anyone with a chronic illness who faces end of life issues that may be complicated by psychiatric or mental health disorders.

Psychiatrists working with patients with HIV should be aware of the legal and ethical issues they may face, as well as their own legal, ethical, and professional obligations.

Case study: Management of an HIV patient on a psychiatric ward

George is a 35-year-old single man who lives with a friend. He has a long history of bipolar disorder complicated by nonadherence. He hates feeling blunted by the medication and enjoys the highs of the manic state. Three years ago, after a psychiatric admission, he tested positive for HIV.

George is brought to the emergency room in a manic state marked by sexual promiscuity, and is admitted. Staff on the inpatient unit are concerned about his sexual disinhibition. He is being very seductive with female patients in emotionally vulnerable states.

Can George be denied admission based on his HIV-serostatus and the potential risk he represents to other patients?

No. Most professional organizations have adopted resolutions against discrimination based on HIV status (see American Psychiatric Association, 1993; Canadian

HIV and Psychiatry. A Training and Resource Manual, Second Edition, ed. Kenneth Citron, Marie-Josée Brouillette, and Alexandra Beckett. Published by Cambridge University Press. © Cambridge University Press 2005.

Psychiatric Association, 1996). People with HIV are entitled to the same standard of care as other patients. Although George is known to be HIV-seropositive, he is not necessarily the only person at risk in a psychiatric hospital environment. Other hospitalized patients may also be infected without being aware of it. Psychiatric wards should have in place measures designed to decrease the transmission of HIV infection, whether or not staff are aware that a patient has HIV.

"Based on the assumption that all patients and staff should be considered potentially at risk for transmitting or receiving HIV infection, universal precautions, as outlined in current Centers for Disease Control and Prevention standards, should be employed at all times for any psychiatric patient of any age. HIV infection by itself does not require individual rooms or toilet facilities, and such patients should participate in all aspects of inpatient treatment programs as their medical condition permits (*APA, 1993*)"

Can George's HIV status be disclosed to other patients?

Patients have a right to confidentiality; their serostatus cannot be disclosed to others. There are few acceptable exceptions to physicians' and healthcare professionals' duty to keep confidential the information they receive about a person's body, life, and secrets. Patients' trust in physicians is essential for their treatment, their healing, and their growth in personal stability and responsibility.

Disclosing George's HIV status would likely make him feel betrayed, which would interfere with his treatment. It could also have a negative effect on the trust of other patients on the ward.

Although the professional obligation to protect confidentiality is strong, it is not absolute. Physicians may find themselves in situations where they are caught between their obligation to keep secret information patients have entrusted to them and their sense of a need to warn specific other persons who are endangered by their patients' behavior. Protecting the health or life of another human being may be an ethical justification for breaking confidentiality. The Code of Medical Ethics of several professional organizations specifies that doctors may divulge information they normally should keep confidential under the following conditions:

- when the patient authorizes it
- when the law permits or requires it
- when there are imperative and justifiable motives relating to the health of the physician's patient or of the community
- in the case of a commanding higher objective.

A commanding higher objective (i.e., higher than the duty to protect confidentiality) may require a clinician to disclose confidential information if his or her patient is carrying a contagious infection that could endanger not only a specific individual, but the health of the community. Disclosure in instances of this kind may also be accompanied by more coercive measures, such as enforced treatment (e.g., for treatment of tuberculosis resistant to a number of available antibiotics).

There may also be occasions in the workplace when the higher purpose of protecting citizens' lives may require a clinician to disclose that a patient is afflicted with a condition that could diminish that person's ability to function and endanger others. For example, the lives of many people depend upon the ability of people employed as airline pilots or railroad engineers to do their jobs.

In the case of HIV infection, the need to protect the health and life of a spouse or sexual partner of the person with HIV could be a commanding higher objective and justify a clinician's decision to break confidentiality. This would be particularly true if the clinician were the only person, other than the patient with HIV, with the knowledge needed to warn the endangered spouse or partner. However, even in this particular situation, breaking confidentiality should be an action of last resort. The HIV-infected person is the one who has the right and the responsibility to warn a spouse or partner. The clinician should sensitively work with a person with HIV to help him or her grow up to the responsibility of informing a spouse or partner.

The clinician should not underestimate the price someone with HIV may have to pay when living up to the demands of personal responsibility. The social, familial, emotional, and financial costs of being honest with a spouse or partner about one's HIV infection can be very high.

If a clinician believes it is necessary to take the action of last resort and to break confidentiality, it would be prudent first to seek the advice of a trusted colleague.

How can the hospital protect other patients and staff from the risk of being infected by George?

All healthcare institutions should have adopted universal precautions by now. In addition, on psychiatric wards, the following strategies should be considered:

- monitor the behavior of all patients to avoid escalation
- if a patient engages or threatens to engage in activities that put others at potential risk for HIV infection, take appropriate measures to control the behavior (e.g., medication, isolation, physical restraints)
- given the fact that needle sharing and sexual activities between patients can occur outside the unit, assess off-ward privileges carefully
- provide regular education for all patients about HIV transmission and strategies they can use to protect themselves.

Given that sexual behavior can happen on a psychiatric unit despite adequate supervision, some units make condoms available to patients. Although this measure is controversial, it is supported by harm reduction principles. It is ethically more important to help people avoid transmitting HIV infection than to withhold a means of protection because it may give a wrong message about sex among patients. Psychiatric units should be more concerned about sending a wrong message about safer sex and HIV prevention.

In the midst of an epidemic of such proportion, why is there such a strong emphasis on confidentiality and protection of the rights of the individual?

A strong emphasis on confidentiality, protection of privacy, and the defense of human rights is an ethical response to the stigma, discrimination, and marginalization associated with HIV infection.

Stigmatization has branded people with HIV as being different from other people and dangerous to the health of others. Discrimination has deprived people with HIV of rights, liberties, opportunities, and goods to which others have unquestioned access. Marginalization has tended to exclude people with HIV from the common spaces people share in a community.

An emphasis on confidentiality and privacy is necessary to protect the human dignity of people with HIV and help them maintain their own sense of self-worth and personal dignity.

Much of the legal and ethical debate around HIV infection focuses on the perceived conflict between society's right to protect itself against the spread of disease and the right of infected people to confidentiality and civil liberties. In fact, this perceived antagonism is misleading for the following reasons:

- Most people who transmit the virus are not aware of their HIV infection.
- The public health approach to the HIV epidemic is based on serological testing, contact tracing, and adherence to measures aimed at decreasing the transmission of the virus. The success of these measures depends on the willingness of individuals to participate. The discrimination and stigma affecting those with HIV compromise this approach. When people perceive their confidentiality is not ensured or anticipate discrimination, they may refuse testing. Conversely, when they feel their confidentiality is protected and their rights are respected, they are more likely to agree to be tested and take steps to prevent transmission. In this way, measures intended to protect the individual also protect society.
- Because so many people are not aware of their HIV status, the responsibility for protection ultimately has to rest with everyone, not just with people who are infected. Strong coercive measures applied to people who are infected may create an illusion of protection that detracts from the personal responsibility to protect oneself (Elliott, 2000).

George's stay on the unit is uneventful. After 3 weeks, he is ready for discharge.

What steps can be taken when patients are discharged to reduce the risk of transmission associated with future episodes of illness?

Before a patient with a psychiatric illness is discharged, the clinician should review with him or her:

- the risks associated with unprotected sexual activities
- steps individuals can take to reduce the risk
- strategies that will help them maintain safer practices.

The clinician reviews with George the risks associated with unprotected sexual activities both for others and for himself (see medical overview). George was already well aware of this information. As his high-risk activities tend to occur exclusively in the context of a manic decompensation, George agrees to be followed more closely as an outpatient and to take his medications. In addition, his friend is involved in the follow-up and advised to call the psychiatrist when he notices the early signs of mania.

Case study: A patient who poses a risk to others

Laura is a 25-year-old woman who has abused cocaine for several years and is involved in prostitution to support her addiction. She eventually enters a residential detoxification program, then attends several months of outpatient follow up. As part of her rehabilitation program, she attends computer courses and eventually finds a job.

In the process of applying for insurance, she is tested for HIV and found to be positive. In the following weeks, she relapses into cocaine use and goes back to prostitution. If clients are willing to pay more money for unprotected sex, she obliges.

She attends her first visit with an HIV physician who is alarmed by the fact that she is having unprotected sex with several partners. Laura knows about HIV and the risk of transmitting it, but justifies her behavior, saying, "One of them infected me, I will get back at them". She accepts a referral to psychiatry to help her deal with her distress about the new diagnosis.

Can Laura's partners be notified of her diagnosis?

Partner notification is part of a broader HIV/AIDS public health and prevention program. The goal of partner notification in HIV/AIDS is twofold:

- to prevent HIV transmission
- to reduce the morbidity and mortality associated with HIV/AIDS.

The objectives of partner notification are to:

- inform the contacts of their possible exposure to HIV
- assist them in evaluating their risk of having acquired HIV
- assist them in making informed decisions about HIV testing
- alert them to the possibility of secondary transmission to their own partners or to their offspring
- enable them to make timely decisions about treatment if they have been infected.

Partner notification should only be undertaken when appropriate support is available for both the index person and the partners who are being notified. While public health experts argue that partner notification is acceptable only if it can be done while still maintaining the confidentiality of the index person (should the person want to remain anonymous), several major medical associations stipulate that present and past partners should be notified without the patient's permission, even if it means breaching confidentiality. Before breaching confidentiality, psychiatrists should reflect on any underlying personal values and assumptions. When clinicians decide to breach confidentiality to protect a third party, their decision may be affected in part by the patient's race, sex, and sexual preference (Schwartzbaum *et al.*, 1990). Partners can be notified in three different ways:

- Index patient notifies partner. When a patient (index person) decides to notify some or all partners, she or he should be coached in the best way to tell them about possible exposure. Before notifying a partner, the index person should be encouraged to consider possible consequences (e.g., the partner may become violent, the partner may divulge the information to other people, affecting the index person's confidentiality).
- Physician notifies partner.
- Public health worker notifies partner.

Partner notification is a complex process. The psychiatrist should clarify who is responsible for partner notification. An HIV specialist who is or will become involved with the patient may have more experience with this task.

In Laura's particular scenario, the main difficulty is that most partners are not identifiable.

What is the clinical approach to a patient with HIV who puts others at risk?

The first step is for the clinician to create and maintain a therapeutic alliance. In some patients, particularly those with a history of abuse, this may take considerable effort. Pressuring patients who are not able or ready to hear prevention messages will not convince them to change. Instead, the clinician should focus the discussion on the patient's feelings and needs.

Once the alliance is established, the psychiatrist can explore the difficulties that interfere with the patient's ability to adhere to strategies designed to decrease the risk of transmission, or the motivations that cause them to put others at risk. It may be that the patient's ability to make the desired behavior change is adversely affected by lack of information, denial, economic imperatives, use of substances, mental illness, fear of rejection or of violence, sadness, anger, lack of social skills, different health beliefs, hopelessness, or lack of a sense of self-efficacy.

Moving upward out of a long spiral of decline, degradation, and loss of sense of self-worth takes a lot of time, a lot of care, and a lot of simple acceptance by other human beings. As the person who feels abandoned works with a professional who knows how to care, his or her biography may change and emerge. As the patient responds to the treatment, care, and unexpected experiences of human and professional kindness and concern, he or she may discover horizons of hope that support behavior change.

In the first meeting with Laura, the psychiatrist focuses on establishing a therapeutic alliance by exploring the difficulties that Laura has encountered in her life as well as talking about her initial success in the drug rehabilitation program. The clinician also pays attention to her immediate need for money and shelter. At the second meeting, Laura breaks down into tears, talking about her shattered dreams. She is angry and fearful about the future. The clinician encourages her to reconnect with the detox program, which she does, and refers her to a group for women living with HIV.

What are some countertransference issues in working with patients who put others at risk?

A clinician who is unable to persuade a patient to quickly stop behaviors that are putting others at risk may experience a sense of anger and frustration. These feelings may tempt the clinician to adopt a hard-line approach, which puts more emphasis on trying to protect society than on helping the patient through the process of change. Although the hard-line approach may be well intentioned, it is likely to be counterproductive. For example, it may lead the patient to drop out of follow-up or to refuse to cooperate with efforts to notify partners. The desire to confront the problem must be balanced with the need to maintain the alliance.

The best way to ensure that countertransference does not interfere with productive work is to discuss difficult cases with other team members. A physician working alone may find it helpful to consult with a colleague experienced in HIV work and discuss any unforeseen consequences of his or her clinical stance.

What can be done about patients who will not change their behaviour and seem to disregard the safety of others?

There is little evidence that criminal prosecution and penalty serve any significant rehabilitative function. Counseling and support are considered more effective means of rehabilitating a person who has engaged in high-risk activities. Only a concerted approach involving mental health resources, social services, and cultural and community groups can address these complex situations. Most clinicians favor a stepwise approach from the least coercive to the most coercive:

- First, try to establish an alliance. Is there a professional who is more likely to be able to do so with this particular patient?
- Explore the reasons that interfere with the desired change in behavior.
- If, after careful consideration, the clinician decides the patient needs to be confronted, who is the best person to do that? Keep in mind that you may

want to preserve certain key relationships in the interest of continued follow-up. For example, the clinician may arrange for a more peripheral team member to "sacrifice" his or her relationship with the patient in order to allow other caregivers to continue their work with him.

How coercive the approach can be depends on the society in which the patient lives. The physician should contact the public health authorities for guidance and information about the law in their area.

Over the next several months, Laura attends the outpatient rehabilitation program. Her relapses into drug use are few and far between. She attends the women's groups where she discusses her dream to have children and how this has been affected by her HIV infection. She receives support from the group and develops some friendships that carry her through difficult times.

Case study: End of life issues

Marc is a 40-year-old man who lives with his male partner of many years, Andrew. Marc is referred to psychiatry because of anxiety over his health. He has been HIV-seropositive for several years, but has always responded well to antiretroviral treatment. However, over the past few months, his viral load has been steadily increasing and he is resistant to most alternative treatments. Although his physician is still trying to get the HIV infection under control, his health is declining and they both know that this does not augur well for the future.

Marc's parents are both deceased and left their children a substantial inheritance. Marc is estranged from his only brother who does not accept his sexual orientation or his partner. After the death of the parents, the brother tried by several means to get more than his share of the inheritance.

In addition to his concerns about his own future, Marc is very concerned about ensuring Andrew's welfare after his death. In particular, he is afraid that his brother will try to prevent Andrew from inheriting.

What are the legal issues that Marc should be addressing?

It is not unusual for people with HIV to be in relationships that are poorly protected by the law. For example, there have been several instances in which distant relatives have been given the decision-making capacity for someone with HIV who has become incompetent – instead of the person's same-sex partner of several years. In addition, many jurisdictions do not guarantee same-sex partners access to their deceased partners' retirement savings.

For this reason, all people with HIV and particularly those living in nontraditional situations should have:

- a will

- a durable medical power of attorney that will be valid once the person becomes incompetent.

The psychiatrist asks Marc whether he has completed these legal documents. Initially, Marc is surprised and replies that he "is not dying yet". However, in the course of therapy, he realizes that this is the best way to ensure that his wishes are respected. He and his partner have avoided talking about death so far. The clinician encourages Marc to open up the discussion and, in particular, to mention to his partner what his choices would be in the event his health deteriorates and to consider writing a living will. He and Andrew meet with a notary and complete a will and a durable medical power of attorney.

Are there any particular considerations for people with advanced HIV disease who want to write a will?

The validity of a will may be contested on several grounds, including the claim that the testator lacked testamentary capacity or was under undue influence. If people are in advanced stages of HIV when they write their will, the validity may be challenged on grounds of mental incapacity related to dementia secondary to HIV infection. To avoid this, the person with HIV may consider having a psychiatrist assess his or her competency to write a will, as close as possible to the time when the legal document is drawn up.

To assess testamentary capacity, the psychiatrist must:

- determine from informed, objective sources the nature of the testator's assets and, if possible, the names and relationship to the testator of all potential heirs
- ask the testator to describe his assets, articulate his understanding of what a will is, and explain who the people named in it are. Particular attention should be paid to any content of the testamentary document that is likely to be challenged.
- determine the nature, extent, and general consequences of mental illness, if any
- assess the possible exertion of undue influence (control and manipulation of the testator's emotions, beliefs, and behavior)
- conduct a complete mental status examination and, if in doubt, obtain neuro-psychological testing (Spar and Garb, 1992).

Unfortunately, Marc no longer responds to medications and his condition continues to decline to the point where he is bedridden. He sometimes talks to Andrew about the fact that he is no longer satisfied with the quality of his life and wants to die. However, at other times, he is able to find pleasure in the company of friends and still enjoys reading. He develops pneumonia and requires admission to hospital.

The course of Marc's admission is marked by a succession of medical complications. After agreeing for several weeks to investigations and treatments, Marc now requests that all active treatment be discontinued, clearly knowing that this will lead to death. Andrew, although saddened, confirms that Marc has been considering this decision for several weeks now, and that it is in line with all prior discussions they have had on the topic. The attending physician requests an assessment of competence to make medical decisions.

How does a clinician determine a patient's competence to make medical decisions?

Competence is a legal concept that can only be formally determined through legal proceedings. All adult patients are considered competent to make decisions about medical care unless a court declares them incompetent. However, in practice, physicians make some assessment of the patient's decision-making capacities.

Although there is no universally accepted definition of competence, Applebaum and Grisso (1998) have proposed that the patient must have:

- the ability to express a sustained preference
- the ability to understand what is being explained about his condition, proposed treatments, and alternatives
- the ability to appreciate that the information explained applies to his or her own situation (this includes the presence of insight)
- the ability to reason.

Competency has both a cognitive and an affective component. Affective states may influence competence by influencing the weight given to treatment risks and benefits. More than one evaluation session may be necessary to complete the process. A patient's competency may fluctuate as a function of the natural course of the illness, response to treatment, psychodynamic factors, metabolic status, or the effect of medications. In addition, patients will often not articulate their most important concerns on the initial visit and interventions themselves may be part of the diagnostic process (Applebaum and Grisso, 1998). The presence of cognitive impairment per se does not necessarily imply incompetence as long as the patient retains the abilities listed above.

What are some of the psychosocial factors that may affect competence to refuse life-saving measures?

Although a comprehensive review of psychosocial factors that influence desire for death in medically ill patients is beyond the scope of this chapter, competence to refuse treatment, especially life-sustaining treatment, must be assessed in the broader context of the patient's life.

Several authors stress the importance of adopting a psychodynamic perspective when assessing a request to die (Applebaum and Roth, 1981; Muskin, 1998). "The idiosyncratic meaning for the patient of any suggested procedure is a function of each patient's unique matrix of previous experiences" (Applebaum and Roth, 1981).

When evaluating a patient who makes requests to hasten his or her death, the clinician should evaluate the person's decision-making capacity and explore the impact that major mental illness, character traits, and psychological defense mechanisms have on the competency, durability, and authenticity of these requests. Cohen suggests that the psychiatric assessment should include discussion, when at all possible, with a patient's family, friends, and even community leaders. "The decision to hasten death should be contextualized within a range of values encompassing the patient's own belief system as well as the belief system of others with whom the patient is close" (Cohen et al., 2000). It is possible, however, that a patient confronted with the reality of a terminal illness may feel differently about decisions than he did when in good health (Zaubler and Sullivan, 1996).

As part of the assessment of decision-making capacity, the psychiatrist will want to assess for:

- the presence of depression and hopelessness
- the presence of organic mental disorders
- poorly controlled pain and physical suffering
- social support
- financial resources (especially in private medical settings)
- the presence of anger, the wish to die as a revenge
- the need to regain a sense of control
- the presence of guilt and desire for self-punishment
- the quality of the relationship with the physician.

The person's decision may change when proper attention is paid to some of these factors. For example, depression and pain can be amenable to treatment, and interpersonal conflicts can be resolved. Respite may be arranged when natural caregivers are exhausted. Exploring dynamic issues has both diagnostic and therapeutic dimensions. Assessing a person's decision-making capacity requires the elaboration of a differential diagnosis approach, appropriate investigation, and reassessment of the patient after therapeutic intervention (Applebaum and Roth, 1981). The sensitive art of communicating with the dying is both difficult and complex. It is difficult because the care of dying people, who may also be suffering intensely, may provoke feelings of hopelessness, helplessness, failure, or demoralization within a doctor. It may be difficult for a doctor experiencing these feelings to avoid reinforcing in patients a sense of helplessness and of diminished self-worth, which may be expressed in a patient's demand for death. The art of communicating with suffering and dying people is also complex because the interaction between doctor and dying patient shapes and limits what each hears from and says to the other. A patient's request for euthanasia may come from the patient's individual despair. However, that request may also come from the patient's sense that others have lost all hope for him.

If some psychiatric observers are correct in reporting that the legal availability of euthanasia as a medical option results in physicians' loss of knowledge about dealing with suicidal thoughts in the gravely ill, physician–patient conversations that would thoroughly explore the origin and meaning of the suicidal ideation, and help a patient discover her adaptive and coping strengths, may simply never occur (Modestin, 1987; Hamilton and Hamilton, 2000; Varghese and Kelly, 2001).

What are some of the factors specifically related to HIV infection that can complicate a competency assessment?

The nature of the impairment found in HIV-associated dementia can complicate a competency assessment in people with advanced HIV disease. As discussed in Chapter 2, HIV-associated dementia affects subcortical functions such as executive functions to a much greater extent than cortical functions. Executive functions include the cognitive abilities needed to assess a situation, make decisions, and act accordingly, and play a crucial role in decision-making capacity.

The assessment of executive functions is easily overlooked in routine mental status examination. A patient may be able to articulate coherent sentences, even though there is severe impairment of the underlying decision-making capacity. In addition, a patient's self-assessment of cognitive status is not reliable (van Gorp *et al.*, 1991). Unless the executive functions are formally tested or a reliable history is gathered from outside sources, the clinician can easily be misled into finding a patient competent. An assessment of executive functions may reveal a history of poor judgment and self-care. As shown by Schindler *et al.* (1995) in their cohort of patients with frontal-lobe dementia with impairment in executive functions, these patients are unable to translate their understanding and appreciation of their condition into actual planning and execution of coordinated, organized behavior.

Because the widely used mini-mental state examination (MMSE) is not sensitive in picking up dysfunction in executive functions, psychiatrists may wish to become familiar with alternative screening examinations that identify cognitive symptoms more likely to be present with advanced HIV infection. For more information on tests that are more sensitive than the MMSE, please consult Chapter 2.

Marc is evaluated by a psychiatrist over the course of a week. He is interviewed alone and with his partner. The results on testing of executive functions are within the normal range. There is no depression, delirium, or significant pain. The relationship between Marc, his partner and the attending physician is devoid of significant conflicts. Marc is found to be competent to refuse treatment and palliative measures are instituted. He dies soon after.

An interview with Andrew 4 months after Marc's death reveals that he remains at peace with Marc's decision and the quality of the care he received until the end of his life. As had been anticipated, Marc's brother is most unhappy with the content of Marc's will and is contesting it. Andrew's lawyer is confident that, with all the steps that had been taken when the will was drawn, its content will be respected.

Conclusion

The ethical aspects of HIV infection have been markedly influenced by the fact that the infection struck predominantly stigmatized populations. Whereas those infected through contaminated blood and blood products were seen as the "innocent victims" and elicited sympathy, the reaction was quite different for those whose infection resulted from "sinful" behavior. While society demanded protection from this disease, public health authorities recognized that the best way to decrease transmission was, in fact, to educate the population, protect those who were infected, and encourage people at risk to be tested for HIV and change the behaviors that put them at risk. Nevertheless, the tension in society between the preventive and the punitive approach continues and flares up intermittently, particularly when the exceptional case of malicious and deliberate infection receives media coverage.

When faced with these complex issues, the clinician is not exempt from experiencing strong emotional reactions. The best way to ensure that clinical decisions are not unduly influenced by prejudices is to have a safe forum in which to vent emotions before moving on to analyze possible scenarios that could accomplish the ultimate goal of protecting both patient and society.

REFERENCES

American Psychiatric Association. AIDS policy: Policy Guidelines for Inpatient Psychiatric Units. *American Journal of Psychiatry*, **150**(5) (1993): 853. (Available as a living document at www.psych.org/aids2/aids_state12.cfm).

Applebaum, P. S. and Grisso, T. Assessing patients' capacities to consent to treatment. *New England Journal of Medicine*, **319** (1998): 1635–8.

Applebaum, P. S. and Roth, H. Clinical issues in the assessment of competency. *American Journal of Psychiatry*, **138** (1981): 1462–77.

Canadian Psychiatric Association. CPA position statement on HIV disease. *Canadian Journal of Psychiatry*, **41**(1996): 595.

Cohen, L. M., Steinberg, M. D., Hails, K. C. *et al.* Psychiatric evaluation of death-hastening requests. *Psychosomatics*, **41**(2000): 199–203.

Elliott, R. *Criminal Law and HIV/AIDS: Strategic Considerations.* A Discussion Paper. (2000). (Available as a living document at www.aidslaw.ca).

Hamilton, N. G. and Hamilton, C. A. Therapeutic response to assisted suicide request. *Issues in Law and Medicine*, **16**(2)(2000): 167–76.

Modestin, J. Countertransference reactions contributing to completed suicide. *British Journal of Medical Psychology*, **60** (1987): 379–85.

Muskin, P. The request to die: role for a psychodynamic perspective on physician-assisted suicide. *Journal of the American Medical Association*, **279** (1998): 323–8.

Schindler, B. A., Ramchandani, D., Matthews, M. K. and Podell, K. Competency and the frontal lobe. *Psychosomatics*, **36** (1995): 400–4.

Schwartzbaum, J. A., Wheat, J. R. and Norton, R. W. Physician breach of patient confidentiality among individuals with human immunodeficiency virus (HIV) infection: patterns of decision. *American Journal of Public Health*, **80**(7) (1990): 829–34.

Spar, J. E. and Garb, A. S. Assessing competency to make a will. *American Journal of Psychiatry*, **149** (1992): 169–74.

Varghese, F. T. and Kelly, B. Countertransference and assisted suicide. *Issues in Law and Medicine*, **16**(3) (2001): 252.

van Gorp, W. G., Satz, P., Hinkin, C. *et al.* Metacognition in HIV-1 seropositive asymptomatic individuals: self-ratings versus objective neuropsychological performance. *Journal of Clinical and Experimental Neuropsychology*, **13** (1991): 812–19.

Zaubler, T. S. and Sullivan, M. D. Psychiatry and physician-assisted suicide. *Psychiatric Clinics of North America*, **19**(3)(1996): 413–27.

SUGGESTED FURTHER READING

Block, S. D. and Billings, J. A. Patient requests for euthanasia and assisted suicide in terminal illness. *Psychosomatics*, **36**(1995): 445–7.

Centers for Disease Control and Prevention standards (Available as a living document at http://www.cdc.gov)

General Medical Council, UK. Serious Communicable Diseases (1997). (available at http://www.gmc-uk.org/global_sections/sitemap_frameset.htm)

American Psychiatric Association. Position statement on confidentiality, disclosure, and protection of others. *American Journal of Psychiatry*, **150**(5)(1993): 852. (Also available at www.psych.org/aids2/aids_state3.cfm)

19

Psychiatrist as caregiver

Thomas N. Kerrihard, M.D.

Director, Psychiatry and Mental Health Services, AIDS Healthcare Foundation, Los Angeles, CA, USA

Introduction

HIV medicine and the people it affects have changed over the past 20 years, and so have the demands on the HIV psychiatrist. In this era of highly effective antiretroviral therapy (HAART), the death rate among people with HIV has decreased. However, advances in HIV medicine have not necessarily lessened the burden of mental health issues, but rather only changed the focus of care. The HIV psychiatrist faces new demands and challenges, and may struggle with these new pressures on emotional, interpersonal, and professional levels.

Case study: The demands of HIV psychiatry

Dr. Lewis works part-time as a consulting psychiatrist in a busy inner-city HIV clinic that serves 1500 patients. He is the only psychiatrist on the staff and works with the primary HIV clinicians to help manage the mental health disorders of the clinic's patients. Dr. Lewis' caseload is full and he is often overbooked. He is frequently asked to squeeze in extra patients who present with urgent psychiatric crises.

Mark is a patient referred to Dr. Lewis for an urgent evaluation due to behavioral problems within the clinic. He has been demanding at times in the past, and today has been yelling at staff and insisting on seeing a provider despite not having an appointment and no identifiable medical urgency. Mark is well known for poor attendance at his scheduled appointments. He has a known crystal methamphetamine addiction and a long history of poor adherence to his antiretroviral medications. His health has been getting worse. He has a rising viral load and low CD4 cell count.

Mark has seen Dr. Lewis for sporadic appointments but never consistently attended his routine appointments. In the past, Mark has admitted to engaging in unsafe sexual practices, including unprotected anal intercourse, especially while on a binge of crystal methamphetamine. He does not feel it is necessary to inform his sexual partners of his HIV status, stating that "in this day and age, everyone knows how to protect themselves and is responsible for their own behavior." The referring medical clinician is frustrated in caring for Mark and expresses this frustration to the psychiatrist, stating, "His problems are

---

HIV and Psychiatry. A Training and Resource Manual, Second Edition, ed. Kenneth Citron, Marie-Josée Brouillette, and Alexandra Beckett. Published by Cambridge University Press. © Cambridge University Press 2005.

all mental. I can't help him." Dr. Lewis is feeling overwhelmed with the case. He does not feel an alliance with the patient and feels he is disappointing the primary medical clinician. Over the years, after repeatedly confronting difficult patients and experiencing poor outcomes, Dr. Lewis has been growing increasingly discontent with his job at the clinic and has considered changing positions.

What are the sources of the psychiatrist's discontent?

Working as a psychiatrist with patients with HIV comes with an array of unique pressures and demands that can become overwhelming and result in an unpleasant, unrewarding work environment – if the clinician does not take precautions. Faced with large caseloads and the need to see many patients for brief visits, the psychiatrist may become increasingly dissatisfied with the quality of care he or she is able to provide. As caseloads get too large, patient care can be compromised, and the psychiatrist's perceptions of stress and job dissatisfaction are magnified.

The psychiatrist can also begin to feel disconnected from the primary medical team. Poor communication among team members and/or lack of multidisciplinary case discussions can ultimately lead to poorly managed, difficult patients who create stress for all caregivers. Difficult patients are often triaged to the psychiatrist or other mental health professionals, which leads to fragmented care and a more dissatisfied patient who feels his primary needs are not being addressed. Primary HIV clinicians who do not understand the complexity of psychiatric disorders may have unrealistic expectations of the psychiatrist and transfer some of their own frustration onto the psychiatrist.

Patients with addiction issues can be frustrating for caregivers who may come to resent the patients for their poor adherence to their treatment plan. Psychiatrists, too, may disapprove of patients' behavior (e.g., Mark's unsafe sexual practices). The psychiatrist can develop feelings toward patients that ultimately interfere with optimal treatment of their psychiatric, substance abuse, and medical issues.

The sources of stress for those working in medical settings have been examined by various authors (Roeske, 1981; Simpson and Grant, 1991; Deckard et al., 1994; Catalan et al., 1996; Bellani et al., 1996; Bennett et al., 1994; Miller, 1996; Miller and Gillies, 1996; Lederberg, 1998; Vachon, 1998). Common stressors identified (Simpson and Grant, 1991; Vachon, 1998; Demmer, 2002) include:

- team communication problems
- work overload/large caseloads
- role ambiguity
- administrative communication problems
- inadequate resources and staffing

- difficult to manage patient/family
- difficult communication with patient/family
- poor office space
- poor salaries.

Several stressors appear to be more specific to providing care for people with HIV (Bellani *et al.*, 1996; Miller and Gillies, 1996; Demmer, 2002), including:

- common comorbidity of medical, psychiatric, and substance abuse disorders
- fear of contagion and occupational risk
- societal attitudes towards AIDS
- issues involving sexuality and alternative lifestyles
- confidentiality requirements
- unpredictable nature of the disease
- witnessing the physical and mental deterioration of patients
- dealing with multiple patient deaths
- overidentification/countertransference issues.

How can the psychiatrist approach his own countertransference issues with a patient?

It is important for a psychiatrist to know when both positive and negative countertransference issues are interfering with patient care. Some patients are so well liked that their psychiatrist may find it difficult to identify potentially worrisome signs and symptoms suggestive of underlying medical or psychiatric pathology that warrants aggressive treatment. For example, a beloved patient may be significantly depressed and suicidal but prefer to please his providers with his smiling and pleasant demeanor, and the psychiatrist may choose not to evaluate his depression in depth.

Of equal concern is the "disliked" patient who is perceived as a burden and unappreciative of the psychiatrist's or medical team member's time and expertise. Patients who abuse drugs often fall into this category, especially if they present with angry, demanding, or agitated behavior. The psychiatrist should be aware of his or her own feelings toward the patient and identify when these feelings are affecting clinical judgments and treatment plans. Personal feelings for patients are common and appropriate but clinical judgment should not be heavily influenced by subjective impressions. If a psychiatrist recognizes that his admiration or disdain for a patient is intense and optimal treatment is impaired, he or she needs to find ways to step back and readdress the clinical issues. This can sometimes be achieved by:

- the process of introspection and/or psychotherapy
- seeking supervision from a senior colleague
- seeking peer-consultation on a case
- organizing a case conference on the patient

- relying on standardized protocols for managing certain behavioral and psychological presentations
- as a final resort, referring the patient to another psychiatrist for care.

Ultimately, it is not how the psychiatrist feels about the patient that is most important in their care, it is how he or she behaves towards the patient. Groves (1978) emphasized this point and suggests that the difficulty of managing difficult patients lies in the additional burden of having to deny or disown the intense hateful feelings kindled by the patient. He suggests that a physician's negative reactions can constitute important clinical data about the patient's psychology, which can help the psychiatrist understand and manage the patient more appropriately.

What are the potential long-term consequences of the psychiatrist's discontent?

Long-term exposure to stressful work conditions and personally challenging situations can lead to professional burnout. Although professional burnout has been researched extensively, the way it is defined has varied from one study to another. Burnout has been defined as a state of mental and/or physical exhaustion caused by excessive and prolonged stress (Girdin *et al.*, 1996) and as "compassion fatigue" which is viewed by some as a form of secondary traumatization. Some authors hypothesize that care providers who suffer burnout can develop similar symptoms to those that they treat. They can develop a form of posttraumatic stress disorder, which is associated with too much exposure to patients in need (Figley, 1995). In general, most studies suggest that less experienced workers are more susceptible to burnout than experienced workers (Bennet, 1994; Gueritault-Chalvin *et al.*, 2000; Demmer, 2002).

Burnout can compromise patient care, as well as personal self-care. Common signs and symptoms of professional burnout (Musick, 1997; Vachon, 1998) include:

- fatigue
- depression
- anxiety
- insomnia
- depersonalization
- anger
- irritability
- isolation
- under or over eating
- frequent tardiness
- poor concentration
- avoidance of patients
- low motivation at work
- interpersonal conflicts at work

- poor job performance
- complaints from coworkers
- multiple medical complaints with frequent "sick days"
- feelings of diminished personal accomplishment
- feelings of inadequacy and insecurity
- general sense of job dissatisfaction
- relationship distress outside of work
- alcohol and drug abuse.

What personal interventions are important for professional self-care?

When a psychiatrist identifies signs and symptoms of professional burnout, he or she should take personal steps to improve the situation. Often it is helpful to inform a supervisor of the problems. This can not only lead to potential organizational problem solving and professional relief, but the very act of acknowledging one's limitations and need for help can be very liberating. Other gestures toward personal self-care include:

- limiting the number of hours spent at work to those that are usual and customary
- taking vacation and/or time off from work
- exploring ways to make the work environment more social and pleasurable
- taking breaks during the workday
- undertaking pleasurable activities during one's time away from work
- integrating healthy eating habits and regular exercise
- exploring stress reduction techniques and exercises.

Engaging in personal psychotherapy can also be extremely useful. Psychotherapy may help the psychiatrist identify inappropriately adopted notions of self and work in the larger context of self-esteem. If the work conditions are too stressful or if supervisors and the organization are unresponsive to the psychiatrist's concerns, he or she can also choose to leave the position.

Managing stress requires a conscious effort on the part of every clinician. There are numerous ways to cope with stress and care for oneself, including (Vachon, 1998):

- acknowledge your own worth
- keep physically fit
- eat well
- get enough rest and sleep
- take time to relax and enjoy activities
- undertake outside activities
- explore spiritual enrichment
- improve communication and conflict resolution skills
- don't stress about being stressed
- learn relationship techniques

- learn to say no appropriately
- develop control over one's practice
- practice good time management skills
- be realistic about your workload expectations
- develop a personal philosophy of illness, death, and one's role in these processes.

What organizational interventions are important for professional self-care?

Much can be done at an organizational or institutional level to reduce work-related stress. To begin with, stressful clinical issues should be shared with colleagues and not managed alone. Stress can be relieved by informal sharing of information, turning to supervisors for advice, calling on colleagues, organizing official case conference forums, or organizing regular professional or peer supervision (Lederberg, 1998).

The complexity of HIV cases is a strong argument for routine case conferences, based on a multidisciplinary team approach. Multidisciplinary teams provide a mechanism where various professionals can compare their experience with a patient and identify new perspectives. When a whole team agrees on a unified approach to a complicated case, it reduces the stress on any one member of the team and allows team members to turn to each other when feeling overwhelmed. This approach also helps communicate one consistent message to the patient.

Organizing education forums for staff on mental health and substance abuse disorders, and treatment options can be very helpful in the overall treatment of psychiatric patients with HIV. Frequently, frustration directed toward the psychiatrist has its roots in staff feeling unprepared and uneducated about mental illness. By educating HIV primary-care physicians, nursing staff, and other support staff, the psychiatrist often gains their support and patience in managing these patients. The staff is also better informed and more likely to make timely referrals, which may help reduce crises in the clinic.

To reduce the stress associated with difficult patients, organizations can also develop formal "policies and procedures" for different clinical presentations. These may include policies and procedures for agitated patients, suicidal patients, substance-abusing patients, or threatening patients. These policies can provide a unified, consistent approach which psychiatrists and other staff can use to deal with "difficult" patients. The policies may outline the staff members who need to be involved when a patient's behavior becomes challenging, and specific steps for limit-setting and chart documentation. Having formal policies and procedures reduces the personal liability that any one professional may feel when managing a case alone.

Institutions can also implement patient contracts, which outline the patient's responsibility to function in the clinic setting in a way that provides a safe and secure work environment. Some institutions have patients sign a set of rules and regulations during their initial clinic intake. These rules outline behavioral standards for the clinic, including institutional policies for dealing with threatening behavior and substance intoxication in the clinic setting.

Peer support groups have been found beneficial for medical staff working with challenging populations (Lederberg, 1998). Support groups, which are led by nonpartisan facilitators, allow physicians and other staff members to express their frustrations without fear of professional repercussions. The support that develops can permeate beyond the support group and into the workplace. Staff support groups can provide the setting where new levels of personal and professional communication and problem solving occur.

Case study: Coping with poor outcomes

John is a 42-year-old male with advanced AIDS and a longstanding history of major depression. John has been working with his psychiatrist, Dr. Wang, for 3 years, and they have developed a mutually respectful relationship. Except for a few times in past years when John relapsed in his addiction to alcohol and heroin, he has been stable on his psychiatric medications and adherent with his antiretroviral medications. Dr. Wang looks forward to John's monthly appointments and over the years has followed John through a few crises, including the break up of a 10-year relationship, the death of his mother from cancer, and John's addiction to alcohol and heroin, which started at age 19. John recently had a close friend die of AIDS and progressive multifocal leukoencephalopathy (PML) and, over the past few months, has started to feel less stable. John presents with depression and expresses fears about dying like his friend. His health has had its ups and downs, but most recently he had a stable CD4 cell count of 45 cells/mm^3 and a viral load in the 20 000 units/ml range. His primary HIV physician is working on getting John on a research drug trial, which could hopefully improve his medical condition. Unexpectedly one day, John is found dead in his apartment. An autopsy reveals that he died from an overdose of alcohol and heroin.

How does the death of the patient affect the psychiatrist?

Psychiatrists can have a broad range of reactions to a patient's death. The personal impact is likely to be greater when the psychiatrist has had a longer-standing relationship with the patient. The loss of a close patient can seem like the loss of a close friend. When patient deaths are too frequent, unexpected or difficult, even seasoned staff will react with tension and the need to escape (Lederberg, 1998). Although death from AIDS was commonplace a few years ago, death now can sometimes be shocking and unpredictable. In fact, the more unpredictable the death, the more difficulty family and care providers have processing it. Since HIV has become a "manageable illness," the event of a death is much harder for physicians to accept. HIV physicians and HIV psychiatrists often feel responsible when a patient dies: if they had done enough, the patient would still be alive. This situation is not helped by the expectation that caregivers will continue working, and digest their emotional responses (Lederberg, 1998).

The death of a patient by drug overdose also raises the possibility of a suicide. Was John getting so depressed that he purposely took an overdose to end his life? Did Dr. Wang miss some important clues that could have saved John's life? Had Dr. Wang done everything possible to care for John's depression and substance abuse issues? Questions of professional competence are often at the core of a psychiatrist's distress after a patient's death. It is normal for physicians to second guess and feel insecure about their actions. Some physicians feel inadequate in their ability to keep up with the immense body of knowledge comprising modern psychiatric care, and these feelings may underlie their sense of insecurity.

Psychiatrists' reactions to their patients' suicides have been summarized into two varieties: spontaneous personal reactions and restitutive responses that are indicative of the therapist's role in society (Litman, 1965). Personal reactions include loss, feelings of defeat and despair, guilt (especially about possible omissions), anger and partial identification with the dead person. The clinicians' restitutive responses included fear that others would blame them and that they were professionally inadequate (Litman, 1965).

Guilt is a common emotional reaction to patient suicide. In Chembob's (1988) national survey of 259 psychiatrists, feelings of guilt after a patient's suicide were negatively correlated with years of practice. Denial is undoubtedly a common defense among surviving psychiatrists. Litman stated that denial was the most frequent defense in the postsuicidal period, which was expressed in such ways as refusing to believe that the death was suicidal or forgetting facets of the case (Litman, 1965).

Grief is an expected reaction to suicide, but for some this grief may reach proportions that interfere with the therapist's ability to function personally and professionally. Maltsberger described three types of pathological grief which he labeled the melancholic, the atonement, and the avoiding types (Maltsberger, 1992). According to Maltsberger, in their severe forms, these three pathological grief reactions may result in psychiatrist suicide (melancholic), in severe anger directed elsewhere (atonement), or in finding a scapegoat to hold responsible for the patient's death (avoiding).

A patient's death may ultimately resonate with the psychiatrist's own sense of immortality. Many of us find death difficult to comprehend and resist reminders of our fragility. The unease that a psychiatrist perceives after a patient's death, especially one close in age, may be based in the physician's own discomfort with death and inability to comprehend its indiscriminate nature.

How can the psychiatrist cope with the poor outcome?

Psychiatrists need to approach poor clinical outcomes on two levels: personal and professional (Bellani, *et al.*, 1996; Miller, 1996; Lederberg, 1998; Vachon, 1998).

On the personal level, Dr. Wang may need to grieve the loss of his patient, for whom he had developed an alliance and affection. Grief in a situation like this can be healthy and appropriate. The grieving process is an individual one and may require an expression of sadness, a gesture of remembrance, participation in a funeral service, an acknowledgement among peers, or simply time and contemplation. Some institutions facilitate this by offering memorial programs on a routine basis or support groups for staff. Some psychiatrists may choose to access their own sources of religious or spiritual support when affected by a patient's death.

The grieving process can also be based in feelings of insecurity, fear, or unprocessed previous loss. A patient's death can take on a meaning independent of the actual case and based in the psychiatrist's unresolved experiences. The psychiatrist may internalize a patient's death in an unhealthy manner. If this is the case, Dr. Wang may need to reflect on his own limitations as a psychiatrist and come to terms with the unpredictable nature of his work. Each psychiatrist needs to feel good about the work he does for patients. If a psychiatrist is feeling inadequate, he or she can address these feelings through personal exploration, peer consultation, professional therapy, or steps involving professional improvement. Time away from work, peer support, or professional therapy can also help psychiatrists through this process.

On the professional level, psychiatrists can use a number of institutional or professional approaches to help themselves process a patient's death. Case reviews or psychological autopsies can be a useful and constructive way to learn from a case and take time to acknowledge the meaningfulness of the relationship. Some professionals value peer support groups or simply talking with colleagues about their personal and professional relationship to a case (O'Brien, 1998). Some institutions have regular memorial services, which allow the professional a moment of reflection. Supervisors can provide an immense source of support if they take the time to acknowledge the good work that a psychiatrist had done on a case, despite its unfortunate outcome.

Conclusion

The stresses on HIV psychiatrists are not likely to ease. In fact, budget difficulties in medical systems may create increasing demands on psychiatrists. The psychiatrist who can adapt to the increasing demands of the job has a strong sense of self-esteem. He or she is able to communicate effectively with administrative supervisors and other members of the team. He or she also has a strong social support system and the ability to accurately assess his or her own talents without being egotistical. The psychiatrist must also build a life that is full of joy and meaning, and then create time for these activities (Musick, 1997).

While much of the literature has focused on the negative aspects and difficulties of offering care to people with HIV/AIDS (Barbour, 1994), it is important to acknowledge the rewards of this type of work. Clinicians who work with patients with HIV have identified the following factors as sources of satisfaction (Barbour, 1994; Horsman and Sheeran, 1995; Demmer, 2002):

- being able to help
- easing someone's burden
- serving the community
- doing something worthwhile
- developing relationships with patients
- providing nonjudgmental care to a stigmatized population
- providing comfort and support
- providing education to patients, staff, and others
- obtaining feedback from patients and their families.

See the reference section for a list of organizations studying physician stress and offering seminars and consultations for individual doctors and practices (Musick, 1997).

REFERENCES

Barbour, R. S. The impact of working with people with HIV/AIDS: a review of the literature. *Social Science and Medicine*, **39** (1994): 221–32.

Bellani, M. L., Furlan, F., Gnecchi, M. *et al.* Burnout and related factors among HIV/AIDS health care workers. *AIDS Care*, **8**(2) (1996): 207–21.

Bennett, L. and Kelaher, M. Longitudinal predictors of burnout in HIV/AIDS health professionals. *Australian Journal of Public Health*, **18** (1994): 334–6.

Bennett, L., Ross, M. W., and Sunderland, R. The relationship between recognition, rewards and burnout in AIDS caring . *AIDS Care*, **8**(2) (1996): 145–53.

Catalan, J., Burgess, A., Pergami, A. *et al.* The psychological impact on staff of caring for people with serious diseases: the case of HIV infection and oncology. *Journal of Psychosomatic Research*, **40**(4) (1996): 425–35.

Chembob, C. M., Hamada, R. S., Bauer, G. *et al.* Patient's suicides: frequency and impact on psychiatrists. *American Journal of Psychiatry*, **145** (1988): 224–8.

Deckard, G., Meterko, M. and Field, D. Physician burnout: an examination of personal, professional, and organizational relationships. *Medical Care*, **32**(7) (1994): 747–54.

Demmer, C. Stressors and rewards for workers in AIDS service organizations. *AIDS Patient Care and STDs*, **16**(4) (2002): 179–87.

Figley, C. R. (ed.) Compassion fatigue as secondary traumatic stress disorder: an overview. In *Compassion Fatigue: Coping with Secondary Traumatic Stress Disorder in Those who Treat the Traumatized*. New York, NY: Brunner/Mazel, 1995.

Girdin, D. A., Everly, G. S. and Dusek, D. E. *Controlling Stress and Tension*. Needham Heights, MA: Allyn and Bacon, 1996.

Groves, J. E. Taking care of the hateful patient. *New England Journal of Medicine*, **298**(16) (1978): 883–7.

Gueritault-Chalvin, V., Kalichman, S., Demi, A. and Peterson, J. L. (2000). Work-related stress and occupational burnout in AIDS caregivers: test of a coping model with nurses providing AIDS care. *AIDS Care*, **12** (2000): 149–61.

Horsman, J. M. and Sheeran, P. Health care workers and HIV/AIDS: a review of the literature. *Social Science and Medicine*, **41** (1995): 1535–67.

Lederberg, M. S. Oncology staff stress and related interventions. In *Psycho-oncology*, J. Holland, ed., pp. 1035–48. New York, NY: Oxford University Press, 1998.

Litman, R. E. When patients commit suicide. *American Journal of Psychotherapy*, **19** (1965): 570–6.

Maltsberger, J. T. The implication of patients suicide for the surviving psychotherapist. In *Suicide and Clinical Practice*, D. Jacobs, ed., pp. 169–182. Washington, DC: American Psychiatric Press, 1992.

Miller, D. HIV/AIDS health worker stress and burnout: introduction and overview. *AIDS Care*, **8**(2) (1996): 133–5.

Miller, D. and Gillies, P. Is there life after work? Experiences of HIV and oncology health staff. *AIDS Care*, **8**(2) (1996): 167–182.

Musick, J. L. How close are you to burnout? American Academy of Family Physicians web site, 1997. (Available as a living document at www.aafp.org/fpm/970400fm.lead.html).

O'Brien, S. R. Staff wellness program promotes quality care. *American Journal of Nursing*, **98**(6) (1998): 16B.

Roeske, N. C. Stress and the physician. *Psychiatric Annals*, **11**(7) (1981): 10–32.

Simpson, L. A. and Grant, L. Sources and magnitude of job stress among physicians. *Journal of Behavioral Medicine*, **14**(10) (1991): 27–42.

Vachon, M. L. S. The stress of the professional caregiver. In *The Oxford Textbook of Palliative Medicine*, D. Doyle, G. W. C. Hanks, and N. MacDonald, eds., pp. 919–29. New York: Oxford University Press, 1998.

ORGANIZATIONS SPECIALIZING IN PHYSICIAN STRESS

Center for Professional Well-Being
Colony West Professional Park
21 W. Colony Place, Suite 150

Durham, NC 27705
919-489-9167

Center for Professional and Personal Renewal
540 N. Santa Cruz Ave., Suite 208
Los Gatos, CA 95030
800-377-1096

Gigi Hirsch, MD and Associates
1 Memorial Drive, 15th floor
Cambridge, MA 02142

Menninger Leadership Center
P.O. Box 829
Topeka, KS 66601-0829
800-288-5357

WEBSITES WITH INFORMATION ON PHYSICIAN BURNOUT

http://www.doctorspage.net/satisf.asp
http://workhealth.org/index.html
http://www.texmed.org/cme/phn/

Appendix I
HIV counseling guidelines for physicians

Pretest counseling

A person's request for HIV testing should be honored.

- Explore risk history and discuss reasons for the test.
- Assess the person's risk of having been exposed to or of being infected with HIV.
- Provide information about HIV infection and testing, including the meaning of positive, negative, and indeterminate test results, and the impact of the window period. Discuss risk reduction and explore specific ways in which the person can avoid or reduce risk-producing behavior.
- Identify testing options available in the region, specifically nominal, non-nominal and anonymous testing.
- Discuss the potential benefits and harms of being tested and of being found HIV-positive.
- Discuss the confidentiality of test results in relation to office or clinical procedures, communicating results to other healthcare officials, provincial reporting requirements and partner notification.
- Discuss the stress related to waiting for test results and possible reactions to learning the results.
- Assess the window period by identifying the most recent risk event and plan an appropriate time for testing. Obtain and record informed consent, whether provided in writing or verbally, before testing is conducted.
- Arrange a return appointment after a predetermined interval for a face-to-face visit to inform the patient of his or her test results.

A person has the right to decline testing.

Post-test counseling

HIV test results are given only in person.

- Assess the patient's understanding of the test result.

HIV and Psychiatry. A Training and Resource Manual, Second Edition, ed. Kenneth Citron, Marie-Josée Brouillette, and Alexandra Beckett. Published by Cambridge University Press. © Cambridge University Press 2005.

- Encourage the patient to express feelings and reactions.

Negative and indeterminate result
- Discuss any need for repeat testing.
- Review the ways in which HIV is transmitted.
- Review risk-producing behavior and assess the patient's commitment to risk-reducing strategies.

Positive result
- Assess the psychological response to being HIV positive.
- Plan how the patient can overcome adverse psychological reactions to being found HIV positive.
- Arrange additional psychological and social support services as needed.
- Provide reassurance about the person's immediate safety.
- Arrange for medical follow-up.
- If possible, review transmission modes and risk-reduction strategies.
- Arrange for partner notification, if necessary.

Other important issues (emphasize early if poor follow-up is likely)

- Discuss health, reproductive and treatment issues.
- Review importance of partner testing and notification and offer assistance if the person needs it.
- Reiterate the patient's right to privacy and confidentiality with respect to medical information.
  "Counselling guidelines for HIV testing," by permission of the publisher, © 1995 Canadian Medical Association.

Index

risk assessment
  substance abuse, 139–40
  see also HIV risk assessment
risperidone, 51
  applications, 49, 80
  in delirium treatment, 132
  in psychosis treatment, 103
  side effects, 72
ritonavir, 18, 57
  drug–drug interactions, 59–60, 60–1, 67, 68
    with antidepressant drugs, 74, 75
    in bipolar disorder therapy, 77
    with clozapine, 81
    with psychostimulants, 76
    with recreational drugs, 69, 72
  metabolism, 59
  side effects, 72
RNA, and HIV infection, 4–5
Robins, E., homosexuality studies, 205
role-play, 238
RPR (rapid plasma reagin) test, 16

safe sex
  adherence issues, 155, 155–6
  and anxiety, 155
  couples, 237–8
  and homophobia, 212
  Latina women, 269
  and self-esteem, 212
  workshops, 269
  see also unsafe sex
Saghir, M., homosexuality studies, 205
St. John's Wort, drug–drug interactions, 58–61, 66–7
San Francisco Department of Health (US), Forensic
    Aids Project, 285
saquinavir, metabolism, 59
schizophrenia, case studies, 138–9, 144, 147
sedating psychotropic drugs, in sleep disorder
    treatment, 133
selective serotonin reuptake inhibitors (SSRIs),
    79–80, 82
  drug–drug interactions, 74
selegiline, 46
self-care (professional) *see* professional self-care
self-esteem
  and lipoatrophy, 221
  and safe sex, 212
  and sexual behavior, 156
self-harm, 110
  assessment, 111–12, 118
    goals, 112
  background factors, 112
  case studies, 111, 113
  risk factors, 112–13
  see also suicidal behavior

self-image
  case studies, 220
  see also body image
Senegal
  HIV prevalence, prison inmates, 283
  HIV prevention programs, 2
serial 7 subtractions, 93
serostatus *see* HIV status
sertraline, 97, 99
  applications, 257
  drug–drug interactions, 74
sexual abstinence, 149
  case studies, 237
sexual abuse
  in boarding schools, 276
  case studies, 144
sexual activity
  and HIV risk, 145
  and HIV status, 219–20
  HIV transmission, 2–3
  same-sex, 139, 145, 149
sexual behavior
  and aggression, 156
  and alcohol abuse, 178
  attitudes, 160
  and emotional expression, 156
  in hospitals, 295–6
  and rejection, 156
  and self-esteem, 156
sexual desire
  loss of, 219–20
  male homosexuals, 209–10
    case studies, 209–10
sexual health, women with HIV, 223–4
sexual inhibition
  case studies, 209–10
  and male homosexuality, 210–11
sexual orientation
  determinants, 205–6
  and gender identity compared, 206
  see also bisexuality; gender identity;
      heterosexuality; homosexuality
sexual politics, 156
sexual risk taking, assessment, 139
sexuality
  case studies, 222
  couples, HIV effects, 237–8
  Native American concepts, 275–6
  splitting-off, 209–10
  see also bisexuality; heterosexuality; homosexuality
sexually transmitted diseases (STDs), assessment, 140
shame
  effects on psychological development, 207–8
  male homosexuals, 207, 208
shingles *see* varicella-zoster virus (VZV)